Clinical Management of Chronic Pain

Clinical Management of Chronic Pain

Editor

Mariateresa Giglio

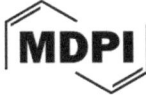

Basel • Beijing • Wuhan • Barcelona • Belgrade • Novi Sad • Cluj • Manchester

Editor
Mariateresa Giglio
Aldo Moro University
Bari
Italy

Editorial Office
MDPI AG
Grosspeteranlage 5
4052 Basel, Switzerland

This is a reprint of articles from the Special Issue published online in the open access journal *Journal of Clinical Medicine* (ISSN 2077-0383) (available at: https://www.mdpi.com/journal/jcm/special_issues/A5173P9619).

For citation purposes, cite each article independently as indicated on the article page online and as indicated below:

Lastname, A.A.; Lastname, B.B. Article Title. *Journal Name* **Year**, *Volume Number*, Page Range.

ISBN 978-3-7258-2443-4 (Hbk)
ISBN 978-3-7258-2444-1 (PDF)
doi.org/10.3390/books978-3-7258-2444-1

© 2024 by the authors. Articles in this book are Open Access and distributed under the Creative Commons Attribution (CC BY) license. The book as a whole is distributed by MDPI under the terms and conditions of the Creative Commons Attribution-NonCommercial-NoDerivs (CC BY-NC-ND) license.

Contents

Javier Picañol Párraga and Aida Castellanos
A Manifesto in Defense of Pain Complexity: A Critical Review of Essential Insights in Pain Neuroscience
Reprinted from: *J. Clin. Med.* **2023**, *12*, 7080, doi:10.3390/jcm12227080 1

Marimée Godbout-Parent, Tristan Spilak, M. Gabrielle Pagé, Manon Choinière, Lise Dassieu, Gwenaelle De Clifford-Faugère and Anaïs Lacasse
The Calm after the Storm: A State-of-the-Art Review about Recommendations Put Forward during the COVID-19 Pandemic to Improve Chronic Pain Management
Reprinted from: *J. Clin. Med.* **2023**, *12*, 7233, doi:10.3390/jcm12237233 21

Bruno Veloso Fracasso, Renato Bender Castro, Marcos Leal Brioschi and Taís Malysz
Exploring Facial Thermography Patterns in Women with Chronic Migraine
Reprinted from: *J. Clin. Med.* **2023**, *12*, 7458, doi:10.3390/jcm12237458 34

Philippe Rigoard, Maxime Billot, Renaud Bougeard, Jose Emilio Llopis, Sylvie Raoul, Georgios Matis, et al.
Improved Outcomes and Therapy Longevity after Salvage Using a Novel Spinal Cord Stimulation System for Chronic Pain: Multicenter, Observational, European Case Series
Reprinted from: *J. Clin. Med.* **2024**, *13*, 1079, doi:10.3390/jcm13041079 52

Giacomo Farì, Rachele Mancini, Laura Dell'Anna, Vincenzo Ricci, Simone Della Tommasa, Francesco Paolo Bianchi, et al.
Medial or Lateral, That Is the Question: A Retrospective Study to Compare Two Injection Techniques in the Treatment of Knee Osteoarthritis Pain with Hyaluronic Acid
Reprinted from: *J. Clin. Med.* **2024**, *13*, 1141, doi:10.3390/jcm13041141 64

Ferdinand Bastiaens, Jessica T. Wegener, Raymond W. J. G. Ostelo, Bert-Kristian W. P. van Roosendaal, Kris C. P. Vissers and Miranda L. van Hooff
Clinical Patient-Relevant Outcome Domains for Persistent Spinal Pain Syndrome—A Scoping Review and Expert Panels
Reprinted from: *J. Clin. Med.* **2024**, *13*, 1975, doi:10.3390/jcm13071975 77

Elena Ammendola, Silvia Giovanna Quitadamo, Emmanuella Ladisa, Giusy Tancredi, Adelchi Silvestri, Raffaella Lombardi, et al.
YAP Ultralate Laser-Evoked Responses in Fibromyalgia: A Pilot Study in Patients with Small Fiber Pathology
Reprinted from: *J. Clin. Med.* **2024**, *13*, 3078, doi:10.3390/jcm13113078 90

Mariana Cruz, Maria Inês Durães, Patrícia Azevedo, Célia Carvalhal, Simão Pinho and Rute Sampaio
Perspectives on Creating a Chronic Pain Support Line in Portugal: Results of a Focus Group Study among Patients and Healthcare Professionals
Reprinted from: *J. Clin. Med.* **2024**, *13*, 5207, doi:10.3390/jcm13175207 103

Giuseppe Forte, Francesca Favieri, Vilfredo De Pascalis and Maria Casagrande
To Be in Pain: Pain Multidimensional Questionnaire as Reliable Tool to Evaluate Multifaceted Aspects of Pain
Reprinted from: *J. Clin. Med.* **2024**, *13*, 5886, doi:10.3390/jcm13195886 116

Marcelina Jasmine Silva
Treating Anxiety-Based Cognitive Distortions Pertaining to Somatic Perception for Better Chronic Pain Outcomes: A Recommendation for Better Practice in the Present Day and the Cyber Age of Medicine
Reprinted from: *J. Clin. Med.* **2024**, *13*, 5923, doi:10.3390/jcm13195923 . . . . **127**

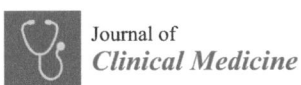

Review

A Manifesto in Defense of Pain Complexity: A Critical Review of Essential Insights in Pain Neuroscience

Javier Picañol Párraga * and Aida Castellanos

Laboratory of Neurophysiology, Biomedicine Department, Faculty of Medicine and Health Sciences, Institute of Neurosciences, University of Barcelona, 08036 Barcelona, Spain
* Correspondence: xpicanol@tecnocampus.cat

Abstract: Chronic pain has increasingly become a significant health challenge, not just as a symptomatic manifestation but also as a pathological condition with profound socioeconomic implications. Despite the expansion of medical interventions, the prevalence of chronic pain remains remarkably persistent, prompting a turn towards non-pharmacological treatments, such as therapeutic education, exercise, and cognitive-behavioral therapy. With the advent of cognitive neuroscience, pain is often presented as a primary output derived from the brain, aligning with Engel's Biopsychosocial Model that views disease not solely from a biological perspective but also considering psychological and social factors. This paradigm shift brings forward potential misconceptions and over-simplifications. The current review delves into the intricacies of nociception and pain perception. It questions long-standing beliefs like the cerebral-centric view of pain, the forgotten role of the peripheral nervous system in pain chronification, misconceptions around central sensitization syndromes, the controversy about the existence of a dedicated pain neuromatrix, the consciousness of the pain experience, and the possible oversight of factors beyond the nervous system. In re-evaluating these aspects, the review emphasizes the critical need for understanding the complexity of pain, urging the scientific and clinical community to move beyond reductionist perspectives and consider the multifaceted nature of this phenomenon.

Keywords: pain; chronic pain; nociception; sensory neuron; pain neuroscience education

Citation: Párraga, J.P.; Castellanos, A. A Manifesto in Defense of Pain Complexity: A Critical Review of Essential Insights in Pain Neuroscience. *J. Clin. Med.* **2023**, *12*, 7080. https://doi.org/10.3390/jcm12227080

Academic Editor: Mariateresa Giglio

Received: 2 October 2023
Revised: 10 November 2023
Accepted: 10 November 2023
Published: 14 November 2023

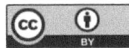

Copyright: © 2023 by the authors. Licensee MDPI, Basel, Switzerland. This article is an open access article distributed under the terms and conditions of the Creative Commons Attribution (CC BY) license (https://creativecommons.org/licenses/by/4.0/).

1. Introduction

Pain is the chief reason for emergency medical consultations [1]. Beyond this immediate concern, the escalating incidence of chronic pain in recent decades has emerged as a major health challenge. It is now recognized as a primary contributor to disability and work-related absenteeism, reflecting profound socioeconomic implications [2,3]. The taxonomy of chronic pain remains under scrutiny, especially regarding whether it should be considered merely as a symptomatic manifestation that lasts more than 3 months or acknowledged as a distinct pathological condition [4]. In fact, the category "Chronic Pain" is included in the ICD-11 (International Classification of Diseases) comprising seven different groups of chronic pain [5]. This distinction plays a pivotal role in shaping discussions around its therapeutic strategies and the necessity for patient-specific interventions.

In the realm of chronic pain management, in some conditions, a discernible paradox emerges: Despite the proliferation of medical interventions, the prevalence of pain disorders persists unmitigated [6]. Considering the modest outcomes associated with many pharmacological regimens and the recalcitrant nature of pain across an individual's lifespan, there is an evident gravitation towards investigating non-pharmacological interventions that promise cost-effectiveness and notable improvements in patient quality of life [7,8].

Notably, contemporary clinical guidelines for diverse chronic pain conditions advocate for the integration of therapeutic education, structured physical activity, and cognitive-behavioral therapy as foundational therapeutic avenues [9–11]. Within this context, the past decade has witnessed an augmented focus on pain neuroscience education, conceived to equip patients with a coherent comprehension of their condition. This strategy seeks to dispel prevailing uncertainties, curtail fear-avoidance tendencies, and fortify patient self-efficacy, among others [12].

With advancements in cognitive neuroscience, there emerges an interpretation that posits pain primarily as a brain-derived output. In a figurative context, pain pedagogy underscores pain as a cerebral appraisal [13]. This viewpoint aligns with the tenets of Engel's Biopsychosocial Model, positing that disease manifestation is not merely a consequence of biological underpinnings but is intricately interwoven with psychological and social factors [14].

This shift in paradigm has introduced nuanced complexities, potentially leading to misconceptions that bear substantial ramifications for patients, educators, and researchers in practical settings. Consequently, within this review, we endeavor to re-examine the intricate mechanisms underpinning pain, emphasizing the necessity to eschew reductionist interpretations of this multifaceted phenomenon.

Highlighting the seminal findings of recent years that challenge long-held assumptions in both clinical and research domains: Is pain experience a cerebral phenomenon? Have we conflated nociception with pain? Is the chronification of pain solely attributable to central mechanisms? Have we misunderstood central sensitization syndromes? Is there a specific neuromatrix dedicated to pain processing? Have we overlooked critical elements beyond the nervous system?

2. Pain and Brain: A Mereological Fallacy We Should Abandon

The nascent period of neuroscience and the exploration of cortical studies engendered certain "cerebrocentric" tendencies. In this paradigm, the brain was posited as the sole agent and thus the focal point of pain. This notion pervaded the pedagogy of pain, forging viewpoints profoundly shaped by the currents of functionalism and connectionism. This led to the propagation of aphorisms such as "pain is an output of the brain" or "pain is an opinion of the brain" [13]. A conception that emerged from connectionist analogies describes that the brain processes information through neural networks, similar to how a computer would use its circuitry to perform computations. Continuing with this, the brain would take stimuli as inputs, producing outputs in the form of behaviors and perceptions [15]. This all culminates with the hypothesis by several authors that when the brain perceives a threat (or potential threat), it decides to produce pain for the protection of the organism. Where "the impact of pain is dependent on the value of the perceived threat" [16], rescuing an "evaluativist" vision of pain [17].

It is true that this perspective may be backed by some evidence, where several authors uphold this connectionist hypothesis when facing a threat. For example, connectivity prior to a stimulus can modulate and determine the perception of pain [18], dopamine and the reward system (relevant in motivational states) influence the perception of pain [19], the insula plays an important role in the chronification of pain [20], complex emotions such as nostalgia modulate the perception of pain through thalamocortical mechanisms [21], and brain activity may monitor and modulate the relevance and degree of pain [22], among a host of other studies focused on brain research in pain contexts through neuroimaging. However, are these data examples truly supportive of the mentioned narrative?

We must be cautious in how this evidence is interpreted and avoid falling into excessively "brain-centric" reasoning, as this reduces a complex human and subjective experience to merely the consequence of an organ, thereby falling into the known mereological fallacy [23]. A concept that describes the error of attributing characteristics and subjective experiences to single components of a whole. In fact, some authors highlight this fallacy as "the central error of many cognitive neuroscientists" [24]. Pain is more understandable when we assign it to the whole itself and to the emergent properties that arise from the interactions of the components of a complex system. This is not limited to pain but applies to biology itself, also viewed epistemologically from the perspective of complex systems [25,26]. Ascribing aspects solely to the brain, disregarding the organism, constitutes a fallacy, falling into speculation rather than empirical evidence and fact-checking.

Building upon this discourse, we have now come to recognize that even pain typically ascribed to central mechanisms often embodies alterations or involvement within peripheral systems. Consider, for example, phantom limb pain—an aftermath of amputation—which has historically been perceived through a predominantly brain-centered lens, attributing this condition to cortical reorganization [27]. However, the significant role that peripheral factors play in both the onset and maintenance of this pain has often been insufficiently acknowledged [28]. These consist of the interplay of peripheral neuromas, the influence of ectopic discharges, and the sensitization of dorsal root ganglia, among others [29]. In fact, interventions aimed at the periphery can also yield effective results in mitigating phantom limb pain [30]. Therefore, the binary discourse debating whether phantom limb pain is a bottom-up or top-down process is not as straightforward, and the pivotal contribution of peripheral mechanisms to changes in cortical reorganization, among other factors, should not be underestimated.

Fibromyalgia presents another salient example of a condition characterized by widespread chronic pain. Owing to its apparent nonspecific nature, it has over recent decades been relegated to a controversial catch-all category, laden with labels and stigma, where the condition seemed reduced to "psychosomatization". This perspective perhaps still persists today in Western societies [31]. However, fibromyalgia is now more widely recognized, and neuroimaging studies have revealed significant alterations in the brain areas that have been identified as key regions in the pain experience, as described by Melzack. Along with the popularization of the concept of central sensitization, this led to a portrayal of fibromyalgia as a condition of purported "pain amplification" and hypersensitivity, where, once again, the brain ultimately decides to elicit it [32]. These terms and conceptions continue to provoke rigorous analysis and debate in the field today. Moreover, this point of view inadvertently ignores the other side of the story. If we consider peripheralist perspectives, it is known that the peripheral nervous system can play an essential role in the production and maintenance of pain [33]. For example, there is a potential link between fibromyalgia and pathological changes in small nerve fibers, characterized by a reduction in the density of both myelinated and unmyelinated fibers [34], low-grade systemic inflammation which can affect nociception itself [35–37], changes in gut microbiota [38], and microvascular alterations, among other factors [39].

These examples of two contexts commonly attributed to cortical reorganization cast doubt on the occasional reductionist tendency within the field of pain. However, it is not solely a matter of the peripheral nervous system interacting with the central system but also the myriad contributors that continuously modulate its activity. This underscores the importance of other factors such as the immune system and hormonal variables [40].

In this context, it is imperative to approach dichotomous perspectives with caution. Within the biomedical domain, we must circumvent the fundamental missteps that have historically ensnared other disorders, as exemplified by the serotonergic hypotheses associated with depression [41]. In our area of study, adherence to simplistic metaphors, such as an imbalance between excitation and inhibition, may lead to an oversimplified belief that medical intervention targeting one pathway could suffice to ameliorate the condition. Nonetheless, the contentious application of opioids and antidepressants, accompanied by their long-term effects, is an example that reflects a nuanced complexity that transcends any binary categorization [42–44]. The current predicament surpasses the realm of specific pharmaceuticals, presenting us with a debatable issue of healthcare medicalization and/or over-medicalization that also demands critical scrutiny [45]. Concurrently, the burgeoning trends in cognitive-behavioral modalities must not neglect the vast expanse of biomedical knowledge, acknowledging that the experience of pain transcends mere cerebral interpretation, a perspective that has to consider the under-treatment of pain that is present in some contexts [46].

Ultimately, caution is necessary to avoid the mereological fallacy in the field of pain, where hypotheses postulating that the perceived threat compels the brain to produce pain are, to some extent, unfalsifiable; hence, many of them are unscientific. Such perspectives should not detract from the body of knowledge that has been accrued in the field of pain science today.

3. Discerning the Ambiguity between Pain and Nociception: A Crucial Source of Misnomers

The International Association for the Study of Pain (IASP) diligently examines its ontology and epistemology, meticulously crafting logical terms and definitions published by the association [47]. However, when confronted with terms not adequately defined by the IASP, a scenario of epistemic gaps emerges, potentially leading to confusion [48]. In this light, pain neuroscience education has gained prominence as a prevalent clinical approach in recent years [49]. Within such a framework, statements such as "pain is not nociception" or "pain is not tissue damage" have been frequently reiterated. Nevertheless, the amalgamation of inherent simplicity and continual repetition may instigate both the bias of plausible simplicity and the availability bias, where simplified and repetitively echoed statements become accepted truths without question [50,51]. These biases can significantly influence decision-making processes not just in clinical settings but also within scientific contexts [52].

This sets the stage where these assertions run the risk of generating confusion and misinterpretations. As a result, we must confront an essential question: Are we oversimplifying these distinctions to the point where we risk creating fallacies?

On the one hand, the International Association for the Study of Pain (IASP) acknowledges the inherent complexity that characterizes pain, defining it as an unpleasant sensory and emotional experience associated with actual or potential tissue damage, or described in terms of such damage [47]. Therefore, pain is connected to a highly individual experience, characterized by unique properties shaped by qualia [53]. This concept, which has been popularized in the fields of philosophy of science and mind, encapsulates the subjective and idiosyncratic qualities of perception. It highlights the intricacy involved in comprehending pain, echoing the so-called hard problem of consciousness: The enigma of how, why, and at what point a subjective experience originates from physical processes within our bodies [54].

This phenomenon is also inseparable from the exploration of the interrelation between mental phenomena and their substrates [55]. Hence, pain as a qualia cannot merely be reduced to nociception but rather requires considering the subject's subjective experience with the accompanying high degree of interindividual variability.

Nociception, on the other hand, is conceived as the neural substrate linked to harmful or potentially harmful elements. This term is specifically defined by the IASP as the neural process of encoding noxious stimuli [56]. Despite the clarity of the primary distinction between the terms—pain and nociception—a plethora of misinterpreted concepts persist. It must be remembered that pain is not a "concrete thing", and the representation of it is heavily influenced by language [48]. In this context, countless misnomers are encountered at both the scientific and clinical levels: Names or terms applied incorrectly that ultimately lead both research and clinical practice astray [57]. Notable misnomers include concepts like pain thresholds, pain processing, pain amplification, pain fibers or pathways, and pain hypersensitivity, among others [48]. Rather than providing clarification, these concepts contribute to confusion in the field of pain-related medical education.

In addressing this topic, a substantial part of pain pedagogy leans towards reductionism, often resorting to thought experiments and contentious, debatable case studies. One such case involves a situation where a man presented to the emergency room with severe pain despite the absence of any apparent noxious stimulus [58]. The case recounts an incident where a man suffered an accident at work involving a large nail that fell onto his foot. This accident caused him intense pain, but upon removing his boot, the nail was found lodged between his toes without any evident tissue damage. This scenario prompts the question: Does it genuinely illustrate the existence of pain without nociception and/or damage?

The reality remains that the evidence supporting this assertion is far from compelling, and these perspectives run the risk, erroneously, of leading patients and clinicians back to a psychogenic phenomenon. Untested thought experiments and anecdotal evidence distance us from a reality that we must keep in mind: Nociceptive activity remains one of the strongest predictors of the experience of pain [59,60]. Demonstrating the empirical manifestation of pain without underlying nociceptive activity is truly challenging. It is crucial to maintain a critical stance and rethink new propositions that have emerged in the past decade, such as pain without nociception. Once again, this assumption deviates from evidence-based substantiation and should be approached with caution, at least for now.

However, it is true that the relationship between nociception and the perception of pain is not linear. Nociceptive information is modulated by a variety of factors. In this context, cognitive factors, such as attentional processes, expectations, and placebo, can greatly influence the final perception of pain [61]. Emotional states [62], uncertainty [63], descending inhibitory and facilitatory modulation [64], and other sensory inputs, as proposed by the Gate Control Theory [65], are among the many factors that can also play an important role.

Within this context, specifically concerning therapeutic pain education, a debate may arise between the utility and accuracy of language [66]. We find ourselves coexisting with concepts we have had to abandon in recent years despite their seeming usefulness, precisely because of the inherent nocebo effect they carry. In an effort to improve pain management, new conceptualizations that encompass advancements in the understanding of pain were proposed. However, in agreement with Cohen et al., language is all we have in some respects, and utility should not overshadow the precision required by the complexity of pain—particularly considering that pain may not be a "thing" with inherently active properties or characteristics [67].

Hence, all of these aspects bring nuance to the traditional notions we hold, indicating the inherent complexity of both nociception and pain. While these concepts are not synonymous, they are not so distinct as to be separated by a clear-cut line in pain pedagogy. Moreover, it is crucial to acknowledge the profound importance of language, as it plays a guiding role in shaping our understanding.

4. Starting from the Periphery: Does Pain Modulation Begin in the Central Nervous System?

From a reductionist standpoint, it can be observed that the study of pain has encompassed both cerebrocentric and peripheralist perspectives. Initially, the understanding in this field was markedly shaped by the Cartesian viewpoint, a paradigm that propelled a significant leap forward in the physiology of pain by Descartes proposing that pain emanated from nociceptive projections directed towards the pineal gland [68]. As time progressed, the focal point of study gradually transitioned towards the central nervous system.

At present, it is acknowledged with considerable certainty that noxious (or potentially noxious) stimuli, whether originating internally or externally, are transduced to nerve impulses. This transduction is facilitated largely due to the pivotal role of nociceptors and some mechanoreceptors, which are endowed with a vast array of ion channels specialized in sensing and reacting to various environmental factors, such as temperature, mechanical stress, or pro-inflammatory conditions, among numerous others [69].

Within this complex system, there are ion channels vital for nociception: those that facilitate the transduction of specific stimuli through the influx of calcium and/or sodium (TRP family, P2X, ASIC, PIEZO, etc.), voltage-dependent channels that hold significant relevance in the genesis and propagation of action potentials (Nav, Cav, etc.), and channels that govern potassium discharge (Kv, Kir, K2P, KaCa, KNa, etc.), among others (5-HT3, HCN channels, TMEM16, TKr, etc.) [70]. Furthermore, these nociceptors are essentially pseudounipolar neurons, with their somas situated within the dorsal root ganglia, a structure integral to nociception. However, it must be emphasized that the scenario is more complex than it seems, and based on their individual characteristics, various types of nociceptors can be identified.

Based on myelination levels, most nociceptors are categorized as C fibers, which have small diameters and low myelination, conducting impulses at speeds between 0.4 and 1.4 m/s. In contrast, A fibers feature higher myelination and faster conduction speeds ranging from 5 to 30 m/s [71]. However, it is clear that the complexity goes beyond mere myelination levels and is also determined by their specialized roles, governed by differences in expression patterns. Within this context, several nociceptors have been identified, each exhibiting different sensitivities and functionalities. For instance, there are non-peptidergic mechanonociceptors that seem to respond solely to mechanical stimuli (MrgprD$^+$), alongside peptidergic nociceptors sensitive to harmful cold temperatures (TRPM8$^+$). Furthermore, some peptidergic nociceptors are responsive to both noxious heat and, likely, mechanical stimuli, identified by markers, such as TRPV1, TRKA, and CGRP. Additionally, A fiber mechanoreceptors without free nerve endings play a crucial role in mechanonociception. These include receptors mediating pin-prick pain, characterized by TRKA, CGRP, and Npy2r presence, as well as those facilitating painful mechanical sensitivity (TRKA and CGRP$^+$) [72]. However, this classification is complex, encompassing silent nociceptors that become active in the presence of inflammation [73], as well as low-threshold C fibers serving as mechanoreceptors, facilitating the pleasant touch [74].

In light of the information discussed, the activity of nociceptors is intrinsically intertwined with the immune system's operations. This correlation is prominently illustrated through the events of peripheral sensitization, a condition delineated by the IASP as a state of "Increased responsiveness and diminished threshold of nociceptive neurons in the periphery to the stimulation of their receptive fields" [56]. In an effort to elucidate the neurobiological mechanics of this phenomenon, previous investigations have revealed a plethora of mediators in the extracellular milieu, alongside a sophisticated cross-talk with the immune system. This interaction is capable of triggering signaling cascades that ultimately augment the sensitization of nociceptors, enhancing their responsiveness to external and internal stimuli [75].

Beyond the essential characterization of peripheral phenomena and peripheral sensitization, there are recent and significant implications that should not be overlooked in this field. Indeed, in a popularized and simplified manner, it has been established that the integration of information and modulation of nociception commence at the spinal cord level, grounded on the Gate Control Theory, which hinges on the action of inhibitory interneurons [65]. This assumption might be steered by the apparent absence of inhibitory interneurons and synapses in the periphery.

However, recent propositions suggest that intrinsic GABAergic signaling is in operation within the dorsal root ganglion (DRG) itself, potentially serving as the "first peripheral gate" at the axonal bifurcation of the DRGs [76,77]. The discourse extends beyond merely addressing GABAergic modulation in the DRGs; it additionally underscores the importance of the peripheral opioid and endocannabinoid systems [78,79]. This includes their active roles at the terminals, where they appear to mediate a substantial portion of the analgesic effects of synthetic cannabinoids, notably through the engagement of CB1 receptors [80]. Furthermore, observations point to a diminished release of inflammatory mediators in states of peripheral sensitization, a process mediated through CB2 receptors in the immune system [81]. This delineates an area of research that demands further intricate exploration and deciphering.

Furthermore, a frequently neglected facet regarding the significance of the periphery resides in the inherent spontaneous activity of sensory afferents, which might be intricately linked with a sustained feedback interaction with the central nervous system (CNS), fostering a persistent somatosensory alteration. Indeed, this peripheral activity could play a pivotal role in sustaining central sensitization [82]. Despite the prevailing assumption that pain is perpetuated by central mechanisms in pathophysiological contexts, emerging evidence suggests that peripheral hyperexcitability and spontaneous activity might be intricately connected to pain [83,84]. These occurrences are closely associated with membrane potential instabilities (MPIs), manifesting as membrane potential oscillations or spontaneous depolarizing fluctuations, potentially serving as a theoretical model for ectopic discharges and repetitive firing, among other phenomena [85]. It seems that both MPIs and spontaneous activity might be correlated with the spontaneous opening of channels permeable to Na^+ and/or Ca^{2+} [83–87].

Additionally, recent findings illuminate the complexity of peripheral cross-talk, including the transfer of mitochondria from macrophages to nociceptors as a modulation strategy for inflammation [88], the role of cytokines such as the macrophage migration inhibitory factor in the previously mentioned spontaneous activity [89], the critical communication between satellite glial cells and the DRGs [90], and the regulation of nociceptor sensitization through top-down mechanisms, including the engagement of the HPA axis in the peripheral nociceptors regulation [91].

Therefore, we encounter evidence that underscores pivotal aspects in understanding nociception, which ought to be emphasized: (1) the inherent dynamic adaptability of the peripheral nervous system to transition between various states, (2) the ongoing discourse regarding whether the subjective perception of different experience of pain stems from the processing and integration of all sensory inputs or, alternatively, from the specific neural activity of various subtypes of sensory afferents, (3) the critical role of continuous communication between the immune system and the nervous system operating as a cohesive unit, (4) the chronification of pain is not solely rooted in alterations within the central nervous system, and (5) both the integration and modulation of nociception are ubiquitous phenomena. Consequently, this perspective challenges a cerebrocentric view of pain emergence, wherein the significance of the peripheral contributions cannot be dismissed.

5. Central Sensitization as a Focus of Confusion: Weaving Threads of Uncertainty

The spinal cord plays a pivotal role in transmitting and processing information. Peripheral nociceptors send information to the dorsal horn, where second-order neurons receive and transmit it in an ascending manner to cortical areas. However, within the dorsal horn, a complex network of excitatory and inhibitory interneurons utilizes glutamate and GABA (among others) as key neurotransmitters to modulate the transmission of nociceptive signals, ensuring precise and accurate modulation [92]. Additionally, descending projections from higher brain regions, including the periaqueductal gray matter, rostroventral medulla, dorsal reticular nucleus, and ventrolateral medulla, exert regulatory control over nociception. These descending pathways critically modulate nociception, contributing to the overall pain experience [93].

The synapses formed between nociceptive afferents and second-order ascending neurons are located in key regions of the dorsal horn. In fact, Rexed classified spinal cord neurons into different laminae (I–X) based on their size, shape, and structure [94]. Specifically, laminae I, II, and III play a crucial role in the processing of nociceptive information, receiving inputs from unmyelinated polymodal C fibers and thinly myelinated Aδ fibers [95].

Within these laminae, intricate neural circuits are formed, where components of the posterior horn are interconnected with multiple interneurons and primary afferents. The proposal of the Gate Control Theory by Melzack and Wall emphasized the importance of these circuits [65]. In this aspect, injury or inflammation, for instance, can lead to the development of hyperalgesia, allodynia, and spontaneous pain. These processes are believed to involve changes at the level of these dorsal horn synapses, including synaptic plasticity (long-term potentiation, LTP), reduction in inhibitory GABAergic/glycinergic neurotransmission, and alterations in the properties of mechanoreceptive afferents, among other mechanisms [96]. Therefore, this area is essential for understanding nociception.

Along the same line of inquiry, it was Woolf who conceptualized and characterized the phenomenon of central sensitization in preclinical studies. This intricate phenomenon involves enduring modifications in the excitability of second-order neurons within the spinal cord, elicited by heightened afferent activity, thereby intricately altering the somatosensory system itself [97]. The profound implications of this concept were further underscored by the seminal discovery of long-term potentiation (LTP) in the hippocampus by Bliss and Lomo, where synchronous high-frequency input was found to engender synaptic efficacy enhancement [98]. Subsequently, analogous mechanisms were unearthed in the spinal cord with the discovery of long-term depression (LTD) [99].

Today, LTP is recognized as an indispensable mechanism underpinning our comprehension of central sensitization [100]. The substrates underlying this synaptic plasticity are profoundly activity-dependent, intricately governed by glutamatergic neurotransmission and the modulation of post-synaptic AMPA and NMDA receptors, among other factors. Indeed, the neurobiological underpinnings of central sensitization extend far beyond mere adjustments in synaptic efficacy (particularly those confined to activity-dependent modifications). They encompass comprehensive transformations in neural circuitry, manifested by an augmented release of neurotransmitters from the presynaptic neuron, a down-regulation in inhibitory signaling, modulations in membrane excitability, adaptations in microglial responsiveness, and astrocytic disturbances, among a multitude of other nuanced alterations.

The progressive comprehension of central sensitization has emphatically underscored the clinical significance and pragmatic repercussions of these biological underpinnings in the realm of pain perception, a clinical viewpoint defended by Woolf [101]. Concurrently, Yunus, within the context of clinical research, pioneered and substantiated the perspective that various diffuse clinical presentations (such as fibromyalgia, myofascial pain syndrome, chronic fatigue, and irritable bowel syndrome, among others) exhibited considerable commonalities in the absence of discernable tissue origin. This observation prompted him to introduce the concept of "central sensitization syndromes" (CSS), constructing a theoretical model that was predicated on the phenomenon of "central sensitization" [102]. Nevertheless, the association drawn between central sensitization and CSS was an extrapolation from deductive reasoning. In fact, it was postulated that the atypical responses of subjects to thermal stimuli (among others), coupled with discernable neuroimaging alterations in reaction to these stimuli, indirectly hinted at the central sensitization mechanisms proposed by Woolf.

Abiding by the foundational principles of logic, the presented argument does not withstand a valid or scientifically robust line of reasoning. It reveals a potential flaw in deduction, where strong general premises based on preclinical studies with animal models (central sensitization) lead to specific conclusions in another distinct area (clinical presentations). Within this deductive framework, there can be an occasional failure to contemplate all potential models when addressing a problem.

Thereby leading to the inference of conclusions that remain in the realm of possibility rather than being definitively correct or accurate [103]. Ergo, the application and tacit acceptance of these premises (central sensitization as the main mechanism of CSS) remain notably contentious. In fact, at present, we lack a definitive method to establish and demonstrate the presence of central sensitization in human subjects.

Moreover, recent systematic reviews suggest that purported central sensitization questionnaires do not entirely align with sensory aspects. However, they demonstrate a substantial correlation with psychological constructs, such as depression, catastrophizing, anxiety, stress, and kinesiophobia, among others [104]. Furthermore, other reviews that incorporate neuroimaging studies from diverse pathological contexts fail to support the concept of CSS. In these studies, it is observed that, notwithstanding a commonly amplified response to stimuli, the assorted phenotypes remain indistinguishable in their classification. This underlines that marked heterogeneity is observed in individual differences, both across different syndromes and within the same syndrome [105].

Notwithstanding the aforementioned, over the course of time, the hypothesis that central sensitization underlies chronic pain has surreptitiously transitioned into an assumption. This shift seems to dismiss the fact that central sensitization has been delineated within laboratory environments, employing electrophysiological experiments that facilitate the recording of neural activity through a range of paradigms.

Thus, the mystified concept of centralized pain resulting from central sensitization became ingrained in clinical practice, research, and education [106,107].

In a similar vein, these interpretations and classifications gained traction within the field of pediatrics, encapsulating constructs such as amplified pain syndrome. This sweeping categorization includes non-specific headaches, generalized musculoskeletal pain, and various types of abdominal discomfort, among others. All of these conditions exhibit a hypothetic unifying feature: central sensitization [108]. These challenges reemerge due to persistent epistemological confusion, where the purported hypersensitivity integral to central sensitization is not directly attributed to pain itself. Instead, it could arguably and speculatively (at least in humans) refer to phenomena that modulate nociception, ultimately influencing the painful experience. Despite the latter, these pathophysiological scenarios continue to be perceived as manifestations of central sensitization, thereby inducing hypersensitivity. This leads us to a circular argument: "The primary pathophysiological feature is a sensitized central nervous system that results in an enhancement in the processing of pain and sensory stimuli" [107,108]. Upon close scrutiny, it seems that the pain is ascribed to sensitization that heightens hyperexcitability, consequently intensifying pain—an argument that paradoxically uses itself to explain its premise [108].

However, these presuppositions pertaining to central sensitization have found broad acceptance in the domain of clinical taxonomy, thus endorsing premises that are currently inaccurate. The objective of this review is not to dispute the potential role of central sensitization as a mechanism underpinning chronic pain states; rather, it challenges the notion of CS serving as the primary etiopathogenesis in an array of contexts. Concurrently, it underscores the necessity for a discerning stance on generalizations—a fundamental pitfall that needs to be rectified in scientific endeavors. Just as the recourse to circular arguments for elucidating intricate pathologies should be avoided. At this juncture, it is incumbent upon us to critically examine our inferences and adopt more appropriate provisional concepts, while exploring and corroborating the factors substantiated in pathologies of such profound complexity. In the same context, it is vital to acknowledge that central sensitization, as characterized in animal models, is not merely a process of synaptic plasticity. Indeed, its neurobiological underpinnings extend to encompass the neural circuitry at large [101].

6. Cortical Processing: Does the Pain Neuromatrix Really Exist? A Controversial Simplification

The information derived from nociceptors is conveyed to higher cortical areas through various ascending pathways within the anterolateral system, facilitating its processing through the coordinated interaction of distinct brain regions. This system encompasses the spinothalamic tract, spinoreticular tract, and spinotectal tract and was evidenced by previous investigations utilizing post-mortem and neurosurgical studies, which also proposed a discernible functional division within the spinothalamic tract [109]. Wherein a lateral and medial pathway exists, exhibiting differential transmission and processing of nociceptive information [110,111].

Within this framework, the lateral system has traditionally been recognized as a principal contributor to the sensory-discriminative aspects of pain, encompassing aspects such as localization, intensity, and duration [112]. This system involves the lateral thalamic nuclei, somatosensory cortices S1 and S2, as well as the insular cortex, which collectively contribute to the integration of sensory afferences [109]. Conversely, the medial system has been proposed as a comparatively slower pathway responsible for the processing of affective components of pain [112]. It encompasses structures like the medial thalamic nuclei, anterior cingulate cortex, prefrontal cortex, and key structures like the amygdala [113].

Clinical cases and lesion paradigms provide support for distinct functional roles of these areas in relation to pain, as evidenced by how localized lesions in the anterior cingulate cortex (ACC) induce alterations in affective pain components [114], while lesions in somatosensory areas impact the sensory-discriminative components of pain [115,116]. A particular instance exemplifying this role differentiation is pain asymbolia, a specific type of depersonalization. In such cases, individuals experience a dissociation wherein the pain perceived is not acknowledged as their own [117]. Such dissociative cases present two opposite poles: a division between the sensory facets of pain and the affective-emotional constituents, and vice versa [118].

In this aspect, it is important to clarify a fundamental distinction between essential percepts: pain and suffering as closely interconnected entities, albeit not synonymous [119]. Suffering can occur independently of pain, just as pain can be experienced without implicit suffering. These phenomena likely differ in their underlying biological correlates, which is crucial for understanding pain. In this aspect, pain is considered an acute stressor [120], and prolonged pain can lead to alterations in the correlates of pain unpleasantness, analogous to the effects of chronic stress [121,122]. For instance, studies have demonstrated that in healthy individuals, pain-related brain activity involves the ACC and anterior insula [123]. Conversely, chronic pain appears to engage cognitive areas of the insula and other corticolimbic regions associated with emotional processing [124,125]. Paradoxically, suffering can modulate our susceptibility to pain perception, with psychosocial factors such as catastrophizing, helplessness, and excessive rumination influencing pain experiences [126,127].

The growing availability of neuroscientific techniques like fMRI, PET, SPECT, and EEG, among others, has shed light on the significant role of cortical processing in pain perception. Former perspectives based on localizationism suggested the existence of specific and specialized regions responsible for pain perception [128], proposing the notion of a "pain center". However, contemporary evidence suggests that pain does not stem from the activation of a single center but involves the coordinated engagement of multiple brain structures. This led to the hypothesis of a "pain neuromatrix", a network of specific structures responsible for processing nociceptive information and generating the experience of pain [129].

However, this concept was originated by Melzack, who initially proposed the existence of a neuromatrix consisting of widespread neural networks that include somatosensory, limbic, and thalamocortical components. Together, these components contribute to the sensory-discriminative, affective-motivational, and cognitive-evaluative aspects of the pain experience [130]. Moreover, Melzack's theory introduced the concept of a neurosignature, suggesting that pain is determined by the synaptic architecture of the neuromatrix, influenced by both genetic and sensory factors [130]. Importantly, the neuromatrix theory of Melzack was not limited to a specialized network solely dedicated to pain processing but plays a crucial role in perceptual outputs.

Many other researchers have further developed and characterized this theoretical model, leading to the emergence of the pain neuromatrix [131]. This term arose due to the observed correlation between perceived pain intensity and the magnitude of response within the structures of the pain neuromatrix [132]. Additionally, the pain neuromatrix areas demonstrate modulatory capabilities influenced by those factors that can reduce pain perception [133]. Consequently, the concept of a pain-processing network gained momentum in pain research, and some authors even consider the pain neuromatrix as a potential biomarker and an objective measure of pain perception [134,135]. However, these perspectives suggesting that pain is the exclusive percept emerging from this network have generated debate [136]. Therefore, it remains crucial to question whether those suggesting specific activation of the pain neuromatrix have robust experimental evidence to support their claims.

Looking at the other side of the argument, there are observations that challenge this model [129,131,136,137]. A significant portion of neural activity within the pain neuromatrix in response to nociceptive stimuli appears to be nonspecific to nociception itself [129]. Notably, certain points emerge: (i) no primary cortical area has been exclusively identified to process thalamocortical nociceptive input; (ii) no cortical column exhibiting preferential response to nociceptive stimuli has been described; (iii) specific nociceptive neurons have been reported across different areas, but their distribution is extensive, and their characterization is based on a high activation threshold. It is noteworthy that many of these neurons can also be activated by other sensory modalities, such as visual stimuli perceived as "threatening"; (iv) the relationship between perceived pain intensity and neuromatrix activation is nonlinear; and (v) the influence of context and novelty on neuromatrix activation has been emphasized [129,136]. These findings challenge the notion of specificity in exclusively eliciting pain. In fact, authors like Patrick Wall suggest that continuing to search for such specific cells is an act of faith [138]. Thus, it raises doubts about whether the information processed within these areas is intrinsically linked to pain or rather to the salience and relevance of sensory stimuli. It is plausible that some nociceptive projections may be involved in predicting and evaluating consequences, indicating a nonspecific role in pain perception.

The preceding discussion prompts the consideration of theoretical models that challenge the notion of a specific neuromatrix for pain. From an alternative perspective, the emphasis shifts towards the importance of the matrix in detecting the salience of sensory stimuli [136]. This view aligns with the nonlinearity often observed in the experience of pain, and the "pain neuromatrix" is conceptualized as a system involved in the detection, attentional orientation, and response to highly relevant sensory events within a specific context. This cortical system is believed to play a fundamental role in detecting events that are significant for bodily integrity, regardless of the sensory modality involved. Additionally, it is proposed that this system contributes to the construction of a multimodal cortical representation of the body and its immediate spatial surroundings, serving as a potential defensive system for the organism [136].

This salience hypothesis aligns with insights provided by other researchers in understanding the underlying mechanisms of reward and aversiveness at the cortical level, offering a more comprehensive perspective on the dynamic interplay between these constructs [139].

The unpleasantness of pain constitutes a crucial component in its understanding, and there is evidence to suggest that complex conditions such as chronic pain may share neurobiological foundations with addictive disorders [140]. Within this framework, functional magnetic resonance imaging studies have indicated that the impact of a reward diminishes in the presence of a threat, and conversely, the perception of a threat is attenuated in the presence of a reward. These findings support the notion that reward and threat processing are not inherently independent but rather engage in a competitive process. Key structures, including the anterior insula, ventral tegmental area, putamen, and striatum, are implicated in detecting and evaluating salient stimuli. This competitive system is hypothesized to enable the identification of stimuli crucial for the organism's survival and adaptation [139].

Nonetheless, these models could overlook the unceasing predictive ability of complex organisms, a vital factor for survival. Recent developments in the computational realm of cognitive neuroscience and machine learning are introducing pain as a heuristic and probabilistic mechanism [141,142]. Indeed, the incorporation of pain probabilistic mechanism paves the way for effective maneuvering in a world saturated with uncertainty, a concept phenomenologically defined as "A state where a given depiction of the world cannot be employed as a compass for guiding subsequent behavior, cognitive processing, or emotional response" [143].

It is therefore noteworthy to emphasize the emergence of a Bayesian approach to comprehending pain [144]. In fact, perception itself follows a probabilistic model to some extent, allowing for the management of ambiguity and the filling of informational gaps with prior knowledge. Thus, the perception of pain extends beyond the mere processing of sensory information, incorporating predictions based on past learning experiences. In fact, the concept of chronic pain has been described by some researchers as aberrant Bayesian inferences [145], highlighting the role of predictive processes in shaping the experience of ongoing pain. Within this context, it is essential to recognize the fundamental role of learning processes in the understanding of pain. Evidence suggests that both classical and operant conditioning mechanisms significantly contribute to the complex phenomenon of pain [146–148]. Moreover, studies have demonstrated the capacity to evoke nocifensive behaviors by exploring specific engrams, which represent the intricate configuration of neural connections associated with a particular memory [149]. These learning processes also modulate nocebo and placebo effects arising in pain treatment through expectations, where prior conditioning and/or suggestion can influence both the exacerbation and alleviation of the patient's pain experience [150–152].

Referencing the Bayesian Model within the context of pain indirectly references one of many modern theories of consciousness (ToC), specifically the comprehension of consciousness through predictive processing [115,153]. This approach suggests a framework for the systematic mapping of neural mechanisms onto certain domains of consciousness. Within this context, key dichotomies must be noted when discussing different theories of consciousness [154]. These include (i) global states versus local states, where the former is understood as levels of consciousness and the latter correlates with conscious contents or qualia; (ii) phenomenological properties versus functional properties, each having a unique objective; and (iii) the selection of a local state (why a subject possesses a specific local state) versus the experiential characterization of local states (why a specific local state is tied to a particular experience).

In essence, various theories of consciousness align with one or some of these perspectives, yet there remains a lack of a single, comprehensive theoretical model that satisfactorily accounts for consciousness in its broadest form. Regardless, these theories are crucial for pain understanding. Some of them emphasize higher-order processing (High-order theories) [155], while others focus on a physical substrate capable of emulating a virtual workspace (Global-workspace theories) [156].

There are theories that underscore mathematical quantification, depicting the degree of information produced by a collection of elements and its irreducibility to the information generated by its constituent parts (Integrated-information Theory) [157], or the ones related to top-down processing, such as predictive theories [153] or re-entry theories, which suggest that information does not solely flow in one direction, from sensory areas to more complex processing areas. Instead, they propose a reverse information flow from higher to lower regions, serving as an essential re-entry in consciousness and perception [158].

Even though these represent different viewpoints, they typically share a common factor leading to a focus on a concept often mentioned but rarely delved into deeply: "information". Numerous hypotheses are framed in terms of information and abstraction, and this gives rise to a question: What is this entity termed as information?

While information is intangible, it remains a constant presence in organisms, ranging from the simplest to the most intricate levels. In the realm of neuroscience, information is conceptualized as a dynamic process encompassing the encoding, transmission, and decoding of diverse and innumerable neural activity patterns. This understanding is grounded in the application of the Information Theory, a theoretical backbone for many contemporary scientific disciplines that centers around the mathematical quantification of information [159,160]. This theory serves as one of the most reliable pathways for deciphering the neural code and stems from the principle of applied probability in information transmission within communication systems. It determines the distribution of possible outputs according to specific signals [161]. However, the implementation of Information Theory within neuroscience poses significant complexity. Neural modeling must not only consider the stimulus but also all preceding states. In this context, a stimulus can be depicted as a vector of various parameters, each symbolizing a preceding state of the stimulus that is pertinent to the response under scrutiny. For instance, in the case of a stimulus capable of taking on eight different values and a response contingent upon seven previous states, there would emerge 16,777,216 (8^7) distinct stimulus conditions [162]. Thus, it is evident that the application of Information Theory carries immense value for understanding Neuroscience, and by extension, the nature of pain.

In this aspect, it is critical to acknowledge the significant heterogeneity inherent in the neural correlates of the pain experience and the overarching abstract concept of information, which presents challenges in terms of external validity and the potential for generalization within scientific research [137]. The issue extends beyond the mere absence of a universally accepted biomarker or neuromarker; it involves the intricate task of authentically characterizing an inherently idiosyncratic event that exhibits not only interindividual variations but also intraindividual differences influenced by contextual factors. Philosophical perspectives in the realm of mind theory have ventured towards eliminativism in this regard. Yet, scientific inquiry necessitates a form of generalization that can achieve equilibrium, acknowledging the commonalities we discern while still honoring the unique individual variances [137].

In conclusion, the concept of a specific "Pain Neuromatrix" has been both defended and challenged over recent years. This stark divide showcases the intricate nature of pain and how it is processed by our neural networks. Modern research suggests that the perception of pain is likely not tied to a single neural network but instead emerges from a multifaceted network responding to important sensory stimuli. This view emphasizes the key role of sensory stimuli in the pain experience. Additionally, innovative models like the Bayesian Model propose a novel perspective on pain, framing it as a probabilistic and inferential process, where perception is shaped not only by present sensory information but also by past experiences. The study of cortical processing and pain shines a light on the complex interaction between pain and consciousness. This understanding is crucial for guiding future research and holds significant potential for enhancing the clinical management of chronic pain.

7. Summary

The investigation into pain has uncovered intricacies that challenge conventional and reductionist views we might have held to date. With the advent of neurosciences, we might have fallen into misconceptions that have permeated various fields. In this regard, pain was conceived as a product of the brain, thereby succumbing to the mereological fallacy—a fallacy that should be avoided when studying complex phenomena dependent on emergent properties arising from interactions within system components (Figure 1).

Consequently, there is a prevalent confusion between pain's multidimensionality (qualia or the individual experience of pain) with the neurophysiology of nociception. However, caution is imperative. While they are not identical concepts, they are intricately related; it is challenging to evidence pain without nociception.

Align with this, to explain the perpetuation of chronic pain, the focus has been on underlying central mechanisms. This trend has often overshadowed the crucial role of the peripheral nervous system, where substantial evidence suggests its active involvement in pain chronification. This goes beyond the communication between the peripheral and central nervous systems but also the cross-talk between the nervous system and other systems. This perspective challenges views that overemphasize the brain as the primary pain generator, underscoring the importance of peripheral contributions.

Similarly, central sensitization has been proposed as a mechanism responsible for pain chronification, characterized by an increase in the hyperexcitability of the second neuron in the dorsal horn. Yet, its significance in some domains has become an umbrella term to justify vague clinical contexts. In clinical taxonomy, it is crucial to critically assess its role as the primary etiopathogenesis of clinical presentations. Central sensitization has been described in basic research and, therefore, is contentious when generalized to clinical contexts. Presently, there is no evidence demonstrating central sensitization as described by Woolf in human subjects, and current evaluation tools for humans, such as central sensitization questionnaires, show controversial correlations with sensory aspects. On the other hand, quantitative sensory testing could provide patient sensory data that might suggest, or not, the presence of central sensitization, as these are not a direct measure of the neurophysiological phenomena. Thus, it seems more appropriate to suggest that it enables the evaluation of nociceptive signal modulation rather than directly indicating central sensitization itself. Therefore, it is vital to adopt more suitable concepts, given the complex nature of widespread pain pathologies.

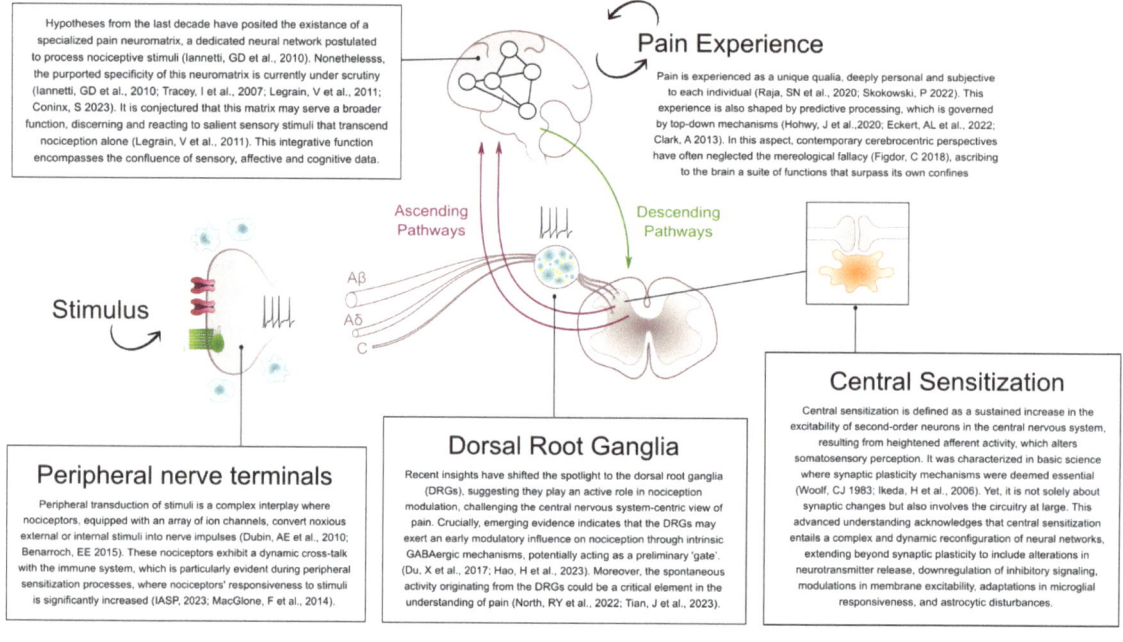

Figure 1. Schematic overview of the principal elements addressed in this narrative review.

Finally, in the past decade, pain awareness has been attributed to a possible specific neuromatrix composed of various brain regions. The specificity of this "Pain Neuromatrix" has been debated, highlighting the inherent complexity of pain.

Recent research against this theory suggests that rather than processing pain-associated information, it processes salient sensory information significant to the organism without an evident specificity. Contemporary theories, in line with consciousness models, propose pain from a Bayesian Model that perceives pain consciousness from a probabilistic and inferential approach, influenced by both current sensory information and past experiences. In this light, we cannot detach pain experience from consciousness research. Comprehending pain as an experience necessitates a deep understanding of the complexities inherent in consciousness.

In summary, the study of pain and nociception is an expansive and multifaceted field that necessitates an approach recognizing the interplay among diverse systems. This understanding is paramount for guiding future research and enhancing the clinical management of chronic pain.

Author Contributions: Conceptualization and writing—original draft preparation, J.P.P.; writing—review and editing, A.C. All authors have read and agreed to the published version of the manuscript.

Funding: This research received no external funding.

Institutional Review Board Statement: Not applicable.

Informed Consent Statement: Not applicable.

Data Availability Statement: Data sharing not applicable.

Conflicts of Interest: The authors declare no conflict of interest.

References

1. Todd, K.H.; Ducharme, J.; Choiniere, M.; Crandall, C.S.; Fosnocht, D.E.; Homel, P.; Tanabe, P.; PEMI Study Group. Pain in the emergency department: Results of the pain and emergency medicine initiative (PEMI) multicenter study. *J. Pain.* **2007**, *8*, 460–466. [CrossRef] [PubMed]
2. Lee, H.; Hübscher, M.; Moseley, G.L.; Kamper, S.J.; Traeger, A.C.; Mansell, G.; McAuley, J.H. How does pain lead to disability? A systematic review and meta-analysis of mediation studies in people with back and neck pain. *Pain* **2015**, *156*, 988–997. [CrossRef] [PubMed]
3. Vos, T.; Flaxman, A.D.; Naghavi, M.; Lozano, R.; Michaud, C.; Ezzati, M.; Shibuya, K.; Salomon, J.A.; Abdalla, S.; Aboyans, V.; et al. Years lived with disability (YLDs) for 1160 sequelae of 289 diseases and injuries 1990–2010: A systematic analysis for the Global Burden of Disease Study 2010. *Lancet* **2012**, *380*, 2163–2196. [CrossRef] [PubMed]
4. Raffaeli, W.; Tenti, M.; Corraro, A.; Malafoglia, V.; Ilari, S.; Balzani, E.; Bonci, A. Chronic Pain: What Does It Mean? A Review on the Use of the Term Chronic Pain in Clinical Practice. *J. Pain Res.* **2021**, *14*, 827–835. [CrossRef] [PubMed]
5. Treede, R.D.; Rief, W.; Barke, A.; Aziz, Q.; Bennett, M.I.; Benoliel, R.; Cohen, M.; Evers, S.; Finnerup, N.B.; First, M.B.; et al. A classification of chronic pain for ICD-11. *Pain* **2015**, *156*, 1003–1007. [CrossRef]
6. Deyo, R.A.; Mirza, S.K.; Turner, J.A.; Martin, B.I. Overtreating chronic back pain: Time to back off? *J. Am. Board Fam. Med. JABFM* **2009**, *22*, 62–68. [CrossRef]
7. Bushnell, M.C.; Frangos, E.; Madian, N. Non-pharmacological Treatment of Pain: Grand Challenge and Future Opportunities. *Front. Pain Res.* **2021**, *2*, 696783. [CrossRef]
8. Tang, S.K.; Tse, M.M.Y.; Leung, S.F.; Fotis, T. The effectiveness, suitability, and sustainability of non-pharmacological methods of managing pain in community-dwelling older adults: A systematic review. *BMC Public Health* **2019**, *19*, 1488. [CrossRef]
9. Foster, N.E.; Anema, J.R.; Cherkin, D.; Chou, R.; Cohen, S.P.; Gross, D.P.; Ferreira, P.H.; Fritz, J.M.; Koes, B.W.; Peul, W.; et al. Prevention and treatment of low back pain: Evidence, challenges, and promising directions. *Lancet* **2018**, *391*, 2368–2383. [CrossRef]
10. Macfarlane, G.J.; Kronisch, C.; Dean, L.E.; Atzeni, F.; Häuser, W.; Fluß, E.; Choy, E.; Kosek, E.; Amris, K.; Branco, J.; et al. EULAR revised recommendations for the management of fibromyalgia. *Ann. Rheum. Dis.* **2017**, *76*, 318–328. [CrossRef]
11. National Institute for Health and Care Excellence (NICE). *Chronic Pain (Primary and Secondary) in Over 16s: Assessment of All Chronic Pain and Management of Chronic Primary Pain*; National Institute for Health and Care Excellence (NICE): London, UK, 2021; NICE Evidence Reviews Collection; ISBN 978-1-4731-4067-7. Available online: https://www.nice.org.uk/guidance/ng193 (accessed on 25 May 2023).
12. Watson, J.A.; Ryan, C.G.; Cooper, L.; Ellington, D.; Whittle, R.; Lavender, M.; Dixon, J.; Atkinson, G.; Cooper, K.; Martin, D.J. Pain Neuroscience Education for Adults With Chronic Musculoskeletal Pain: A Mixed-Methods Systematic Review and Meta-Analysis. *J. Pain* **2019**, *20*, 1140.e1–1140.e22. [CrossRef] [PubMed]
13. Butler, D.S.; Moseley, G.L. *Explain Pain*, 2nd ed.; Noigroup Publications: Adelaide, Australia, 2013.
14. Engel, G.L. The need for a new medical model: A challenge for biomedicine. *Science* **1977**, *196*, 129–136. [CrossRef] [PubMed]
15. McClelland, J.L.; Cleeremans, A. Connectionist models. In *The Oxford Companion to Consciousness*; Bayne, T., Cleeremans, A., Wilken, P., Eds.; Oxford University Press: Oxford, UK, 2009.
16. Moseley, G.L.; Brhyn, L.; Ilowiecki, M.; Solstad, K.; Hodges, P.W. The threat of predictable and unpredictable pain: Differential effects on central nervous system processing? *Aust. J. Physiother.* **2003**, *49*, 263–267. [CrossRef]
17. Bain, D. Evaluativist Accounts of Pain's Unpleasantness. In *The Routledge Handbook of the Philosophy of Pain*; Corns, J., Ed.; Routledge: London, UK, 2017; pp. 40–50.
18. Ploner, M.; Lee, M.C.; Wiech, K.; Bingel, U.; Tracey, I. Prestimulus functional connectivity determines pain perception in humans. *Proc. Natl. Acad. Sci. USA* **2010**, *107*, 355–360. [CrossRef] [PubMed]
19. Mitsi, V.; Zachariou, V. Modulation of pain, nociception, and analgesia by the brain reward center. *Neuroscience* **2016**, *338*, 81–92. [CrossRef]
20. Labrakakis, C. The Role of the Insular Cortex in Pain. *Int. J. Mol. Sci.* **2023**, *24*, 5736. [CrossRef]
21. Zhang, M.; Yang, Z.; Zhong, J.; Zhang, Y.; Lin, X.; Cai, H.; Kong, Y. Thalamocortical Mechanisms for Nostalgia-Induced Analgesia. *J. Neurosci.* **2022**, *42*, 2963–2972. [CrossRef]
22. Kim, J.; Kang, I.; Chung, Y.-A.; Kim, T.-S.; Namgung, E.; Lee, S.; Oh, J.K.; Jeong, H.S.; Cho, H.; Kim, M.J.; et al. Altered attentional control over the salience network in complex regional pain syndrome. *Sci. Rep.* **2018**, *8*, 7466. [CrossRef]
23. Figdor, C. The Nonsense View. In *Pieces of Mind: The Proper Domain of Psychological Predicates*; Oxford University Press: Oxford, UK, 2018.
24. Harré, R. Behind the Mereological Fallacy. *Philosophy* **2012**, *87*, 329–352. [CrossRef]
25. Bich, L. Autonomous Systems and the Place of Biology Among Sciences. Perspectives for an Epistemology of Complex Systems. In *Multiplicity and Interdisciplinarity. Contemporary Systems Thinking*; Minati, G., Ed.; Springer: Cham, Switzerland, 2021. [CrossRef]
26. Ma'ayan, A. Complex systems biology. *J. R. Soc. Interface* **2017**, *14*, 20170391. [CrossRef]

27. Flor, H.; Elbert, T.; Mühlnickel, W.; Pantev, C.; Wienbruch, C.; Taub, E. Cortical reorganization and phantom phenomena in congenital and traumatic upper-extremity amputees. *Exp. Brain Res.* **1998**, *119*, 205–212. [CrossRef] [PubMed]
28. Collins, K.L.; Russell, H.G.; Schumacher, P.J.; Robinson-Freeman, K.E.; O'Conor, E.C.; Gibney, K.D.; Yambem, O.; Dykes, R.W.; Waters, R.S.; Tsao, J.W. A review of current theories and treatments for phantom limb pain. *J. Clin. Investig.* **2018**, *128*, 2168–2176. [CrossRef] [PubMed]
29. Vaso, A.; Adahan, H.M.; Gjika, A.; Zahaj, S.; Zhurda, T.; Vyshka, G.; Devor, M. Peripheral nervous system origin of phantom limb pain. *Pain* **2014**, *155*, 1384–1391. [CrossRef]
30. Borghi, B.; D'Addabbo, M.; White, P.F.; Gallerani, P.; Toccaceli, L.; Raffaeli, W.; Tognù, A.; Fabbri, N.; Mercuri, M. The use of prolonged peripheral neural blockade after lower extremity amputation: The effect on symptoms associated with phantom limb syndrome. *Anesth. Analg.* **2010**, *111*, 1308–1315. [CrossRef] [PubMed]
31. Quintner, J. Why Are Women with Fibromyalgia so Stigmatized? *Pain Med.* **2020**, *21*, 882–888. [CrossRef] [PubMed]
32. Nijs, J.; George, S.Z.; Clauw, D.J.; Fernández-de-las-Peñas, C.; Kosek, E.; Ickmans, K.; Fernández-Carnero, J.; Polli, A.; Kapreli, E.; Huysmans, E.; et al. Central sensitisation in chronic pain conditions: Latest discoveries and their potential for precision medicine. *Lancet Rheumatol.* **2021**, *3*, e383–e392. [CrossRef]
33. Martínez-Lavín, M. Centralized nociplastic pain causing fibromyalgia: An emperor with no cloths? *Clin. Rheumatol.* **2022**, *41*, 3915–3917. [CrossRef]
34. Grayston, R.; Czanner, G.; Elhadd, K.; Goebel, A.; Frank, B.; Üçeyler, N.; Malik, R.A.; Alam, U. A systematic review and meta-analysis of the prevalence of small fiber pathology in fibromyalgia: Implications for a new paradigm in fibromyalgia etiopathogenesis. *Semin. Arthritis Rheum.* **2019**, *48*, 933–940. [CrossRef]
35. Coskun Benlidayi, I. Role of inflammation in the pathogenesis and treatment of fibromyalgia. *Rheumatol. Int.* **2019**, *39*, 781–791. [CrossRef]
36. Olausson, P.; Ghafouri, B.; Ghafouri, N.; Gerdle, B. Specific proteins of the trapezius muscle correlate with pain intensity and sensitivity-an explorative multivariate proteomic study of the trapezius muscle in women with chronic widespread pain. *J. Pain Res.* **2016**, *9*, 345–356. [CrossRef]
37. Wåhlén, K.; Ernberg, M.; Kosek, E.; Mannerkorpi, K.; Gerdle, B.; Ghafouri, B. Significant correlation between plasma proteome profile and pain intensity, sensitivity, and psychological distress in women with fibromyalgia. *Sci. Rep.* **2020**, *10*, 12508. [CrossRef] [PubMed]
38. Erdrich, S.; Hawrelak, J.A.; Myers, S.P.; Harnett, J.E. Determining the association between fibromyalgia, the gut microbiome and its biomarkers: A systematic review. *BMC Musculoskelet. Disord.* **2020**, *21*, 181. [CrossRef] [PubMed]
39. Coderre, T.J. Contribution of microvascular dysfunction to chronic pain. *Front. Pain Res.* **2023**, *4*, 1111559. [CrossRef] [PubMed]
40. Rittner, H.L.; Brack, A.; Stein, C. Pain and the immune system. *Br. J. Anaesth.* **2008**, *101*, 40–44. [CrossRef]
41. Moncrieff, J.; Cooper, R.E.; Stockmann, T.; Amendola, S.; Hengartner, M.P.; Horowitz, M.A. The serotonin theory of depression: A systematic umbrella review of the evidence. *Mol. Psychiatry* **2022**, *28*, 3243–3256. [CrossRef]
42. Lee, M.; Silverman, S.M.; Hansen, H.; Patel, V.B.; Manchikanti, L. A comprehensive review of opioid-induced hyperalgesia. *Pain Physician.* **2011**, *14*, 145–161. [CrossRef]
43. Ferreira, G.E.; Abdel-Shaheed, C.; Underwood, M.; Finnerup, N.B.; Day, R.O.; McLachlan, A.; Eldabe, S.; Zadro, J.R.; Maher, C.G. Efficacy, safety, and tolerability of antidepressants for pain in adults: Overview of systematic reviews. *BMJ Clin. Res. Ed.* **2023**, *380*, e072415. [CrossRef]
44. Carvalho, A.F.; Sharma, M.S.; Brunoni, A.R.; Vieta, E.; Fava, G.A. The Safety, Tolerability and Risks Associated with the Use of Newer Generation Antidepressant Drugs: A Critical Review of the Literature. *Psychother. Psychosom.* **2016**, *85*, 270–288. [CrossRef]
45. Kaczmarek, E. How to distinguish medicalization from over-medicalization? *Med. Health Care Philos.* **2019**, *22*, 119–128. [CrossRef]
46. Paice, J.A.; Von Roenn, J.H. Under- or overtreatment of pain in the patient with cancer: How to achieve proper balance. *J. Clin. Oncol.* **2014**, *32*, 1721–1726. [CrossRef]
47. Raja, S.N.; Carr, D.B.; Cohen, M.; Finnerup, N.B.; Flor, H.; Gibson, S.; Keefe, F.J.; Mogil, J.S.; Ringkamp, M.; Sluka, K.A.; et al. The Revised International Association for the Study of Pain Definition of Pain: Concepts, Challenges, and Compromises. *Pain* **2020**, *161*, 1976–1982. [CrossRef] [PubMed]
48. Cohen, M.; Weisman, A.; Quintner, J. Pain is Not a "Thing": How That Error Affects Language and Logic in Pain Medicine. *J. Pain* **2022**, *23*, 1283–1293. [CrossRef] [PubMed]
49. Louw, A.; Nijs, J.; Puentedura, E.J. A Clinical Perspective on a Pain Neuroscience Education Approach to Manual Therapy. *J. Man. Manip. Ther.* **2017**, *25*, 160–168. [CrossRef]
50. Saposnik, G.; Redelmeier, D.; Ruff, C.C.; Tobler, P.N. Cognitive Biases Associated with Medical Decisions: A Systematic Review. *BMC Med. Inform. Decis. Mak.* **2016**, *16*, 138. [CrossRef] [PubMed]
51. Feldman, J. The Simplicity Principle in Perception and Cognition. *Wiley Interdiscip. Rev. Cogn. Sci.* **2016**, *7*, 330–340. [CrossRef]
52. Fares, W.H. The 'Availability' Bias: Underappreciated but with Major Potential Implications. *Crit. Care* **2014**, *18*, 118. [CrossRef] [PubMed]
53. Skokowski, P. Sensing Qualia. *Front. Syst. Neurosci.* **2022**, *16*, 795405. [CrossRef]
54. Chalmers, D.J. Facing Up to the Problem of Consciousness. *J. Conscious. Stud.* **1995**, *2*, 200–219.
55. Moreira-Almeida, A.; Araujo, S.F.; Cloninger, C.R. The Presentation of the Mind-Brain Problem in Leading Psychiatry Journals. *Rev. Bras. Psiquiatr.* **2018**, *40*, 335–342. [CrossRef]

56. International Association for the Study of Pain. Terminology. Available online: https://www.iasp-pain.org/resources/terminology/ (accessed on 25 May 2023).
57. Savitha, S.A.; Sacchidanand, S.A.; Gowda, S.K. Misnomers in Dermatology: An Update. *Indian J. Dermatol.* **2013**, *58*, 467–474. [CrossRef]
58. Fisher, J.P.; Hassan, D.T.; Connor, N.O. Minerva. *BMJ* **1995**, *310*, 70. [CrossRef]
59. Reichling, D.B.; Green, P.G.; Levine, J.D. The Fundamental Unit of Pain is the Cell. *Pain* **2013**, *154* (Suppl. S1), S2–S9. [CrossRef]
60. Sneddon, L.U. Comparative Physiology of Nociception and Pain. *Physiology* **2018**, *33*, 63–73. [CrossRef]
61. Tobimatsu, S. Understanding Cortical Pain Perception in Humans. *Neurol. Clin. Neurosci.* **2021**, *9*, 24–29. [CrossRef]
62. Roy, M.; Piché, M.; Chen, J.I.; Peretz, I.; Rainville, P. Cerebral and Spinal Modulation of Pain by Emotions. *Proc. Natl. Acad. Sci. USA* **2009**, *106*, 20900–20905. [CrossRef] [PubMed]
63. Tracy, L.M.; Gibson, S.J.; Georgiou-Karistianis, N.; Giummarra, M.J. Effects of Explicit Cueing and Ambiguity on the Anticipation and Experience of a Painful Thermal Stimulus. *PLoS ONE* **2017**, *12*, e0183650. [CrossRef]
64. Boadas-Vaello, P.; Castany, S.; Homs, J.; Álvarez-Pérez, B.; Deulofeu, M.; Verdú, E. Neuroplasticity of Ascending and Descending Pathways after Somatosensory System Injury: Reviewing Knowledge to Identify Neuropathic Pain Therapeutic Targets. *Spinal Cord* **2016**, *54*, 330–340. [CrossRef]
65. Melzack, R.; Wall, P.D. Pain Mechanisms: A New Theory. *Science* **1965**, *150*, 971–979. [CrossRef]
66. Moseley, G.L.; Pearson, N.; Reezigt, R.; Madden, V.J.; Hutchinson, M.R.; Dunbar, M.; Beetsma, A.J.; Leake, H.B.; Moore, P.; Simons, L.; et al. Considering Precision and Utility When we Talk About Pain. Comment on Cohen et al. *J. Pain.* **2023**, *24*, 178–181. [CrossRef]
67. Cohen, M.; Weisman, A.; Quintner, J. Response to van Rysewyk S and Moseley GL et al.'s Comments on Cohen et al. *J Pain* 2022; 23(8):1283–1293. *J. Pain.* **2023**, *24*, 184–185. [CrossRef]
68. Descartes, R.; Quintás, G. *Traité de l'homme (El Tratado del Hombre)*; Alianza Editorial: Madrid, Spain, 1990.
69. Dubin, A.E.; Patapoutian, A. Nociceptors: The Sensors of the Pain Pathway. *J. Clin. Investig.* **2010**, *120*, 3760–3772. [CrossRef] [PubMed]
70. Benarroch, E.E. Ion Channels in Nociceptors: Recent Developments. *Neurology* **2015**, *84*, 1153–1164. [CrossRef] [PubMed]
71. Djouhri, L.; Lawson, S.N. Abeta-fiber Nociceptive Primary Afferent Neurons: A Review of Incidence and Properties in Relation to Other Afferent A-fiber Neurons in Mammals. *Brain Res. Rev.* **2004**, *46*, 131–145. [CrossRef] [PubMed]
72. Lechner, S. An Update on the Spinal and Peripheral Pathways of Pain Signalling. *e-Neuroforum* **2017**, *23*, 131–136. [CrossRef]
73. Prato, V.; Taberner, F.J.; Hockley, J.R.F.; Callejo, G.; Arcourt, A.; Tazir, B.; Hammer, L.; Schad, P.; Heppenstall, P.A.; Smith, E.S.; et al. Functional and Molecular Characterization of Mechanoinsensitive "Silent" Nociceptors. *Cell Rep.* **2017**, *21*, 3102–3115. [CrossRef]
74. McGlone, F.; Wessberg, J.; Olausson, H. Discriminative and Affective Touch: Sensing and Feeling. *Neuron* **2014**, *82*, 737–755. [CrossRef]
75. Hucho, T.; Levine, J.D. Signaling Pathways in Sensitization: Toward a Nociceptor Cell Biology. *Neuron* **2007**, *55*, 365–376. [CrossRef]
76. Du, X.; Hao, H.; Yang, Y.; Huang, S.; Wang, C.; Gigout, S.; Ramli, R.; Li, X.; Jaworska, E.; Edwards, I.; et al. Local GABAergic Signaling within Sensory Ganglia Controls Peripheral Nociceptive Transmission. *J. Clin. Investig.* **2017**, *127*, 1741–1756. [CrossRef]
77. Hao, H.; Ramli, R.; Wang, C.; Liu, C.; Shah, S.; Mullen, P.; Lall, V.; Jones, F.; Shao, J.; Zhang, H.; et al. Dorsal Root Ganglia Control Nociceptive Input to the Central Nervous System. *PLoS Biol.* **2023**, *21*, e3001958. [CrossRef]
78. Spigelman, I. Therapeutic Targeting of Peripheral Cannabinoid Receptors in Inflammatory and Neuropathic Pain States. In *Translational Pain Research: From Mouse to Man*; Kruger, L., Ed.; CRC Press/Taylor & Francis: Boca Raton, FL, USA, 2010.
79. Sehgal, N.; Smith, H.S.; Manchikanti, L. Peripherally Acting Opioids and Clinical Implications for Pain Control. *Pain Physician* **2011**, *14*, 249–258. [CrossRef]
80. Agarwal, N.; Pacher, P.; Tegeder, I.; Amaya, F.; Constantin, C.E.; Brenner, G.J.; Rubino, T.; Michalski, C.W.; Marsicano, G.; Monory, K.; et al. Cannabinoids Mediate Analgesia Largely Via Peripheral Type 1 Cannabinoid Receptors in Nociceptors. *Nat. Neurosci.* **2007**, *10*, 870–879. [CrossRef] [PubMed]
81. Guindon, J.; Hohmann, A.G. Cannabinoid CB2 Receptors: A Therapeutic Target for the Treatment of Inflammatory and Neuropathic Pain. *Br. J. Pharmacol.* **2008**, *153*, 319–334. [CrossRef] [PubMed]
82. Baron, R.; Hans, G.; Dickenson, A.H. Peripheral Input and its Importance for Central Sensitization. *Ann. Neurol.* **2013**, *74*, 630–636. [CrossRef] [PubMed]
83. Yang, Q.; Wu, Z.; Hadden, J.K.; Odem, M.A.; Zuo, Y.; Crook, R.J.; Frost, J.A.; Walters, E.T. Persistent Pain After Spinal Cord Injury is Maintained by Primary Afferent Activity. *J. Neurosci.* **2014**, *34*, 10765–10769. [CrossRef]
84. North, R.Y.; Odem, M.A.; Li, Y.; Tatsui, C.E.; Cassidy, R.M.; Dougherty, P.M.; Walters, E.T. Electrophysiological Alterations Driving Pain-Associated Spontaneous Activity in Human Sensory Neuron Somata Parallel Alterations Described in Spontaneously Active Rodent Nociceptors. *J. Pain.* **2022**, *23*, 1343–1357. [CrossRef]
85. Velasco, E.; Alvarez, J.L.; Meseguer, V.M.; Gallar, J.; Talavera, K. Membrane Potential Instabilities in Sensory Neurons: Mechanisms and Pathophysiological Relevance. *Pain* **2022**, *163*, 64–74. [CrossRef]
86. Velasco, E.; Alvarez, J.; Meseguer Vigueras, V.M.; Gallar, J.; Talavera, K. Action Potential Firing and Sensory Transduction are Sustained by Membrane Potential Instabilities in Peripheral Sensory Neurons. *Biophys. J.* **2023**, *122*, 417a. [CrossRef]

87. Tian, J.; Bavencoffe, A.G.; Zhu, M.X.; Walters, E.T. Readiness of nociceptor cell bodies to generate spontaneous activity results from background activity of diverse ion channels and high input resistance. *Pain* **2023**. [CrossRef]
88. van der Vlist, M.; Raoof, R.; Willemen, H.L.D.M.; Prado, J.; Versteeg, S.; Martin Gil, C.; Vos, M.; Lokhorst, R.E.; Pasterkamp, R.J.; Kojima, T.; et al. Macrophages Transfer Mitochondria to Sensory Neurons to Resolve Inflammatory Pain. *Neuron* **2022**, *110*, 613–626.e9. [CrossRef]
89. Bavencoffe, A.G.; Spence, E.A.; Zhu, M.Y.; Garza-Carbajal, A.; Chu, K.E.; Bloom, O.E.; Dessauer, C.W.; Walters, E.T. Macrophage Migration Inhibitory Factor (MIF) Makes Complex Contributions to Pain-Related Hyperactivity of Nociceptors after Spinal Cord Injury. *J. Neurosci.* **2022**, *42*, 5463–5480. [CrossRef]
90. Hanani, M.; Spray, D.C. Emerging Importance of Satellite Glia in Nervous System Function and Dysfunction. *Nat. Rev. Neurosci.* **2020**, *21*, 485–498. [CrossRef] [PubMed]
91. Zheng, H.; Lim, J.Y.; Seong, J.Y.; Hwang, S.W. The Role of Corticotropin-Releasing Hormone at Peripheral Nociceptors: Implications for Pain Modulation. *Biomedicines* **2020**, *8*, 623. [CrossRef]
92. D'Mello, R.; Dickenson, A.H. Spinal Cord Mechanisms of Pain. *Br. J. Anaesth.* **2008**, *101*, 8–16. [CrossRef] [PubMed]
93. Heinricher, M.M.; Tavares, I.; Leith, J.L.; Lumb, B.M. Descending Control of Nociception: Specificity, Recruitment and Plasticity. *Brain Res. Rev.* **2009**, *60*, 214–225. [CrossRef]
94. Rexed, B. The Cytoarchitectonic Organization of the Spinal Cord in the Cat. *J. Comp. Neurol.* **1952**, *96*, 414–495. [CrossRef]
95. Todd, A. Neuronal Circuitry for Pain Processing in the Dorsal Horn. *Nat. Rev. Neurosci.* **2010**, *11*, 823–836. [CrossRef] [PubMed]
96. Sandkühler, J. Models and Mechanisms of Hyperalgesia and Allodynia. *Physiol. Rev.* **2009**, *89*, 707–758. [CrossRef]
97. Woolf, C.J. Evidence for a Central Component of Post-Injury Pain Hypersensitivity. *Nature* **1983**, *306*, 686–688. [CrossRef]
98. Bliss, T.V.; Lomo, T. Long-lasting Potentiation of Synaptic Transmission in the Dentate Area of the Anaesthetized Rabbit Following Stimulation of the Perforant Path. *J. Physiol.* **1973**, *232*, 331–356. [CrossRef]
99. Randic, M.; Jiang, M.C.; Cerne, R. Long-term Potentiation and Long-term Depression of Primary Afferent Neurotransmission in the Rat Spinal Cord. *J. Neurosci.* **1993**, *13*, 5228–5241. [CrossRef]
100. Ikeda, H.; Stark, J.; Fischer, H.; Wagner, M.; Drdla, R.; Jager, T.; Sandkuhler, J. Synaptic Amplifier of Inflammatory Pain in the Spinal Dorsal Horn. *Science* **2006**, *312*, 1659–1662. [CrossRef] [PubMed]
101. Woolf, C.J. Central Sensitization: Implications for the Diagnosis and Treatment of Pain. *Pain* **2011**, *152*, S2–S15. [CrossRef] [PubMed]
102. Yunus, M.B. Fibromyalgia and Overlapping Disorders: The Unifying Concept of Central Sensitivity Syndromes. *Semin. Arthritis Rheum.* **2007**, *36*, 339–356. [CrossRef] [PubMed]
103. Johnson-Laird, P.N. Mental Models and Deduction. *Trends Cogn. Sci.* **2001**, *5*, 434–442. [CrossRef]
104. Adams, G.R.; Gandhi, W.; Harrison, R.; van Reekum, C.M.; Wood-Anderson, D.; Gilron, I.; Salomons, T.V. Do "Central Sensitization" Questionnaires Reflect Measures of Nociceptive Sensitization or Psychological Constructs? A Systematic Review and Meta-Analyses. *Pain* **2023**, *164*, 1222–1239. [CrossRef]
105. Walitt, B.; Ceko, M.; Gracely, J.L.; Gracely, R.H. Neuroimaging of Central Sensitivity Syndromes: Key Insights from the Scientific Literature. *Curr. Rheumatol. Rev.* **2016**, *12*, 55–87. [CrossRef]
106. Yunus, M.B. Central Sensitivity Syndromes: A New Paradigm and Group Nosology for Fibromyalgia and Overlapping Conditions, and the Related Issue of Disease Versus Illness. *Semin. Arthritis Rheum.* **2008**, *37*, 339–352. [CrossRef]
107. Clauw, D.J. Fibromyalgia and Related Conditions. *Mayo Clin. Proc.* **2015**, *90*, 680–692. [CrossRef]
108. Weisman, A.; Quintner, J.; Masharawi, Y. Amplified Pain Syndrome—An Insupportable Assumption. *JAMA Pediatr.* **2021**, *175*, 557–558. [CrossRef]
109. Al-Chalabi, M.; Reddy, V.; Gupta, S. Neuroanatomy, Spinothalamic Tract. In *StatPearls*; StatPearls Publishing: Treasure Island, FL, USA, 2022.
110. Bowsher, D. Termination of the Central Pain Pathway in Man: The Conscious Appreciation of Pain. *Brain* **1957**, *80*, 607–622. [CrossRef]
111. Albe-Fessard, D.; Berkley, K.J.; Kruger, L.; Ralston, H.J., III; Willis, W.D., Jr. Diencephalic Mechanisms of Pain Sensation. *Brain Res.* **1985**, *356*, 217–296. [CrossRef] [PubMed]
112. De Ridder, D.; Adhia, D.; Vanneste, S. The Anatomy of Pain and Suffering in the Brain and Its Clinical Implications. *Neurosci. Biobehav. Rev.* **2021**, *130*, 125–146. [CrossRef]
113. Craig, A.D.; Dostrovsky, J. Medulla to Thalamus. In *Textbook of Pain*; Wall, P., Melzack, R., Eds.; Churchill-Livingstone: Edinburgh, UK, 1999; pp. 183–214.
114. Tolomeo, S.; Christmas, D.; Jentzsch, I.; Johnston, B.; Sprengelmeyer, R.; Matthews, K.; Steele, J.D. A Causal Role for the Anterior Mid-Cingulate Cortex in Negative Affect and Cognitive Control. *Brain* **2016**, *139*, 1844–1854. [CrossRef] [PubMed]
115. Hohwy, J.; Seth, A.K. Predictive Processing as a Systematic Basis for Identifying the Neural Correlates of Consciousness. *Philos. Mind Sci.* **2020**, *1*, 3. [CrossRef]
116. Flor, H.; Elbert, T.; Knecht, S.; Wienbruch, C.; Pantev, C.; Birbaumers, N.; Larbig, W.; Taub, E. Phantom-Limb Pain as a Perceptual Correlate of Cortical Reorganization Following Arm Amputation. *Nature* **1995**, *375*, 482–484. [CrossRef] [PubMed]
117. Gerrans, P. Pain Asymbolia as Depersonalization for Pain Experience. An Interoceptive Active Inference Account. *Front. Psychol.* **2020**, *11*, 523710. [CrossRef]
118. Grahek, N. *Feeling Pain and Being in Pain*, 2nd ed.; Boston Review; Bradford Books; MIT Pess: Cambridge, MA, USA, 2007.

119. Stilwell, P.; Hudon, A.; Meldrum, K.; Pagé, M.G.; Wideman, T.H. What is Pain-Related Suffering? Conceptual Critiques, Key Attributes, and Outstanding Questions. *J. Pain* **2022**, *23*, 729–738. [CrossRef]
120. Koolhaas, J.M.; Bartolomucci, A.; Buwalda, B.; de Boer, S.; Flügge, G.; Korte, S.; Meerlo, P.; Murison, R.; Olivier, B.; Palanza, P.; et al. Stress Revisited: A Critical Evaluation of the Stress Concept. *Neurosci. Biobehav. Rev.* **2011**, *35*, 1291–1301. [CrossRef]
121. Blackburn-Munro, G.; Blackburn-Munro, R.E. Chronic Pain, Chronic Stress and Depression: Coincidence or Consequence? *J. Neuroendocrinol.* **2001**, *13*, 1009–1023. [CrossRef]
122. Abdallah, C.G.; Geha, P. Chronic Pain and Chronic Stress: Two Sides of the Same Coin? *Chronic Stress* **2017**, *1*, 2470547017704763. [CrossRef]
123. Kornelsen, J.; McIver, T.A.; Stroman, P.W. Unique Brain Regions Involved in Positive Versus Negative Emotional Modulation of Pain. *Scand. J. Pain* **2019**, *19*, 583–596. [CrossRef]
124. Mathur, V.A.; Moayedi, M.; Keaser, M.L.; Khan, S.A.; Hubbard, C.S.; Goyal, M.; Seminowicz, D.A. High Frequency Migraine is Associated with Lower Acute Pain Sensitivity and Abnormal Insula Activity Related to Migraine Pain Intensity, Attack Frequency, Pain Catastrophizing. *Front. Hum. Neurosci.* **2016**, *10*, 489. [CrossRef]
125. Yang, S.; Chang, M.C. Chronic Pain: Structural and Functional Changes in Brain Structures and Associated Negative Affective States. *Int. J. Mol. Sci.* **2019**, *20*, 3130. [CrossRef]
126. Wade, J.B.; Riddle, D.L.; Price, D.D.; Dumenci, L. Role of Pain Catastrophizing During Pain Processing in a Cohort of Patients with Chronic and Severe Arthritic Knee Pain. *Pain* **2011**, *152*, 314–319. [CrossRef]
127. Edwards, R.R.; Dworkin, R.H.; Sullivan, M.D.; Turk, D.C.; Wasan, A.D. The Role of Psychosocial Processes in the Development and Maintenance of Chronic Pain. *J. Pain* **2016**, *17*, T70–T92. [CrossRef]
128. Piazza, M. Maine de Biran and Gall's Phrenology: The Origins of a Debate About the Localization of Mental Faculties. *Br. J. Hist. Philos.* **2020**, *28*, 866–884. [CrossRef]
129. Iannetti, G.D.; Mouraux, A. From the Neuromatrix to the Pain Matrix (and Back). *Exp. Brain Res.* **2010**, *205*, 1–12. [CrossRef]
130. Melzack, R. From the Gate to the Neuromatrix. *Pain* **1999**, *82*, S121–S126. [CrossRef]
131. Tracey, I.; Mantyh, P.W. The Cerebral Signature for Pain Perception and Its Modulation. *Neuron* **2007**, *55*, 377–391. [CrossRef]
132. Büchel, C.; Bornhovd, K.; Quante, M.; Glauche, V.; Bromm, B.; Weiller, C. Dissociable Neural Responses Related to Pain Intensity, Stimulus Intensity, and Stimulus Awareness within the Anterior Cingulate Cortex: A Parametric Single-Trial Laser Functional Magnetic Resonance Imaging Study. *J. Neurosci.* **2002**, *22*, 970–976. [CrossRef]
133. Hofbauer, R.K.; Rainville, P.; Duncan, G.H.; Bushnell, M.C. Cortical Representation of the Sensory Dimension of Pain. *J. Neurophysiol.* **2001**, *86*, 402–411. [CrossRef] [PubMed]
134. Schweinhardt, P.; Bountra, C.; Tracey, I. Pharmacological FMRI in the Development of New Analgesic Compounds. *NMR Biomed.* **2006**, *19*, 702–711. [CrossRef] [PubMed]
135. Boly, M.; Faymonville, M.E.; Schnakers, C.; Peigneux, P.; Lambermont, B.; Phillips, C.; Lancellotti, P.; Luxen, A.; Lamy, M.; Moonen, G.; et al. Perception of Pain in the Minimally Conscious State with PET Activation: An Observational Study. *Lancet Neurol.* **2008**, *7*, 1013–1020. [CrossRef] [PubMed]
136. Legrain, V.; Iannetti, G.D.; Plaghki, L.; Mouraux, A. The Pain Matrix Reloaded: A Salience Detection System for the Body. *Prog. Neurobiol.* **2011**, *93*, 111–124. [CrossRef]
137. Coninx, S. The Notorious Neurophilosophy of Pain: A Family Resemblance Approach to Idiosyncrasy and Generalizability. *Mind Lang.* **2023**, *38*, 178–197. [CrossRef]
138. Wall, P.D. Independent Mechanisms Converge on Pain. *Nat. Med.* **1995**, *1*, 740–741. [CrossRef]
139. Choi, J.M.; Padmala, S.; Spechler, P.; Pessoa, L. Pervasive Competition between Threat and Reward in the Brain. *Soc. Cogn. Affect. Neurosci.* **2014**, *9*, 737–750. [CrossRef]
140. Elman, I.; Borsook, D. Common Brain Mechanisms of Chronic Pain and Addiction. *Neuron* **2016**, *89*, 11–36. [CrossRef]
141. De Ridder, D.; Vanneste, S. The bayesian brain in imbalance: Medial, lateral and descending pathways in tinnitus and pain: A perspective. *Prog. Brain Res.* **2021**, *262*, 309–334. [CrossRef]
142. Tabor, A.; Thacker, M.A.; Moseley, G.L.; Körding, K.P. Pain: A Statistical Account. *PLoS Comput. Biol.* **2017**, *13*, e1005142. [CrossRef]
143. Harris, S.; Sheth, S.A.; Cohen, M.S. Functional Neuroimaging of Belief, Disbelief, and Uncertainty. *Ann. Neurol.* **2008**, *63*, 141–147. [CrossRef] [PubMed]
144. Eckert, A.L.; Pabst, K.; Endres, D.M. A Bayesian Model for Chronic Pain. *Front. Pain Res.* **2022**, *3*, 966034. [CrossRef] [PubMed]
145. Hechler, T.; Endres, D.M.; Thorwart, A. Why Harmless Sensations Might Hurt in Individuals with Chronic Pain: About Heightened Prediction and Perception of Pain in the Mind. *Front. Psychol.* **2016**, *7*, 1638. [CrossRef] [PubMed]
146. McCarberg, B.; Peppin, J. Pain Pathways and Nervous System Plasticity: Learning and Memory in Pain. *Pain Med.* **2019**, *20*, 2421–2437. [CrossRef]
147. Zhang, L.; Lu, X.; Bi, Y.; Hu, L. Pavlov's Pain: The Effect of Classical Conditioning on Pain Perception and its Clinical Implications. *Curr. Pain Headache Rep.* **2019**, *23*, 19. [CrossRef]
148. Gatzounis, R.; Schrooten, M.G.; Crombez, G.; Vlaeyen, J.W. Operant learning theory in pain and chronic pain rehabilitation. *Curr. Pain Headache Rep.* **2012**, *16*, 117–126. [CrossRef]
149. Stegemann, A.; Liu, S.; Romero, O.A.R.; Oswald, M.J.; Han, Y.; Beretta, C.A.; Gan, Z.; Tan, L.L.; Wisden, W.; Gräff, J.; et al. Prefrontal engrams of long-term fear memory perpetuate pain perception. *Nat. Neurosci.* **2023**, *26*, 820–829. [CrossRef]

150. Blasini, M.; Corsi, N.; Klinger, R.; Colloca, L. Nocebo and Pain: An Overview of the Psychoneurobiological Mechanisms. *Pain Rep.* **2017**, *2*, e585. [CrossRef]
151. Rossettini, G.; Campaci, F.; Bialosky, J.; Huysmans, E.; Vase, L.; Carlino, E. The Biology of Placebo and Nocebo Effects on Experimental and Chronic Pain: State of the Art. *J. Clin. Med.* **2023**, *12*, 4113. [CrossRef]
152. Colloca, L.; Barsky, A.J. Placebo and Nocebo Effects. *N. Engl. J. Med.* **2020**, *382*, 554–561. [CrossRef]
153. Clark, A. Whatever next? Predictive brains, situated agents, and the future of cognitive science. *Behav. Brain Sci.* **2013**, *36*, 181–204. [CrossRef]
154. Seth, A.K.; Bayne, T. Theories of consciousness. *Nat. Rev. Neurosci.* **2022**, *23*, 439–452. [CrossRef] [PubMed]
155. Brown, R.; Lau, H.; LeDoux, J.E. Understanding the higher-order approach to consciousness. *Trends Cogn. Sci.* **2019**, *23*, 754–768. [CrossRef]
156. Mashour, G.A.; Roelfsema, P.; Changeux, J.P.; Dehaene, S. Conscious processing and the global neuronal workspace hypothesis. *Neuron* **2020**, *105*, 776–798. [CrossRef]
157. Tononi, G.; Boly, M.; Massimini, M.; Koch, C. Integrated information theory: From consciousness to its physical substrate. *Nat. Rev. Neurosci.* **2016**, *17*, 450–461. [CrossRef]
158. Lamme, V.A. Towards a true neural stance on consciousness. *Trends Cogn. Sci.* **2006**, *10*, 494–501. [CrossRef]
159. Piasini, E.; Panzeri, S. Information Theory in Neuroscience. *Entropy* **2019**, *21*, 62. [CrossRef]
160. Borst, A.; Theunissen, F.E. Information theory and neural coding. *Nat. Neurosci.* **1999**, *2*, 947–957. [CrossRef]
161. Shannon, C.E. The mathematical theory of communication. *Bell Syst. Tech. J.* **1948**, *27*, 379–423. [CrossRef]
162. Eckhorn, R.; Popel, B. Rigorous and extended application of information theory to the afferent visual system of the cat. *Biol. Cybern.* **1975**, *17*, 7–17. [CrossRef]

Disclaimer/Publisher's Note: The statements, opinions and data contained in all publications are solely those of the individual author(s) and contributor(s) and not of MDPI and/or the editor(s). MDPI and/or the editor(s) disclaim responsibility for any injury to people or property resulting from any ideas, methods, instructions or products referred to in the content.

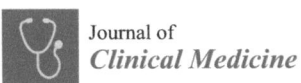 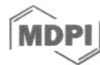

Review

The Calm after the Storm: A State-of-the-Art Review about Recommendations Put Forward during the COVID-19 Pandemic to Improve Chronic Pain Management

Marimée Godbout-Parent [1], Tristan Spilak [1,2], M. Gabrielle Pagé [2,3], Manon Choinière [2,3], Lise Dassieu [2], Gwenaelle De Clifford-Faugère [1] and Anaïs Lacasse [1,*]

[1] Département des Sciences de la Santé, Université du Québec en Abitibi-Témiscamingue (UQAT), Rouyn-Noranda, QC J9X 5E4, Canada; marimee.godbout-parent@uqat.ca (M.G.-P.)
[2] Centre de Recherche, Centre Hospitalier de l'Université de Montréal (CHUM), Montréal, QC H2X 0A9, Canada
[3] Département D'anesthésiologie et de Médecine de la Douleur, Faculté de Médecine, Université de Montréal, Montréal, QC H3T 1J4, Canada
* Correspondence: anais.lacasse@uqat.ca

Abstract: The COVID-19 pandemic has brought its fair share of consequences. To control the transmission of the virus, several public health restrictions were put in place. While these restrictions had beneficial effects on transmission, they added to the pre-existing physical, psychosocial, and financial burdens associated with chronic pain, and made existing treatment gaps, challenges, and inequities worse. However, it also prompted researchers and clinicians to seek out possible solutions and expedite their implementation. This state-of-the-art review focuses on the concrete recommendations issued during the COVID-19 pandemic to improve the health and maintain the care of people living with chronic pain. The search strategy included a combination of chronic pain and pandemic-related terms. Four databases (Medline, PsycINFO, CINAHL, and PubMed) were searched, and records were assessed for eligibility. Original studies, reviews, editorials, and guidelines published in French or in English in peer-reviewed journals or by recognized pain organizations were considered for inclusion. A total of 119 articles were analyzed, and over 250 recommendations were extracted and classified into 12 subcategories: change in clinical practice, change in policy, continuity of care, research avenues to explore, group virtual care, health communications/education, individual virtual care, infection control, lifestyle, non-pharmacological treatments, pharmacological treatments, and social considerations. Recommendations highlight the importance of involving various healthcare professionals to prevent mental health burden and emergency overload and emphasize the recognition of chronic pain. The pandemic disrupted chronic pain management in an already-fragile ecosystem, presenting a unique opportunity for understanding ongoing challenges and identifying innovative solutions. Numerous recommendations were identified that are relevant well beyond the COVID-19 crisis.

Keywords: chronic pain; COVID-19; pandemic; management; care treatment; recommendations; solutions; review

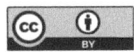

1. Introduction

The global population have seen their health and lives affected by the COVID-19 pandemic and its numerous consequences [1]. In fact, the pandemic has caused a combination of physical consequences (e.g., virus-related dry cough, fever, respiratory difficulties, fatigue [2], long-haul COVID [3]), psychosocial consequences (e.g., psychological distress, limited access to health services, domestic violence [4]), and economic consequences (e.g., business closures, increased unemployment rates, reduced work hours [5]). During the crisis, efforts were rapidly deployed to help people affected by the virus and to control its spread as much as possible [6]. The COVID-19 pandemic and its consequences mentioned above have disproportionately affected vulnerable groups, such as persons marginalized by their social identities, the elderly, people living with disabilities, women, and people with chronic illness [4,7]. For example, the pandemic has exacerbated the physical, psychological, economical, and health challenges that people living with chronic pain (CP) face on a daily basis [8–10]. Even before the COVID-19 pandemic, CP was an under-reported, under-recognized, under-diagnosed, and frequently under-treated disease [11–14]. Several barriers are named as potential sources leading to this suboptimal management, such as the lack of access to multidisciplinary care and the suboptimal integration of multimodal approaches which seek a balance between pharmacological and non-pharmacological treatments [13,15–17]. The restrictions imposed by public health during the COVID-19 pandemic, including lockdowns, the closure of non-essential services, and requirements to stop in-person treatment, have affected the accessibility of treatment, therefore potentially causing significant harm to people living with CP [8,9]. The pandemic has also worsened pre-existing physical, psychological, and financial burdens associated with CP and increased risk factors such as reduced sleep, inactivity, fear, anxiety, and depression [10,18].

COVID-19 has certainly intensified the existing gaps, difficulties, and inequalities in treatment for people living with CP, but has also emphasized the magnitude of the disease and created a sense of urgency in research [8]. In the most urgent time of the pandemic, much research was conducted on the impacts of the pandemic and many recommendations were made by researchers, experts, and healthcare professionals. Considering the current slower COVID-19 transmission rates and the concomitantly ongoing recovery of our healthcare systems from such a trial, it is vital to analyze the research carried out during this period. This is relevant not only to prepare for potential new pandemics, but to harness recommendations issued during the crisis that could help improve pain management well beyond the COVID-19 crisis. Therefore, this study represents a state-of-the-art review, conducted to synthesize concrete recommendations issued during the COVID-19 pandemic (2019–2021) for improving the health and maintaining the care of people living with CP.

2. Methodology

A "state-of-the-art" review [19] was conducted to address the state of knowledge regarding suggested improvements for the management of CP during the first 20 months of the COVID-19 pandemic and to classify the recommendations to be implemented. This type of review is time-bound in terms of literature temporal exhaustiveness and focuses on rapidly but methodically searching the current literature to address contemporary issues; its results focus on knowledge and priorities for future investigation and research [19].

Eligibility criteria. This review considered original studies, reviews, editorials, and guidelines that have been published in peer-reviewed journals or in some reports/statements issues by recognized pain organizations (e.g., International Association for the Study of Pain, Canadian Pain Society), or other grey literature. The articles had to focus on adults (age $\geq$ 18 years old) living with CP (pain that persists for more than 3 months [20]) of non-cancerous origin. They also had to be published in English or in French between December 2019 and July 2021. As an example, this period corresponded to the first three COVID-19 waves of the pandemic in Canada [21]. The present review thus allowed us to harness the recommendations published during the crisis and to put them into perspective with the current situation in healthcare facilities that have slowly recovered from the COVID-19 crisis.

Exclusion criteria. Preclinical studies were excluded, as well as articles specifically addressing molecular aspects of pain, post-COVID syndrome (long COVID), cancer pain or pediatric pain.

Information sources and search strategy. Studies were retrieved on 1 July 2021 by searching the following computerized databases: Medline (Ovid), PsycINFO (Ovid), CINAHL (EBSCOhost), and PubMed (past 7 days). The search on PubMed was made to capture potential new articles indexed on PubMed but not yet on Ovid (as both are windows for Medline but PubMed indexation is sometimes more rapid) [22].

The search strategy was developed in collaboration with an experienced medical librarian of the *Centre Hospitalier de l'Université de Montréal* (CHUM). The strategies were peer-reviewed by another senior information specialist prior to executing using the PRESS Checklist [23]. The search strategy included synonyms for: (1) CP and (2) COVID-19 (File S1). Different types of chronic non-cancer pain conditions (e.g., CP in general, neuropathic pain, fibromyalgia, arthritis, back pain, and migraine) as defined by the International Association for the Study of Pain (IASP) Task Force for the Classification of Chronic Pain [24] were included in the search strategy.

Study selection. All citations were entered in the citation management software Endnote X9® and duplicates were removed by the librarian using the method reported by W. Bramer [25]. A fast process was favoured, so the selection process was achieved by one trained reviewer with medical expertise (TS) rather than two. Firstly, titles and abstracts were screened according to the inclusion criteria. Secondly, full texts of previously selected studies were reviewed to assess their eligibility.

Data Extraction. The data collection process was carried out using a standardized extraction form that was pretested and improved with a sample of 14 studies at the beginning of the extraction process. For each study meeting the eligibility criteria, the following information was retrieved: date of publication, authors, country of data collection (if applicable), the type of article, and concrete recommendations to improve health and maintain care for people living with CP. In order to remain as precise as possible, the recommendations have been extracted keeping the authors' wording. Relevant data were also extracted to allow the classification of recommendations and to check whether they were made for specific populations (e.g., elderly, migraine populations, fibromyalgia, specific cultural groups, etc.). All this information was collected in an Excel® spreadsheet.

Synthesis of results. The various recommendations retrieved from studies were described, combined in tables, and classified into 12 categories. The categories were chosen by consensus after the analysis of all the recommendations issued. When a recommendation could be inserted in more than one category, a choice was made by two of the authors (MG-P and AL) on the most representative category.

3. Results

Flow diagram representing the study selection process is shown in Figure 1. After assessing the articles for eligibility, a total of 119 articles were included in the study. The characteristics of these studies and their respective recommendations to improve health and maintain care for people living with CP are detailed in File S2. From the 119 articles, over 250 concrete recommendations were extracted and then reduced to 150 recommendations to minimize redundancies. Recommendations were then classified into 12 distinct categories: change in clinical practice, change in policy, continuity of care, research avenues to explore, group virtual care, health communication/education, individual virtual care, infection control, lifestyle, non-pharmacological treatments, pharmacological treatments, and social considerations (Figure 2). For the sake of the brevity of this report, two illustrative recommendations from each category were selected by the research team and are presented in Table 1. The complete list of recommendations is presented in File S3.

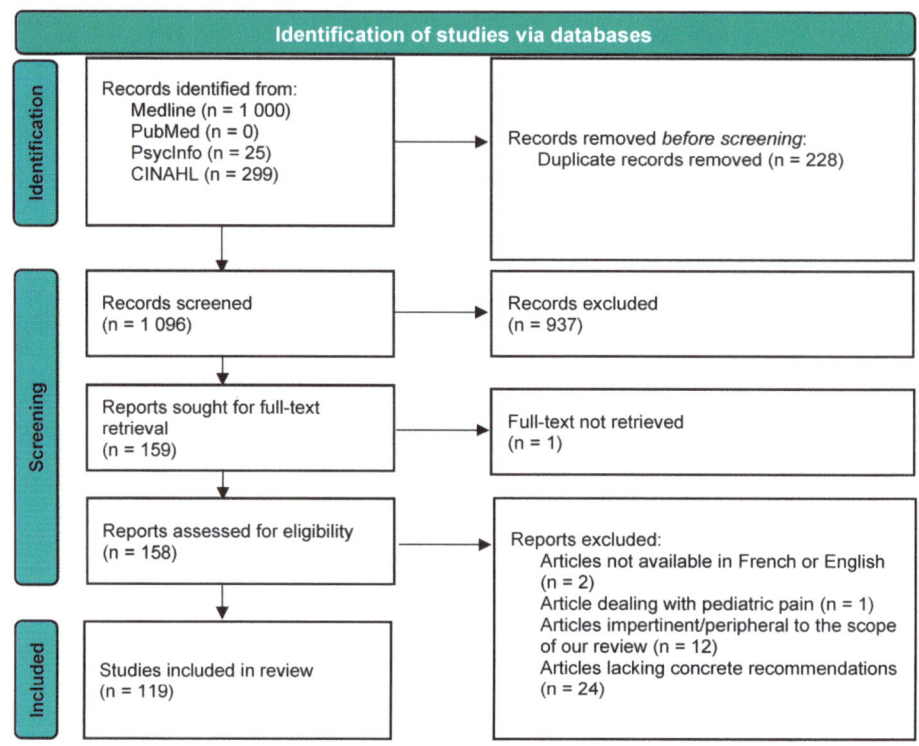

Figure 1. Study selection flow diagram.

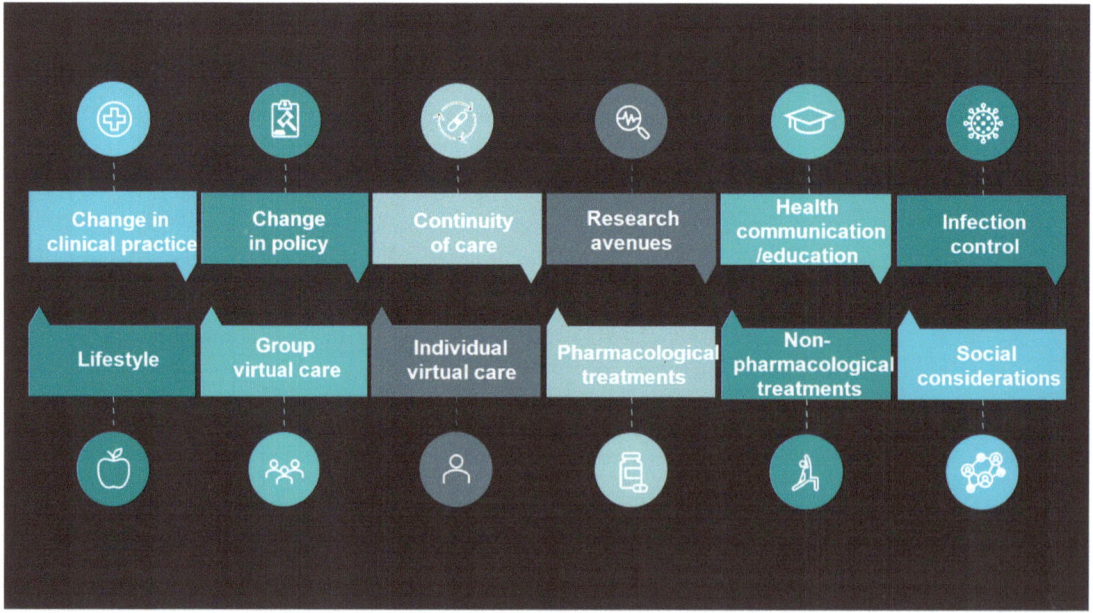

Figure 2. Categories of recommendations.

Table 1. Illustrative recommendations for the 12 different categories.

Recommendation Categories	Recommendations
Change in clinical practice	• Need for increased participation of psychiatrists and psychologists to support psychological distress [26]. • Need for a reinforcement of non-urgent healthcare services and outpatient assistance to redirect CP patients away from overly saturated emergency services in an environment of scarce resources, which can be achieved by means of increased collaboration between multidisciplinary pain treatment facilities and community/primary care healthcare teams. This can include preparing "rescue care" plans, home delivery of medications, and self-administered therapies to keep patients away from emergency departments and limit their exposure to COVID-19 [27,28].
Change in policy	• Need to improve the recognition of CP experience and related physical limitations, through information and advocacy to the public, healthcare professionals, and policymakers [9]. • Urgency that policymakers take action to prevent the pandemic's detrimental effects on mental health of people living with CP, especially the most socially and economically vulnerable. Implementing accessible psychosocial interventions tailored to these vulnerable populations appears essential [9].
Continuity of care	• Need for routine follow-up visits, whether conducted virtually (telehealth options) or in person. These visits can be performed by any member of the healthcare team and should be time-limited, focused, and regularly scheduled. These encounters will allow for assessing current symptoms, adherence to medication regimens, and the presence of any red-flag concerns [29–31]. • Need for CP to be treated as an urgent condition and for healthcare professionals to feel morally and ethically obliged to ensure continued support for CP patients. Some may require urgent pain consultations, interventions, or medication titration and refills, as the deferment of multidisciplinary pain treatment facilities consultations and limited access to primary care can increase morbidity and mortality [32–34].
Research avenues to explore	• Need for studies evaluating the long-term impact of the pandemic on pain-related, emotional, and psychological outcomes in CP patients, and determinants implicated in such outcomes (e.g., coping skills, self-management) [35,36]. • Need for studies evaluating the efficacy of non-pharmacological treatment modalities conducted virtually [37].
Group virtual care	• Evaluate whether the use of synchronous videoconferencing to deliver pain management programs is worthwhile, and if so, how to develop, deliver, and measure outcomes of such programs [38]. • Implementation of group virtual care to benefit patients struggling with loneliness and social isolation, in addition to helping address concerns in overwhelmed clinicians [39].
Health communication/education	• Need to ensure that key information regarding serious infectious diseases is as accurate and transparent as possible with timely updates. Public administration and media should facilitate public awareness and reduce false rumours that can cause widespread panic and unease [40]. • Provide online resources that can disseminate pain education and online self-management programs that can be developed for those living with pain, those close to them, and healthcare professionals [41].
Individual virtual care	• Healthcare professionals and support group organizations should implement individual virtual care options to supplement safe in-person care. Online interventions and knowledge transfer activities could also prioritize informing and empowering people living with CP regarding alternative physical/psychological approaches when the usual ones are not feasible. Harnessing the web could enhance treatment access for people living with CP well beyond the COVID-19 pandemic [8]. • Mobile health apps for headache documentation such as Migraine Buddy, Migraine Coach, and Migraine Monitor have been shown to be useful in improving communication between patients and physicians. A balance between the amount of data collected by the app for clinical purposes and the patient's perception of satisfaction must be assessed. Likewise, physicians should allow for an adjustment period when introducing an app to their patients and ensure that they have been well informed on how to use it [42].

Table 1. *Cont.*

Recommendation Categories	Recommendations
Infection control	• Triage of pain patients may be helpful in terms of differentiating those who may be adequately treated by virtual care versus in-clinic consultations. Triage factors may also include acuity and severity of pain, whether or not the patient has comorbid psychiatric conditions, but also occupational risks of infection (e.g., whether the patient is a first responder) and social situation (e.g., whether the patient is also a caregiver or has children) [43–45]. • Reinforcing patients' and healthcare workers' education on fundamental preventive gestures, such as frequent hand washing, social distancing, and symptom monitoring will aid in reducing transmission of infectious diseases [46].
Lifestyle	• Need for healthcare professionals to provide patients with proper education and guidance on ways to stay physically active at home during future pandemics [47,48]. • Migraine patients could benefit from lifestyle changes associated with intelligent lockdown, such as working from home, scaling down demanding social lives, and freedom to choose how to organize one's time [49].
Non-pharmacological treatments	• Healthcare professionals should take the opportunity to further reinforce the utility of effective nonpharmacologic treatment options including graded exercise, healthy lifestyle, meditation, and meditative movement activities (tai chi and yoga), mindfulness activities, paced diaphragmatic breathing, supportive counselling, cognitive behavioural therapy, biofeedback therapy, sleep hygiene, and ongoing patient education [29]. • Interdisciplinary interventions should be designed in such a way that psychologists and medical care staff work together to minimize the psychological distress of patients with central sensitization pain syndromes [50].
Pharmacological treatments	• Ensuring the availability of pharmacological treatments for CP patients at all times via the establishment of programs in conjunction with local pharmacies is a priority. Identification and implementation of strategies aimed at ensuring continuity of care provision while mitigating the risk of inadequate analgesic treatment, self-medication with potential risk of adverse events, and even treatment discontinuation, are crucial [26,51]. • Prescribe pain drugs for an extended period of time—i.e., filling of prescriptions of controlled substances (opioids and psychotropics) for longer periods than usual (e.g., 60 to 90 days) [52].
Social inequalities	• Need for strategies aimed at the reduction in disparities related to healthcare access, such as improvements in the accessibility of telehealth services (impoverished, rural, digitally illiterate populations) [41,53,54]. • Need for an increased awareness, identification, and reduction in conscious and unconscious biases involved in affecting the management of CP patients from vulnerable and/or minority groups [9,55].

4. Discussion

This state-of-the-art review resulted in 12 categories of concrete recommendations (evidence-based or from different experts) issued during the COVID-19 pandemic. The recommendations consider many areas of healthcare that must be taken into consideration in order to hope for positive changes in CP management. By focusing on the recommendations issued in crisis time, this article provides an opportunity to describe and classify solutions that have been issued to improve the health and maintain the care of people living with CP well beyond the pandemic.

4.1. Virtual Care

The literature underlined that restrictive measures put in place by the government, along with the beginning of the lockdown, created new uncertainties regarding the continuity of healthcare services for the treatment of CP [9]. Moreover, difficulties accessing medical services, medication refills, and non-pharmacological treatments have been reported [8]. Knowing the importance of a multimodal approach for the management of CP, accessibility to non-pharmacological care was a major issue during the pandemic [8]. To address this gap, recommendations were made to provide the opportunity to offer non-pharmacological treatments in a virtual manner. The use of synchronous videoconferencing to deliver pain management programs [38] and the implementation of virtual support groups have been recommended [39]. These group meetings allowed patients to break the isolation brought on by the pandemic [39]. Indeed, some have reported that online support groups played an important role in their psychological well-being during the pandemic [9]. In addition to virtual treatment, communication and education can also be provided through virtual modalities. The development of online pain acceptance programs or self-management programs (e.g., *Agir pour moi* program [56]) could not only help patients, but also clinicians and patients' families [41]. Healthcare professionals and support groups' organizations could also use online modalities for interventions, and knowledge transfer activities regarding alternative physical/psychological approaches, allowing CP patients to still benefit from these kinds of treatment [29]. For example, education on possible exercises to do at home to stay active despite the confinement, meditation exercises, or relaxation techniques could be provided via online modalities, and were recommended as important elements to ensure the continuity of care [47,48]. Despite the importance of increasing the accessibility of virtual care [53,54], studies should be conducted to validate the effectiveness of virtually conducted treatments [37], and special attention should be paid to inequalities in access to care. Indeed, although virtual care can be beneficial for persons living outside of large urban centres, it can be more challenging for individuals with low digital literacy (e.g., members of the elderly population) or people living in isolated geographical areas (i.e., with limited access to the internet). Also, a communication of trust is more difficult to establish with healthcare professionals [9,57]. One Canadian study reported that nearly 15% of patients were not well equipped to receive virtual care [58]. Despite some accessibility challenges, the development of effective non-pharmacological treatments delivered virtually may be essential during any future pandemic, especially when lockdowns are in place. Many multidisciplinary pain treatment facilities in Canada are now well prepared to deliver virtual care and consider virtual care to be sustainable for any future pandemic and well beyond [58]. It is also a good opportunity for healthcare professionals to reinforce the utility of effective non-pharmacological treatment options and their benefits in pain management [29]. The COVID-19 pandemic developments have accelerated the adoption of virtual care and have brought huge benefits (e.g., cost saving for patients [59], improved access and efficiency [60], and greater geographical reach for clinicians [58]), even while still being a work in progress [61].

4.2. Involvement of Different Healthcare Professionals and Mental Health Burden

Long before the pandemic, a multidisciplinary approach was recommended for CP management [15]. As this condition is responsible for many physical, psychological, and emotional consequences, many key players must be involved in order to ensure adequate management (e.g., psychologists, physicians, nurses, pharmacists, and physiotherapists) [11]. The pandemic brought a climate of fear and a considerable increase in the patients' level of stress, anxiety, and depression [62,63]. Considering that the impacts on Considering that the impacts on physical health, and mental health, and well-being may be heightened during times of stress periods [10], it is now clear that the pandemic will have increased psychological distress in the general population [64,65] and people living with CP [9]. Indeed, in a study on a population of people living with rheumatoid arthritis, it was reported that the lockdown had increased pain and impairment of function, both of which were linked to increased rates of depression, anxiety, low self-esteem, insomnia, and other mental health problems [26]. In the light of these observations, it was recommended that the participation of psychiatrists and psychologists in CP management be increased in order to deal with this incoming surge of mental illnesses [26]. Even though psychologists are often involved in tertiary care multidisciplinary teams [66], different barriers prevent patients from being able to consult these specialists for their pain management (e.g., access is limited and patients end up having to consult privately, which can directly cause a financial limit [8], and there is a shortage of trained pain psychologists [67]). Other allied healthcare professionals such as social workers should thus be involved. Since interdisciplinary interventions where staff work together can minimize psychological distress [55], it is, therefore, important that policymakers prevent the pandemic's harmful effects on the mental health of people living with CP and make accessible psychosocial interventions rapidly [9]. Furthermore, accessible psychosocial interventions that take into consideration the most socially and economically vulnerable are required [9], and are recommended to deal with the impacts of the pandemic. Recognizing that mental health challenges existed in people with CP before the pandemic, and that COVID-19-related anxiety may persist, [68] a multidisciplinary approach with psychologists remains relevant beyond the pandemic.

4.3. Involvement of Different Healthcare Professionals and Overcrowded Emergency Departments

In addition to increasing skills to deal with the negative consequences that the pandemic had on people living with CP, collaboration between healthcare professionals could help to decrease the number of patients with CP who attend already-overcrowded emergency departments. This problem was known long before the COVID-19 pandemic, but was exacerbated during this period [69]. The emergency department is usually not the appropriate place to address the complex needs of CP patients where physical, cognitive, behavioural, and psychosocial assessments are required for the comprehensive management of CP [70,71]. The collaboration between multidisciplinary pain treatment facilities and community/primary care healthcare teams seems to be part of the solution [27], and can include preparing "rescue care" plans (timely and appropriate measures to stabilize a patient's condition during emergencies), the home delivery of medications, and self-administered therapies [27,28]. In the past, community healthcare teams have effectively supported efforts to manage epidemics, including the H1N1 and Ebola epidemics [72,73]. Implementing community/primary-care multidisciplinary healthcare teams is important not just during the pandemic, but beyond it as well.

4.4. Recognition of CP and Its Consequences

Despite the many consequences associated with CP, this condition remains stigmatized and under-recognized in clinical practice and in the general population [11,12]. Even before the pandemic, people living with CP already faced many challenges in obtaining a diagnosis and being believed to be legitimate patients by healthcare professionals [74–78]. As the pandemic exacerbated challenges arising from this under-recognition, several new recommendations have been issued to move towards a greater recognition and acceptance of CP. Indeed, the need for an improved recognition of CP and its associated physical limitations has been highlighted, and such an improvement can be achieved by prioritizing continued education and advocacy amongst the public, healthcare professionals, and policymakers. Such advocacy could, for example, push for the provision of material compensation for pain-related disabilities [9] (e.g., assistive devices, transportation, universal insurance coverage for non-pharmacological approaches and services). In the same way, there is a need for CP to be treated as an urgent condition and for healthcare professionals to feel morally and ethically obliged to offer adequate treatments, and to ensure continued support for these patients [32,34]. A better recognition of CP will help advance research, understand the true magnitude of the problem, and consequently improve the chances of patients receiving viable treatment options [79]. In addition, there is a need for a greater awareness, identification, and reduction in conscious and unconscious biases that can affect the care of CP patients from vulnerable and/or minority groups [9,55]. These numerous recommendations echo the work of various large-scale working groups such as Health Canada's Canadian Pain Task Force [13,14,80]. While there is still a long way to go to overcome the under-recognition and stigma surrounding the disease, the recent work and recommendations of the Canadian Pain Task Force and the present review may certainly help move things forward.

Whether through virtual care or the better integration of key healthcare professionals in chronic pain management, several recommendations emerged during the COVID-19 pandemic. The improved management of CP can be hoped only if the stigma decreases and it becomes better recognized.

4.5. Strengths and Limitations

Despite the advantages of a "state-of-the-art review" (e.g., rapid but comprehensive searching of the current literature to state the knowledge and address recommendations or future investigations needed [19]), this type of review does not take into account the quality of the studies from which the data was extracted. For feasibility purposes, only some electronic databases were used in this study (Medline, PsycINFO, CINAHL, and PubMed), which may have led to potential articles being missed. The strength of the recommendations can thus not be assessed. Also, although we conducted the review between December 2019 and July 2021 (during the first three COVID-19 waves in Canada), some information could have been published thereafter and other recommendations may have been missed. This temporal cut-off may have influenced the results. Nevertheless, the present review allows us to harness the recommendations published during the crisis and put them into perspective with the current situation in healthcare facilities that have slowly recovered from the crisis. Most recommendations were formulated at the outset of the pandemic, and we are now better prepared to adapt our healthcare practices and methods of delivering care for CP patients in future crises.

5. Conclusions

The COVID-19 pandemic has undoubtedly exacerbated the existing physical, psychological, and economic burden associated with CP. However, it has also provided a unique opportunity for all stakeholders involved in CP management to collaborate and swiftly devise solutions for better care. Numerous recommendations regarding treatments, clinical practice, policy, and research avenues have been proposed to address existing pain management deficiencies. The pandemic has showcased the potential and effectiveness of virtual care, contributing to its wider acceptance as a treatment method. Critical aspects that have often been overlooked, such as the mental health of individuals living with CP, were reinforced. The ongoing battle to provide equitable, effective treatment and combat stereotypes surrounding CP is far from being over, but the numerous insights shared by the scientific community reinforce awareness and propel us in a promising direction. As the pandemic's hold weakens, it is crucial to make use of the research carried out during this crisis and incorporate it into our healthcare system.

This literature synthesis summarizes recommendations to better prepare for future pandemics and extends our knowledge well beyond the confines of this particular crisis. Future research could be conducted to verify whether the recommendations issued between 2019 and 2021 are applicable to or implemented in the current healthcare system.

Supplementary Materials: The following supporting information can be downloaded at https://www.mdpi.com/article/10.3390/jcm12237233/s1, File S1. Complete search strategies used in the various electronic databases. File S2. Data extracted from the 119 articles (compiled recommendations). File S3. Summary of all the recommendations by category. Refs. [81,82] are listed in supplementary materials File S1.

Author Contributions: Each author listed in the manuscript has participated actively and sufficiently in this study to fulfill all authorship criteria of the International Committee of Medical Journal Editors (ICMJE). A.L., M.G.P., L.D., and M.C. consolidated funding and conceptualized this project. Article screening, data extraction, and classification were conducted by T.S. under the close supervision of A.L. Data interpretation and drafting of the manuscript were achieved by M.G.-P. under the supervision of A.L., assisted by G.D.C.-F. All authors revised the manuscript critically, gave approval of the final version, and agreed to act as guarantors of the work. All authors have read and agreed to the published version of the manuscript.

Funding: This study was funded by the Fonds de développement académique du réseau (FODAR) des Universités du Québec, Projets intersectoriels—Fonds de développement académique. M. Godbout-Parent holds a Canadian Institutes of Health Research (CIHR) doctoral degree scholarship. G. De Clifford-Faugère holds a postdoctoral scholarship from the CIHR and the Fonds de recherche du Quebéc—Santé (FRQS). M.G. Pagé holds a Junior 2 research scholarship from the FRQS.

Institutional Review Board Statement: Not applicable.

Informed Consent Statement: Not applicable.

Data Availability Statement: Provided in Supplementary files.

Acknowledgments: We would like to warmly thank Valérie Jacques, librarian at the Centre Hospitalier de l'Université de Montréal (CHUM), who helped us develop the search strategy for the review and ensured the search for evidence in the appropriate databases. We also want to thank Christine Gauthier, who provided punctual translation and linguistic revision services for the manuscript's preparation.

Conflicts of Interest: The authors report no conflict of interest and no financial interests related to this study. M.G. Pagé received honoraria from Canopy Growth and research funds from Pfizer Canada for projects unrelated to this study. The Chronic Pain Epidemiology Laboratory led by A. Lacasse is funded by the Fondation de l'Université du Québec en Abitibi-Témiscamingue, in partnership with local businesses: the Pharmacie Jean-Coutu de Rouyn-Noranda and Glencore Fonderie Horne (copper smelter).

Abbreviation

Chronic pain (CP); Centre Hospitalier de l'Université de Montréal (CHUM); International Association for the Study of Pain (IASP); Fonds de développement académique du réseau (FODAR); Canadian Institutes of Health Research (CIHR); Fonds de recherche du Québec—Santé (FRQS).

References

1. Clauw, D.J.; Hauser, W.; Cohen, S.P.; Fitzcharles, M.A. Considering the potential for an increase in chronic pain after the COVID-19 pandemic. *Pain* **2020**, *161*, 1694–1697. [CrossRef] [PubMed]
2. Yuki, K.; Fujiogi, M.; Koutsogiannaki, S. COVID-19 pathophysiology: A review. *Clin. Immunol.* **2020**, *215*, 108427. [CrossRef] [PubMed]
3. Davis, H.E.; McCorkell, L.; Vogel, J.M.; Topol, E.J. Long COVID: Major findings, mechanisms and recommendations. *Nat. Rev. Microbiol.* **2023**, *21*, 133–146. [CrossRef] [PubMed]
4. Chu, I.Y.; Alam, P.; Larson, H.J.; Lin, L. Social consequences of mass quarantine during epidemics: A systematic review with implications for the COVID-19 response. *Travel Med.* **2020**, *27*, taaa192. [CrossRef]
5. Béland, L.-P.; Wright, T.; Bordeur, A. *The Short-Term Economic Consequences of COVID-19: Exposure to Disease, Remote Work and Government Response*; Institute of Labor Economics: Bonn, Germany, 2020; pp. 1–92.
6. Deer, T.R.; Sayed, D.; Pope, J.E.; Chakravarthy, K.V.; Petersen, E.; Moeschler, S.M.; Abd-Elsayed, A.; Amirdelfan, K.; Mekhail, N.; Workgroup, A.C. Emergence From the COVID-19 Pandemic and the Care of Chronic Pain: Guidance for the Interventionalist. *Anesth. Analg.* **2020**, *131*, 387–394. [CrossRef]
7. Bambra, C.; Riordan, R.; Ford, J.; Matthews, F. The COVID-19 pandemic and health inequalities. *J. Epidemiol. Community Health* **2020**, *74*, 964–968. [CrossRef]
8. Lacasse, A.; Page, M.G.; Dassieu, L.; Sourial, N.; Janelle-Montcalm, A.; Dorais, M.; Nguena Nguefack, H.L.; Godbout-Parent, M.; Hudspith, M.; Moor, G.; et al. Impact of the COVID-19 pandemic on the pharmacological, physical, and psychological treatments of pain: Findings from the Chronic Pain & COVID-19 Pan-Canadian Study. *Pain Rep.* **2021**, *6*, e891. [CrossRef]
9. Dassieu, L.; Page, M.G.; Lacasse, A.; Laflamme, M.; Perron, V.; Janelle-Montcalm, A.; Hudspith, M.; Moor, G.; Sutton, K.; Thompson, J.M.; et al. Chronic pain experience and health inequities during the COVID-19 pandemic in Canada: Qualitative findings from the chronic pain & COVID-19 pan-Canadian study. *Int. J. Equity Health* **2021**, *20*, 147. [CrossRef]
10. Page, M.G.; Lacasse, A.; Dassieu, L.; Hudspith, M.; Moor, G.; Sutton, K.; Thompson, J.M.; Dorais, M.; Janelle Montcalm, A.; Sourial, N.; et al. A cross-sectional study of pain status and psychological distress among individuals living with chronic pain: The Chronic Pain & COVID-19 Pan-Canadian Study. *Health Promot. Chronic Dis. Prev. Can. Res. Policy Pract.* **2021**, *41*, 141–152. [CrossRef]
11. Kress, H.G.; Aldington, D.; Alon, E.; Coaccioli, S.; Collett, B.; Coluzzi, F.; Huygen, F.; Jaksch, W.; Kalso, E.; Kocot-Kepska, M.; et al. A holistic approach to chronic pain management that involves all stakeholders: Change is needed. *Curr. Meded. Res. Opin.* **2015**, *31*, 1743–1754. [CrossRef]

12. Lalonde, L.; Choiniere, M.; Martin, E.; Levesque, L.; Hudon, E.; Belanger, D.; Perreault, S.; Lacasse, A.; Laliberte, M.C. Priority interventions to improve the management of chronic non-cancer pain in primary care: A participatory research of the ACCORD program. *Pain Res.* **2015**, *8*, 203–215. [CrossRef]
13. Campbell, F.; Hudspith, M.; Anderson, M.; Choiniere, M.; El-Gabalawy, H.; Laliberte, J.; Swidrovich, J.; Wilhelm, L. *Chronic Pain in Canada: Laying a Fondation for Action. A Report by the Canadian Pain Task Force*; Health Canada: Ottawa, ON, Canada, 2019; pp. 1–50.
14. Campbell, F.; Hudspith, M.; Choiniere, M.; El-Gabalawy, H.; Laliberte, J.; Sangster, M.; Swidrovich, J.; Wilhelm, L. *Working Together to Better Understand, Prevent, and Manage Chronic Pain: What We Heard. A Report by the Canadian Pain Task Force*; Report by the Canadian Pain Task Force; Health Canada: Ottawa, ON, Canada, 2020; pp. 1–75.
15. Hylands-White, N.; Duarte, R.V.; Raphael, J.H. An overview of treatment approaches for chronic pain management. *Rheumatol. Int.* **2017**, *37*, 29–42. [CrossRef] [PubMed]
16. Sarzi-Puttini, P.; Vellucci, R.; Zuccaro, S.M.; Cheruhino, P.; Labianca, R.; Fornasar, D. The Appropriate Treatment of Chronic Pain. *Clin. Drug Investig.* **2012**, *32*, 21–33. [CrossRef]
17. Becker, W.C.; Dorflinger, L.; Edmond, S.N.; Islam, L.; Heapy, A.A.; Fraenkel, L. Barriers and facilitators to use of non-pharmacological treatments in chronic pain. *BMC Fam. Pract.* **2017**, *18*, 41. [CrossRef]
18. El-Tallawy, S.N.; Nalamasu, R.; Pergolizzi, J.V.; Gharibo, C. Pain Management During the COVID-19 Pandemic. *Pain Ther.* **2020**, *9*, 453–466. [CrossRef] [PubMed]
19. Grant, M.J.; Booth, A. A typology of reviews: An analysis of 14 review types and associated methodologies. *Health Inf. Libr. J.* **2009**, *26*, 91–108. [CrossRef] [PubMed]
20. Treede, R.-D.; Rief, W.; Barke, A.; Aziz, Q.; Bennett, M.I.; Benoliel, R.; Cohen, M.; Evers, S.; Finnerup, N.B.; First, M.B.; et al. Chronic pain as a symptom or a disease: The IASP Classification of Chronic Pain for the International Classification of Diseases (ICD-11). *Pain* **2019**, *160*, 19–27. [CrossRef] [PubMed]
21. Institut National de Santé Publique (INSPQ). *Ligne du Temps COVID-19 au Québec*; Gouvernement du Québec: Québec, QC, Canada, 2022.
22. Duffy, S.; de Kock, S.; Misso, K.; Noake, C.; Ross, J.; Stirk, L. Supplementary searches of PubMed to improve currency of MEDLINE and MEDLINE In-Process searches via Ovid. *J. Med. Libr. Assoc.* **2016**, *104*, 309–312. [CrossRef] [PubMed]
23. McGowan, J.; Sampson, M.; Salzwedel, D.M.; Cogo, E.; Foerster, V.; Lefebvre, C. PRESS Peer Review of Electronic Search Strategies: 2015 Guideline Statement. *Clin. Epidemiol.* **2016**, *75*, 40–46. [CrossRef]
24. Treede, R.D.; Rief, W.; Barke, A.; Aziz, Q.; Bennett, M.I.; Benoliel, R.; Cohen, M.; Evers, S.; Finnerup, N.B.; First, M.B.; et al. A classification of chronic pain for ICD-11. *Pain* **2015**, *156*, 1003–1007. [CrossRef]
25. Bramer, W.M.; Giustini, D.; de Jonge, G.B.; Holland, L.; Bekhuis, T. De-duplication of database search results for systematic reviews in EndNote. *Med. Libr. Assoc.* **2016**, *104*, 240–243. [CrossRef]
26. Bhatia, A.; Kc, M.; Gupta, L. Increased risk of mental health disorders in patients with RA during the COVID-19 pandemic: A possible surge and solutions. *Rheumatol. Int.* **2021**, *41*, 843–850. [CrossRef] [PubMed]
27. George, J.M.; Xu, Y.; Nursa'adah, B.J.; Lim, S.F.; Low, L.L.; Chan, D.X. Collaboration between a tertiary pain centre and community teams during the pandemic. *Br. J. Community Nurs.* **2020**, *25*, 480–488. [CrossRef] [PubMed]
28. Al-Hashel, J.Y.; Ismail, I.I. Impact of coronavirus disease 2019 (COVID-19) pandemic on patients with migraine: A web-based survey study. *J. Headache Pain* **2020**, *21*, 115. [CrossRef]
29. Mohabbat, A.B.; Mohabbat, N.M.L.; Wight, E.C. Fibromyalgia and Chronic Fatigue Syndrome in the Age of COVID-19. *Mayo Clin. Proc. Innov. Qual. Outcomes* **2020**, *4*, 764–766. [CrossRef]
30. Driver, L.C. Ethical Considerations for Chronic Pain Care During a Pandemic. *Pain Med.* **2020**, *21*, 1327–1330. [CrossRef]
31. Aloush, V.; Gurfinkel, A.; Shachar, N.; Ablin, J.N.; Elkana, O. Physical and mental impact of COVID-19 outbreak on fibromyalgia patients. *Clin. Exp. Rheumatol.* **2021**, *39* (Suppl. S130), 108–114. [CrossRef] [PubMed]
32. Bara, G.A.; de Ridder, D.; Vatter, H.; Maciaczyk, J. Between Scylla and Charybdis: Navigating Chronic Pain Patients Through the COVID-19 and the Opioid Pandemic. *Pain Physician* **2020**, *23*, S469–S472. [CrossRef] [PubMed]
33. Chan, D.X.; Lin, X.F.; George, J.M.; Liu, C.W. Clinical Challenges and Considerations in Management of Chronic Pain Patients During a COVID-19 Pandemic. *Ann. Acad. Med.* **2020**, *49*, 669–673. [CrossRef]
34. Alonso-Matielo, H.; da Silva Oliveira, V.R.; de Oliveira, V.T.; Dale, C.S. Pain in Covid Era. *Front. Physiol.* **2021**, *12*, 624154. [CrossRef]
35. Picchianti Diamanti, A.; Cattaruzza, M.S.; Di Rosa, R.; Del Porto, F.; Salemi, S.; Sorgi, M.L.; Martin Martin, L.S.; Rai, A.; Iacono, D.; Sesti, G.; et al. Psychological Distress in Patients with Autoimmune Arthritis during the COVID-19 Induced Lockdown in Italy. *Microorganisms* **2020**, *8*, 1818. [CrossRef]
36. Gonzalez-Martinez, A.; Planchuelo-Gomez, A.; Guerrero, A.L.; Garcia-Azorin, D.; Santos-Lasaosa, S.; Navarro-Perez, M.P.; Odriozola-Gonzalez, P.; Irurtia, M.J.; Quintas, S.; de Luis-Garcia, R.; et al. Evaluation of the Impact of the COVID-19 Lockdown in the Clinical Course of Migraine. *Pain Med.* **2021**, *22*, 2079–2091. [CrossRef] [PubMed]
37. Grazzi, L.; Rizzoli, P.; Andrasik, F. Effectiveness of mindfulness by smartphone, for patients with chronic migraine and medication overuse during the COVID-19 emergency. *Neurol. Sci.* **2020**, *41*, 461–462. [CrossRef] [PubMed]
38. Walumbe, J.; Belton, J.; Denneny, D. Pain management programmes via video conferencing: A rapid review. *Scand. J. Pain* **2021**, *21*, 32–40. [CrossRef] [PubMed]

39. Thompson-Lastad, A.; Gardiner, P. Group Medical Visits and Clinician Wellbeing. *Glob. Adv. Health Med.* **2020**, *9*, 2164956120973979. [CrossRef]
40. Song, X.-J.; Xiong, D.-L.; Wang, Z.-Y.; Yang, D.; Zhou, L.; Li, R.-C. Pain Management During the COVID-19 Pandemic in China: Lessons Learned. *Pain Med.* **2020**, *21*, 1319–1323. [CrossRef]
41. Karos, K.; McParland, J.L.; Bunzli, S.; Devan, H.; Hirsh, A.; Kapos, F.P.; Keogh, E.; Moore, D.; Tracy, L.M.; Ashton-James, C.E. The social threats of COVID-19 for people with chronic pain. *Pain* **2020**, *161*, 2229–2235. [CrossRef]
42. Noutsios, C.D.; Boisvert-Plante, V.; Perez, J.; Hudon, J.; Ingelmo, P. Telemedicine Applications for the Evaluation of Patients with Non-Acute Headache: A Narrative Review. *Pain Res.* **2021**, *14*, 1533–1542. [CrossRef] [PubMed]
43. Coluzzi, F.; Marinangeli, F.; Pergolizzi, J. Managing chronic pain patients at the time of COVID-19 pandemic. *Minerva Anestesiol.* **2020**, *86*, 797–799. [CrossRef]
44. Puntillo, F.; Giglio, M.; Brienza, N.; Viswanath, O.; Urits, I.; Kaye, A.D.; Pergolizzi, J.; Paladini, A.; Varrassi, G. Impact of COVID-19 pandemic on chronic pain management: Looking for the best way to deliver care. *Best Pract. Res. Clin. Anaesthesiol.* **2020**, *34*, 529–537. [CrossRef]
45. Lo Bianco, G.; Papa, A.; Schatman, M.E.; Tinnirello, A.; Terranova, G.; Leoni, M.L.G.; Shapiro, H.; Mercadante, S. Practical Advices for Treating Chronic Pain in the Time of COVID-19: A Narrative Review Focusing on Interventional Techniques. *J. Clin. Med.* **2021**, *10*, 2303. [CrossRef]
46. Romao, V.C.; Cordeiro, I.; Macieira, C.; Oliveira-Ramos, F.; Romeu, J.C.; Rosa, C.M.; Saavedra, M.J.; Saraiva, F.; Vieira-Sousa, E.; Fonseca, J.E. Rheumatology practice amidst the COVID-19 pandemic: A pragmatic view. *Rheum. Musculoskelet. Dis. Open* **2020**, *6*, e001314. [CrossRef] [PubMed]
47. Roux, C.H.; Brocq, O.; Gerald, F.; Pradier, C.; Bailly, L. Impact of Home Confinement During the COVID-19 Pandemic on Medication Use and Disease Activity in Spondyloarthritis Patients. *Arthritis Rheumatol.* **2020**, *72*, 1771–1772. [CrossRef] [PubMed]
48. van Zanten, J.J.C.S.V.; Fenton, S.A.M.; Brady, S.; Metsios, G.S.; Duda, J.L.; Kitas, G.D. Mental Health and Psychological Wellbeing in Rheumatoid Arthritis during COVID-19—Can Physical Activity Help? *Mediterr. J. Rheumatol.* **2020**, *31*, 284–287. [CrossRef] [PubMed]
49. Verhagen, I.E.; van Casteren, D.S.; de Vries Lentsch, S.; Terwindt, G.M. Effect of lockdown during COVID-19 on migraine: A longitudinal cohort study. *Cephalalgia Int. J. Headache* **2021**, *41*, 865–870. [CrossRef]
50. Serrano-Ibanez, E.R.; Esteve, R.; Ramirez-Maestre, C.; Ruiz-Parraga, G.T.; Lopez-Martinez, A.E. Chronic pain in the time of COVID-19: Stress aftermath and central sensitization. *Br. J. Health Psychol.* **2021**, *26*, 544–552. [CrossRef] [PubMed]
51. Marinangeli, F.; Giarratano, A.; Petrini, F. Chronic Pain and COVID-19: Pathophysiological, clinical and organizational issues. *Minerva Anestesiol.* **2020**, *87*, 828–832. [CrossRef]
52. De Moraes, E.B.; Santos Garcia, J.B.; de Macedo Antunes, J.; Daher, D.V.; Seixas, F.L.; Muniz Ferrari, M.F. Chronic Pain Management during the COVID-19 Pandemic: A Scoping Review. *Pain Manag. Nurs.* **2021**, *22*, 103–110. [CrossRef]
53. George, M.; Danila, M.I.; Watrous, D.; Reddy, S.; Alper, J.; Xie, F.; Nowell, W.B.; Kallich, J.; Clinton, C.; Saag, K.G.; et al. Disruptions in Rheumatology Care and the Rise of Telehealth in Response to the COVID19 Pandemic in a Community Practice-Based Network. *Arthritis Care Res.* **2021**, *73*, 1153–1161. [CrossRef]
54. Muskens, W.D.; Rongen-van Dartel, S.A.A.; Vogel, C.; Huis, A.; Adang, E.M.M.; van Riel, P.L.C.M. Telemedicine in the management of rheumatoid arthritis: Maintaining disease control with less health-care utilization. *Rheumatol. Adv. Pract.* **2021**, *5*, rkaa079. [CrossRef]
55. King, S.A. Race, Ethnicity, and Chronic Pain. *Psychiatr. Times* **2021**, *38*, 25.
56. Réseau Québécois de Recherche Sur la Douleur. Agir Pour Moi. Available online: https://www.gerermadouleur.ca/agir-pour-moi/ (accessed on 4 August 2023).
57. Naveen, R.; Sundaram, T.G.; Agarwal, V.; Gupta, L. Teleconsultation experience with the idiopathic inflammatory myopathies: A prospective observational cohort study during the COVID-19 pandemic. *Rheumatol. Int.* **2021**, *41*, 67–76. [CrossRef] [PubMed]
58. Borg Debono, V.; Neumark, S.; Buckley, N.; Zacharias, R.; Hapidou, E.; Anthonypillai, J.; Faria, S.; Meyer, C.L.; Carter, T.; Parker, N.; et al. Transition to Virtual Care Services during COVID-19 at Canadian Pain Clinics: Survey and Future Recommendations. *Pain Res. Manag.* **2023**, *2023*, 6603625. [CrossRef]
59. Buvik, A.; Bergmo, T.S.; Bugge, E.; Smaabrekke, A.; Wilsgaard, T.; Olsen, J.A. Cost-Effectiveness of Telemedicine in Remote Orthopedic Consultations: Randomized Controlled Trial. *Med. Internet Res.* **2019**, *21*, e11330. [CrossRef] [PubMed]
60. Snoswell, C.L.; Taylor, M.L.; Comans, T.A.; Smith, A.C.; Gray, L.C.; Caffery, L.J. Determining if Telehealth Can Reduce Health System Costs: Scoping Review. *Med. Internet Res.* **2020**, *22*, e17298. [CrossRef]
61. Lynch, M.E.; Williamson, O.D.; Banfield, J.C. COVID-19 impact and response by Canadian pain clinics: A national survey of adult pain clinics. *Can. J. Pain* **2020**, *4*, 204–209. [CrossRef]
62. Banerjee, D.; Kosagisharaf, J.R.; Sathyanarayana Rao, T.S. 'The dual pandemic' of suicide and COVID-19: A biopsychosocial narrative of risks and prevention. *Psychiatry Res.* **2021**, *295*, 113577. [CrossRef]
63. Mendelson, M.; Nel, J.; Blumberg, L.; Madhi, S.; Dryden, M.; Stenven, W.; Venter, F. Long-COVID: An evolving problem with an extensive impact. *S. Afr. Med. J.* **2021**, *111*, 10–12. [CrossRef]
64. Salari, N.; Hosseinian-Far, A.; Jalali, R.; Vaisi-Raygani, A.; Rasoulpoor, S.; Mohammadi, M.; Rasoulpoor, S.; Khaledi-Paveh, B. Prevalence of stress, anxiety, depression among the general population during the COVID-19 pandemic: A systematic review and meta-analysis. *Glob. Health* **2020**, *16*, 57. [CrossRef]

65. Daly, Z.; Slemon, A.; Richardson, C.G.; Salway, T.; McAuliffe, C.; Gadermann, A.M.; Thomson, K.C.; Hirani, S.; Jenkins, E.K. Associations between periods of COVID-19 quarantine and mental health in Canada. *Psychiatry Res.* **2021**, *295*, 113631. [CrossRef]
66. International Association for the Study of Pain (IASP). Pain Treatment Services Guidelines. Available online: https://www.iasp-pain.org/resources/guidelines/pain-treatment-services/?ItemNumber=1381 (accessed on 1 November 2021).
67. Schatman, M.E.; Fortino, M.G. The Problem (and the Answer?) to the Limited Availability of Pain Psychologists: Can Clinical Social Workers Help? *J. Pain. Res.* **2020**, *13*, 3525–3529. [CrossRef] [PubMed]
68. Kwong, A.S.F.; Pearson, R.M.; Smith, D.; Northstone, K.; Lawlor, D.A.; Timpson, N.J. Longitudinal evidence for persistent anxiety in young adults through COVID-19 restrictions. *Wellcome Open Res.* **2020**, *5*, 195. [CrossRef]
69. Depelteau, A.; Racine-Hemmings, F.; Lagueux, E.; Hudon, C. Chronic pain and frequent use of emergency department: A systematic review. *Am. J. Emerg. Med.* **2020**, *38*, 358–363. [CrossRef] [PubMed]
70. Olsen, J.C.; Ogarek, J.L.; Goldenberg, E.J.; Sulo, S. Impact of a Chronic Pain Protocol on Emergency Department Utilization. *Acad. Emerg. Med.* **2016**, *23*, 424–432. [CrossRef]
71. Woodhouse, J.; Peterson, M.; Campbell, C.; Gathercoal, K. The efficacy of a brief behavioral health intervention for managing high utilization of ED services by chronic pain patients. *Emerg. Nurs.* **2010**, *36*, 399–403. [CrossRef]
72. Siekmans, K.; Sohani, S.; Boima, T.; Koffa, F.; Basil, L.; Laaziz, S. Community-based health care is an essential component of a resilient health system: Evidence from Ebola outbreak in Liberia. *BMC Public Health* **2017**, *17*, 84. [CrossRef]
73. Wynn, A.; Moore, M. Integration of Primary Health Care and Public Health During a Public Health Emergency. *Am. Public Health Assoc.* **2012**, *102*, e9–e12. [CrossRef]
74. Choy, E.; Perrot, S.; Leon, T.; Kaplan, J.; Petersel, D.; Ginivker, A.; Kramer, E. A patient survey of the impact of fibromyalgia and the journey to diagnosis. *BMC Health Serv. Res.* **2010**, *10*, 102. [CrossRef] [PubMed]
75. Madden, S.; Sim, J. Acquiring a diagnosis of fibromyalgia syndrome: The sociology of diagnosis. *Soc. Theory Health* **2016**, *14*, 88–108. [CrossRef]
76. Boulton, T. Nothing and Everything: Fibromyalgia as a Diagnosis of Exclusion and Inclusion. *Qual. Health Res.* **2019**, *6*, 809–819. [CrossRef]
77. Lillrank, A. Back pain and the resolution of diagnostic uncertainty in illness narratives. *Soc. Sci. Med.* **2003**, *57*, 1045–1054. [CrossRef]
78. Werner, A.; Malterud, K. It is hard work behaving as a credible patient: Encounters between women with chronic pain and their doctors. *Soc. Sci. Med.* **2003**, *57*, 1409–1419. [CrossRef] [PubMed]
79. International Association for the Study of Pain (IASP). Establishing Recognition for the Chronic Pain Community. Available online: https://foundation.asaecenter.org/research/centennial-research-initiative/iasp-chronic-pain-case-study (accessed on 1 November 2021).
80. Campbell, F.; Hudspith, M.; Choinière, M.; El-Gabalawy, H.; Laliberté, J.; Sangster, M.; Swidrovich, J.; Wilhelm, L. *An Action Plan for Pain in Canada*; Report by the Canadian Pain Task Force; Health Canada: Ottawa, ON, Canada, 2021.
81. Rethlefsen, M.L.; Kirtley, S.; Waffenschmidt, S.; Ayala, A.P.; Moher, D.; Page, M.J.; Koffel, J.B. PRISMA-S: An extension to the PRISMA Statement for Reporting Literature Searches in Systematic Reviews. *Syst. Rev.* **2021**, *10*, 39. [CrossRef] [PubMed]
82. Page, M.J.; McKenzie, J.E.; Bossuyt, P.M.; Boutron, I.; Hoffmann, T.C.; Mulrow, C.D.; Shamseer, L.; Tetzlaff, J.M.; Akl, E.A.; Brennan, S.E.; et al. The PRISMA 2020 statement: An updated guideline for reporting systematic reviews. *Int. J. Surg.* **2021**, *88*, 105906. [CrossRef] [PubMed]

Disclaimer/Publisher's Note: The statements, opinions and data contained in all publications are solely those of the individual author(s) and contributor(s) and not of MDPI and/or the editor(s). MDPI and/or the editor(s) disclaim responsibility for any injury to people or property resulting from any ideas, methods, instructions or products referred to in the content.

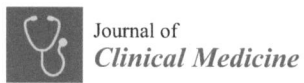
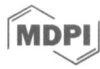

Article

Exploring Facial Thermography Patterns in Women with Chronic Migraine

Bruno Veloso Fracasso [1,*], Renato Bender Castro [2], Marcos Leal Brioschi [3,4] and Taís Malysz [1]

1. Postgraduate Program in Neurosciences, Institute of Basic Health Sciences (ICBS), Federal University of Rio Grande do Sul (UFRGS), Porto Alegre 90035-003, RS, Brazil; tais.malysz@ufrgs.br
2. Independent Researcher, Porto Alegre 90570-020, RS, Brazil
3. Medical Thermology and Thermography Specialization Group, Faculty of Medicine, University of São Paulo (FMUSP), Sao Paulo 01246-903, SP, Brazil; termometria@yahoo.com.br
4. American Academy of Thermology (ATT), Greenville, SC 29607, USA
* Correspondence: brunofracasso@hotmail.com

Abstract: (1) Background: Chronic migraine is a debilitating neurological condition affecting millions worldwide. This study delves into the facial point-of-care (POC) thermographic patterns of women with chronic migraine, aiming to shed light on the condition's pathophysiology and diagnostic potential. (2) Methods: Using infrared POC thermography, the facial temperature distribution of 24 female participants with chronic migraine were analyzed. (3) Results: The findings revealed significant temperature asymmetry in women with right-sided unilateral headaches, particularly in the right frontal and temporal regions. Notably, individuals with bilateral pain did not exhibit thermal pattern differences, suggesting potential diagnostic complexities. While these results offer valuable insights, further research with larger samples is warranted (4) Conclusions: Facial thermography holds promise as an adjunctive tool for migraine diagnosis and understanding its neurophysiological basis; however, cautious interpretation is advised, given the need for validation and expanded investigations. Improved diagnostic criteria and treatment strategies may emerge from this ongoing exploration, ultimately enhancing the quality of life of chronic migraine sufferers.

Keywords: female; headache; humans; migraine disorders; quality of life; pain; temperature; thermography

Citation: Fracasso, B.V.; Castro, R.B.; Brioschi, M.L.; Malysz, T. Exploring Facial Thermography Patterns in Women with Chronic Migraine. *J. Clin. Med.* 2023, 12, 7458. https://doi.org/10.3390/jcm12237458

Academic Editor: Mariateresa Giglio

Received: 31 October 2023
Revised: 28 November 2023
Accepted: 29 November 2023
Published: 1 December 2023

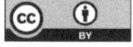

Copyright: © 2023 by the authors. Licensee MDPI, Basel, Switzerland. This article is an open access article distributed under the terms and conditions of the Creative Commons Attribution (CC BY) license (https:// creativecommons.org/licenses/by/ 4.0/).

1. Introduction

Migraine is a disorder characterized by throbbing, unilateral headaches aggravated by physical exertion [1,2]. Globally, this condition affects 1 billion people, imposing substantial and negative impacts not only on those afflicted but also on their families, colleagues, employers, and society due to its widespread prevalence and associated disabilities [3]. According to the Global Burden of Disease 2019 study, migraine ranks as the second leading cause of disability worldwide, with it being the third leading cause of disability among those under 50 years old [4,5]. While headache is the most common symptom of migraine, this condition extends beyond mere pain disorder, encompassing a spectrum of painful and painless symptoms that can occur before, during, and after the headache [6]. Migraine can be conceptualized as a chronic disorder with episodic attacks [7,8], broadly classified into episodic and chronic migraine [2]. According to the International Headache Society's ICHD-3 criteria [2], episodic migraine is diagnosed when headache occurs on fewer than 15 days per month, while chronic migraine is characterized by 15 or more headache episodes monthly. Migraine attacks progress through three phases: the premonitory phase preceding the headache, followed by the headache phase and, eventually, the postdromal phase [9]. In the premonitory phase, dysfunction initiates in the brainstem and modulatory diencephalic systems governing afferent signals [10]. This phase may potentially be subclinical, termed migraine without aura, or manifest symptoms such as vomiting, visual scotomas, and balance disturbances, categorized as migraine with aura [2].

Although it was thought that migraine had a vascular etiology, it is now known that this vascular event is a secondary phenomenon resulting from a complex process involving the central nervous system; after all, Do et al. (2003) point out that strong vasodilation of the cephalic arteries only causes "mild headache" and, furthermore, they state that there is no correlation between the degree of vasodilation and pharmacologically induced headache in healthy individuals [11]. Vincent [12] indicates that migraine involves a genetic alteration of a specific cerebral calcium channel, resulting in a state of hyperexcitability with abnormal cerebral metabolism, rendering the central nervous system more susceptible to stimuli. However, the pituitary adenylate cyclase-activating polypeptide (PACAP) and the activation of its receptor subtypes play a pivotal role in the disorder's pathophysiology. This includes actions within the trigeminovascular system to activate this nociceptive pathway and external involvement in limbic structures and environmental triggers in migraine pathogenesis [13]. In addition to these factors, or perhaps as a precursor to them all, there is an electrophysiological event known as cortical spreading depression present in migraine, whereby the consequences of this phenomenon result in the release of multiple pro-inflammatory agents and excitatory mediators, including nitric oxide, glutamate, and adenosine triphosphate. These agents activate meningeal and perivascular nociceptors of the trigeminal nerve, initiating the headache associated with migraine [14].

Left- and right-sided migraine differ across a wide range of domains, raising the possibility that the pathophysiology of left- and right-maintained may not be identical. In a systematic review, Blum et al. [15] sought to understand the differences between right-sided and left-sided migraine manifestations and found no significant differences in terms of prevalence, symptoms, or triggering factors. However, this same study indicated that complaints of right-sided pain were related to alterations in cutaneous temperature, while left-sided pain correlated with increased parasympathetic activity. The reduction in pain threshold and altered regulation of cutaneous vasoconstriction in migraine may represent two distinct aspects of a hyperexcitable neural network justifying the thermal discrepancy observed in these patient profiles [16].

Corroborating these findings, Antonaci et al. [17] compared frontal and temporal infrared thermography images in healthy individuals and patients with chronic migraine, revealing that this method is reliable for measuring temperature in these regions both at rest and during mental stress. In this context, Dalla Volta et al. [16] proposed an interventional study in migraine employing transcranial direct current stimulation (tDCS) guided by thermography. The intervention was conducted on the hemisphere with the lower temperature in the frontal region, leading to clinical improvement and alterations in facial thermal patterns because of the treatment. Additionally, it is worth noting that one study demonstrated that the administration of sumatriptan during acute attacks reversed the thermal discrepancy in the face, suggesting that the underlying mechanism for the disappearance of the cooler region involves rebalancing the sympathetic and parasympathetic systems (i.e., reducing sympathetic hypertonia and cutaneous microcirculation vasoconstriction) [18]. While this thermal event has not yet been definitively characterized as a migraine epiphenomenon or implicated in its mechanisms, evidence suggests that thermal asymmetry is specific to migraine and tends to diminish with effective treatments.

Therefore, while the literature has suggested that infrared thermography may assist in understanding pathophysiological mechanisms of chronic migraine, aside from identifying specific thermal patterns associated with this condition, aid in differential diagnosis, and offer a means for monitoring treatment outcomes [16,17], it is important to approach these claims with a certain level of caution and consideration. Moreover, facial thermography has been proposed as an objective tool for assessing the effectiveness of therapeutic interventions, potentially allowing for a more personalized and precise approach to monitoring chronic migraine cases [18]. Given these assertions and the potential implications for clinical practice, our study seeks to investigate the existence of distinctive thermographic patterns in women with chronic migraine. This exploration aims to contribute to a deeper understanding of the condition's pathophysiology and its clinical relevance for diagnosis and new treatment insights into this neurological condition.

2. Materials and Methods

This study is a descriptive cross-sectional investigation. Female participants with chronic migraine (lasting at least 3 months), with or without medication use (criteria not considered for data analysis), were recruited according to the International Headache Society's (IHS) criteria as outlined in ICHD-3 [2] through research posters posted on the researchers' social media networks in Canoas, Rio Grande do Sul, Brazil. Data collection occurred at the Functional Science Physiotherapy Clinic in Canoas, Brazil.

This study included women who voluntarily participated from September 2021 to December 2022. Inclusion criteria were as follows: female individuals aged 18 to 50 years, diagnosed with chronic migraine, experiencing at least 15 headache days per month, with a minimum of 8 migraine attacks, following the ICHD-3 criteria [2]. Exclusion criteria were pregnancy, lactation, and fever on the day of data collection. Eligibility criteria data were collected during an initial assessment after obtaining the participant's informed consent through reading and signing the Informed Consent Form.

This research received approval from the Ethics and Research Committee of the Regional University of Alto Uruguai and Missions through CAAE (Certificate of Presentation for Ethical Appreciation) number 35901320.6.0000.5351, approval date 6 November 2020.

Information regarding sample characteristics was collected using a semi-structured questionnaire, including data on age, body mass, height, presence or absence of aura, and menstrual characteristics such as contraceptive use.

Other variables analyzed that helped describe the composition of the sample were pain, motion sickness, panic, agoraphobia, and quality of life. Pain assessment involves the use of a visual analogue scale (VAS) for pain perception according to Rosier, Iadarola, and Coghill's protocol [19]. Motion sickness was assessed based on self-reported nausea associated with dizziness or imbalance, using the Dizziness Handicap Inventory (DHI) [20,21]. Evaluation of panic and agoraphobia was carried out by self-perception of behaviors in everyday situations, employing the Panic and Agoraphobia Scale (PAS) tool [22,23]. Quality of life was assessed using the WHOQOL-BREF tool, which relies on self-perceived activities of daily living affecting an individual's quality of life [24]. The sampling process included the application of all relevant assessment tools after obtaining informed consent from participants. Data collection, conducted by the research team, lasted for 30 min, and involved the completion of eight questionnaires: one for sample profiling and seven for each of the analyzed outcomes, following the order presented above.

Infrared point-of-care (POC) thermography was employed to identify the spatial distribution of heat on the human face, with images captured outside the migraine episode period. In the images, temperature variations were represented by different shades of blue, green, yellow, orange, red, pink, and white, with dark blue representing minimum temperature and white representing maximum temperature, while the other colors indicated intermediate values. Data collection was conducted using an infrared thermographic camera (T400, FLIR Systems© Inc., Boston, MA, USA), with a resolution of 320 × 240 pixels (76,800 pixels), operating within the spectral range of 7.5 to 14 μm far infrared. The sensor exhibited a thermal sensitivity (NETD) of 0.04 °C (40 mK) and a frame rate of 30 Hz, as per Schwartz et al. [25]. The skin emissivity was set to 0.98 for the measurements. The camera was positioned at 1 m from the participant's face in a room with a stable temperature (23 °C ± 1), capturing an anterior view of the face. Data collection was consistently performed at the same time of day (7:00 p.m.). The POC images were analyzed utilizing specialized medical software (Sao Paulo, Brazil), developed by one of the authors (M.L.B.), that enables 3D assessment and multispectral thermovisual overlay for qualitative evaluation, while simultaneously obtaining quantitative data.

To ensure assessment reliability, two different assessors analyzed the images through 15 regions of interest (ROI), each measuring 1.13 cm^2 (6 mm radius), as shown in Figure 1, positioned over the respective thermoanatomical points, adapted from the protocols established by Antonaci et al. [17], Haddad et al. [26], and Zaproudina et al. [27].

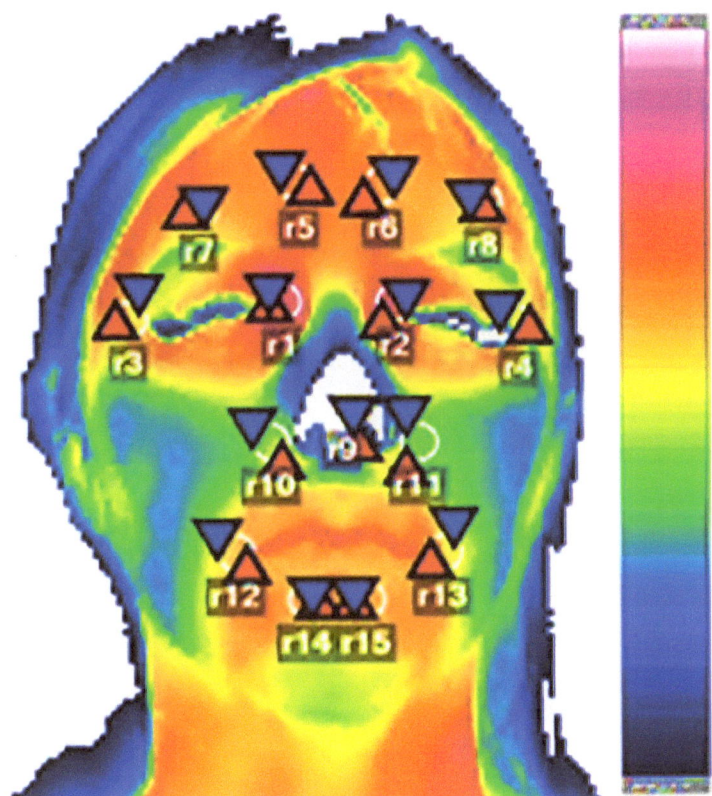

Figure 1. Facial point-of-care thermographic image illustrating the 15 regions of interest (ROI) used in this study. The facial cutaneous thermal distribution corresponds to a color scale displayed on the right side of the image. For this participant, thermographic values ranging from 28 °C (minimum temperature, dark blue) to 37 °C (maximum temperature, white) were identified. Regions of interest analyzed from the thermographic image, where R1 denotes the medial right palpebral corner, R2 medial left palpebral corner, R3 lateral right palpebral corner, R4 lateral left palpebral corner, R5 right frontal, R6 left frontal, R7 right temporal, R8 left temporal, R9 nasal tip, R10 right nasolabial, R11 left nasolabial, R12 right lateral commissure, R13 left lateral commissure, R14 right infralabial, and R15 left infralabial. Within each ROI, there are triangular red markings indicating the maximum temperature and blue markings indicating the minimum temperature.

Through this analysis, the maximum, average, and minimum temperatures of each ROI were identified, enabling a comparison between the right and left hemifaces. Participant data were categorized and analyzed based on pain location (right, left, or bilateral pain).

Statistical analysis was performed using JASP software (v.0.13.1, 2023, Amsterdam, The Netherlands). Interrater agreement was assessed using the Intraclass Correlation Coefficient (ICC), with values equal to or greater than 0.7 considered indicative of good reliability [28]. After verifying data distribution normality, the mean and standard deviation were calculated for thermographic variations in the fifteen regions of interest. Data from the right and left hemifaces were compared using paired t-tests ($p < 0.05$).

To compare the predominant sides, Analysis of Variance (ANOVA) complemented by the Tukey (normal distribution) or Kruskal–Wallis test (asymmetric distribution), was used for numerical variables. For categorical variables, Pearson's chi-square test was applied. Associations between variables on each side were assessed using Pearson or Spearman correlation coefficients. Data normality was assessed using the Shapiro–Wilk test. To compare differences depending on the patient's aura, the Student's t-test was applied. To determine the best cutoff point for differences between temperatures depending on regions of the face, the Receiver Operating Characteristic (ROC) curve was used. The analyses were carried out using IBM SPSS Statistics v.27.0 (Armonk, NY, USA).

3. Results

In this study, 24 women were evaluated, with a mean age of 39.2 ± 7.7 years, weight of 72.2 ± 15.3 kg, height of 1.59 ± 0.04 m, and a body mass index (BMI) of 29 ± 6.1 kg/m^2. Aura, a transient focal neurological symptom, was present in 66.7% of the participants ($n = 16$), while compliance with the ICHD-3 criteria (15 days of headache per month, with at least eight migraine attacks), taking the last month as a reference, was observed in 91.7% ($n = 22$) of participants; however, all participants met the criteria for diagnosing chronic migraine. Hormonal contraceptive use was reported by 33.3% ($n = 8$), and 12.5% ($n = 3$) mentioned being in the postmenopausal period. The participants reported that they had suffered from migraines for 3.5 years.

Regarding pain intensity, based on the Visual Analog Scale (VAS, ranging from 0 to 10), the mean score was 6.7 ± 1.7. When evaluated using the McGill Pain Questionnaire (ranging from 0 to 100), the total pain index was 60.6 ± 14.7. For the assessment of conditions related to nausea and vomiting associated with migraine, the Dizziness Handicap Inventory (DHI) yielded a median score of 34 points (with a maximum score of 100 points indicating the worst-case scenario). The Panic Disorder and Agoraphobia scale showed modest scores, with a median score of 4 points (ranging from 0 to 52 points). In the evaluation of quality of life using the WHOQOL tool, the Physical and Psychological domains yielded lower scores, with means of 53.3 ± 17.8 and 58.9 ± 18.7, respectively. In this context, higher scores on the WHOQOL reflect a better quality of life (Table 1).

Table 1. Clinical Parameters and Quality of Life Scores of the Chronic Migraine Patients ($n = 24$).

Parameter	Measurement Method	Mean (±SD)
Pain Intensity	Visual Analog Scale (VAS, 0–10)	6.7 ± 1.7
Total Pain Index	McGill Pain Questionnaire (0–100)	60.6 ± 14.7
Nausea and Vomiting	Dizziness Handicap Inventory (DHI)	34 (0–100)
Panic Disorder and Agoraphobia	Panic and Agoraphobia Scale (0–52)	4 (0–52)
Quality of Life—Physical Domain	WHOQOL (0–100, higher = better QoL)	53.3 ± 17.8
Quality of Life—Psychological Domain	WHOQOL (0–100, higher = better QoL)	58.9 ± 18.7

Note: SD = standard deviation.

From a descriptive analysis, it was possible to show that women who reported pain on the left had more intense pain (VAS 7.25 + 0.5). When we analyzed the PAS scale, a higher score was seen in those who complained of bilateral pain (PAS9, 20 + 13.39). Nausea and Vomiting, assessed by the DHI, obtained a higher score in participants with complaints on the right (DHI 44.40 + 21.49), similarly, they also had lower overall quality of life scores (WHOQOL 12.98 + 3.79) (Table 2). There was no significant difference between the subgroup scores.

Regarding the analysis of thermographic data, there was agreement between assessors for all analyzed points, with ICC values ranging from 0.97 to 0.99, and $p < 0.001$ for all variables. Thermographic data from different regions of interest (R1 to R15) for participants with complaints of unilateral right-sided pain ($n = 10$), unilateral left-sided pain ($n = 4$), and bilateral pain ($n = 10$) are presented in Table 3, Table 4 and Table 5, respectively.

Table 2. Descriptive analysis of the variables pain, panic and agoraphobia, nausea and vomiting and quality of life, separated by subgroups according to the side of the migraine complaint (RIGHT, LEFT or BILATERAL).

	Mean	SD
VAS RIGHT	6.10	2.42
VAS LEFT	7.25	0.50
VAS BILATERAL	7.10	0.74
PAS RIGTH	8.90	8.52
PAS LEFT	5.25	6.70
PAS BILATERAL	9.20	13.39
DHI RIGHT	44.40	21.49
DHI LEFT	25.00	33.37
DHI BILATERAL	26.80	25.05
WHOQOL RIGHT	12.98	3.79
WHOQOL LEFT	13.76	3.09
WHOQOL BILATERAL	13.93	2.54

Note: SD = standard deviation; VAS = Visual Analog Scale; DHI = Dizziness Handicap Inventory; PAS = Panic and Agoraphobia Scale; WHOQOL = World Health Organization Quality of Life.

Table 3. Temperature Average Values (in °C) Obtained at Thermoanatomical Points in Participants with Right Unilateral Complaints ($n = 10$).

	R1	R2	R3	R4	R5	R6	R7	R8	R9	R10	R11	R12	R13	R14	R15
Mean	34.55	34.41	33.68	33.41	33.66	34.04	33.98	33.70	29.50	33.07	33.41	34.31	34.35	33.85	33.83
SD	1.01	0.85	1.06	0.90	0.77	0.64	0.61	0.72	1.63	0.74	0.95	0.63	0.88	0.94	0.88
Minimum	32.64	33.19	31.90	31.87	32.56	32.68	32.91	32.42	28.06	32.12	32.22	33.56	33.13	32.72	32.71
Maximum	35.94	35.67	35.21	34.69	34.89	35.02	34.88	34.71	32.95	34.38	35.03	35.37	35.84	35.22	34.94

Legend: R1—right medial palpebral corner, R2—left medial palpebral corner, R3—right lateral palpebral corner, R4—left lateral palpebral corner, R5—right frontal, R6—left frontal, R7—right temporal, R8—left temporal, R9—nasal tip, R10—right nasolabial, R11—left nasolabial, R12—right lateral commissure, R13—left lateral commissure, R14—right infralabial, R15—left infralabial, SD—standard deviation.

Table 4. Temperature Average Values (in °C) Obtained at Thermoanatomical Points in Participants with Left Unilateral Complaints ($n = 4$).

	R1	R2	R3	R4	R5	R6	R7	R8	R9	R10	R11	R12	R13	R14	R15
Mean	34.56	34.89	33.53	33.26	33.61	33.41	33.39	33.30	31.45	33.76	33.66	34.52	34.52	33.96	34.01
SD	0.88	0.81	1.10	0.90	0.29	0.30	0.32	0.76	2.69	0.80	1.33	0.75	0.67	1.092	1.02
Minimum	33.49	34.06	32.49	32.53	33.37	33.08	33.00	32.28	28.56	33.10	32.06	33.91	33.88	32.48	32.63
Maximum	35.47	35.73	35.07	34.55	33.99	33.68	33.68	34.10	33.91	34.91	35.22	35.61	35.37	35.02	35.02

Legend: R1—right medial palpebral corner, R2—left medial palpebral corner, R3—right lateral palpebral corner, R4—left lateral palpebral corner, R5—right frontal, R6—left frontal, R7—right temporal, R8—left temporal, R9—nasal tip, R10—right nasolabial, R11—left nasolabial, R12—right lateral commissure, R13—left lateral commissure, R14—right infralabial, R15—left infralabial, SD—standard deviation.

Table 5. Temperature Average Values (in °C) Obtained at Thermoanatomical Points in Participants with Bilateral Complaints ($n = 10$).

	R1	R2	R3	R4	R5	R6	R7	R8	R9	R10	R11	R12	R13	R14	R15
Mean	34.78	34.44	33.65	33.45	33.93	33.85	34.05	34.27	30.81	33.78	33.73	34.55	34.69	34.28	34.28
SD	0.44	0.76	0.73	1.06	0.99	0.96	0.87	0.96	2.59	1.11	1.08	1.07	1.07	0.99	0.98
Minimum	34.01	32.82	32.82	31.91	31.97	32.28	32.78	32.97	28.11	32.01	31.68	31.95	32.27	32.03	32.09
Maximum	35.41	35.61	35.02	35.04	35.42	35.25	35.78	36.45	34.91	35.14	35.10	35.61	35.59	35.50	35.57

Legend: R1—right medial palpebral corner, R2—left medial palpebral corner, R3—right lateral palpebral corner, R4—left lateral palpebral corner, R5—right frontal, R6—left frontal, R7—right temporal, R8—left temporal, R9—nasal tip, R10—right nasolabial, R11—left nasolabial, R12—right lateral commissure, R13—left lateral commissure, R14—right infralabial, R15—left infralabial, SD—standard deviation.

Women with chronic migraine exhibited facial temperatures in the analyzed regions of interest, ranging from $T_{avg} = 28.06$ °C at the tip of the nose (minimum value) to $T_{avg} = 36.45$ °C in the left temporal region (maximum value).

Among the 24 women diagnosed with chronic migraine, 41.67% displayed facial thermal asymmetry, notably in the frontal (R5 vs. R6) and temporal (R7 vs. R8) regions. All the women who exhibited face asymmetry had migraine with aura, and the mean temperature difference between these areas measured 0.3 °C, demonstrating statistical significance only in the group of women with complaints on the right side ($p = 0.023$), as indicated in Table 6.

Table 6. Statistical Comparison of Average Temperature among Thermoanatomical Points in Women with Right-Sided Pain. ($n = 10$).

Right Side	Left Side	p
R1	R2	0.655
R3	R4	0.091
R5	R6	0.023
R7	R8	0.023
R10	R11	0.147
R12	R13	0.772
R14	R15	0.597

Legend: R1—right medial palpebral corner, R2—left medial palpebral corner, R3—right lateral palpebral corner, R4—left lateral palpebral corner, R5—right frontal, R6—left frontal, R7—right temporal, R8—left temporal, R9—nasal tip, R10—right nasolabial, R11—left nasolabial, R12—right lateral commissure, R13—left lateral commissure, R14—right infralabial, and R15—left infralabial.

Comparing temperatures on the right and left sides, participants with bilateral pain ($n = 10$) and left-sided pain ($n = 4$) showed no significant differences ($p > 0.05$). However, those with right-sided unilateral pain had a significant temperature difference in the right frontal (R5: 33.66 °C ± 0.779 vs. R6: 34.04 °C ± 0.647; $p = 0.023$) and temporal (R7: 33.98 °C ± 0.614 vs. R8: 33.70 °C ± 0.720; $p = 0.023$) regions (Table 7).

Table 7. Comparative Analysis of Thermoanatomical Points Between Hemifaces and Their Corresponding Mean, Maximum, and Minimum Thermal Difference Values (ΔT)—groups with unilateral right-sided pain ($n = 10$), unilateral left-sided pain ($n = 4$), and bilateral pain ($n = 10$).

Variables		Predominant Side			p
		Right ($n = 10$)	Left ($n = 4$)	Bilateral ($n = 10$)	
		Mean ± SD	Mean ± SD	Mean ± SD	
R1	Maximum	35.1 ± 0.7	35.0 ± 0.7	35.3 ± 0.3	0.656
	Minimum	33.8 ± 1.3	33.9 ± 1.4	33.9 ± 0.8	0.979
	Average	34.6 ± 1.0	34.6 ± 0.9	34.8 ± 0.4	0.795
R2	Maximum	35.1 ± 0.8	35.1 ± 0.9	35.1 ± 0.6	0.982
	Minimum	33.3 ± 1.2	34.5 ± 0.7	33.3 ± 1.4	0.246
	Average	34.4 ± 0.9	34.9 ± 0.8	34.4 ± 0.8	0.582
R3	Maximum	34.1 ± 0.9	34.1 ± 1.2	34.2 ± 0.5	0.927
	Minimum	33.3 ± 1.1	32.9 ± 1.0	33.1 ± 1.0	0.833
	Average	33.7 ± 1.1	33.5 ± 1.1	33.7 ± 0.7	0.963
R4	Maximum	33.9 ± 0.8	34.0 ± 1.1	34.0 ± 0.7	0.880
	Minimum	32.9 ± 1.1	32.5 ± 0.7	32.6 ± 1.9	0.880
	Average	33.4 ± 0.9	33.3 ± 0.9	33.5 ± 1.1	0.949
R5	Maximum	33.8 ± 0.8	33.7 ± 0.2	34.1 ± 0.9	0.613
	Minimum	33.6 ± 0.8	33.5 ± 0.4	33.8 ± 1.0	0.768
	Average	33.7 ± 0.8	33.6 ± 0.3	33.9 ± 1.0	0.702
R6	Maximum	34.1 ± 0.7	33.6 ± 0.3	34.0 ± 0.9	0.448
	Minimum	33.9 ± 0.6	33.2 ± 0.4	33.7 ± 1.0	0.327
	Average	34.0 ± 0.6	33.4 ± 0.3	33.9 ± 0.9	0.397
R7	Maximum	34.2 ± 0.6	33.7 ± 0.3	34.4 ± 0.8	0.189
	Minimum	33.7 ± 0.7	33.1 ± 0.6	33.7 ± 1.0	0.354
	Average	34.0 ± 0.6	33.4 ± 0.3	34.1 ± 0.9	0.294

Table 7. Cont.

Variables		Predominant Side			p
		Right (n = 10)	Left (n = 4)	Bilateral (n = 10)	
		Mean ± SD	Mean ± SD	Mean ± SD	
R8	Maximum	34.0 ± 0.7	33.5 ± 0.8	34.6 ± 0.9	0.081
	Minimum	33.4 ± 0.8	33.0 ± 0.7	33.8 ± 1.1	0.280
	Average	33.7 ± 0.7	33.3 ± 0.8	34.3 ± 1.0	0.128
R9	Maximum	29.6 ± 1.6	31.8 ± 2.6	31.1 ± 2.6	0.192
	Minimum	29.5 ± 1.6	31.0 ± 3.0	30.5 ± 2.6	0.462
	Average	29.6 ± 1.6	31.4 ± 2.8	30.8 ± 2.6	0.308
R10	Maximum	33.5 ± 0.6	34.2 ± 1.0	34.2 ± 1.1	0.203
	Minimum	32.4 ± 1.2	33.2 ± 0.6	33.2 ± 1.1	0.202
	Average	33.1 ± 0.7	33.8 ± 0.8	33.8 ± 1.1	0.209
R11	Maximum	33.8 ± 0.8	34.2 ± 1.0	34.2 ± 1.1	0.681
	Minimum	32.6 ± 1.5	33.3 ± 1.3	33.2 ± 1.0	0.477
	Average	33.4 ± 1.0	33.7 ± 1.3	33.7 ± 1.1	0.786
R12	Maximum	34.6 ± 0.6	34.8 ± 0.8	34.8 ± 0.8	0.861
	Minimum	33.9 ± 0.8	34.3 ± 0.7	34.2 ± 1.1	0.720
	Average	34.3 ± 0.6	34.5 ± 0.8	34.6 ± 1.1	0.820
R13	Maximum	34.7 ± 0.8	34.8 ± 0.6	35.0 ± 0.9	0.700
	Minimum	34.0 ± 1.1	34.2 ± 0.7	34.3 ± 1.3	0.832
	Average	34.4 ± 0.9	34.5 ± 0.7	34.7 ± 1.1	0.733
R14	Maximum	34.1 ± 0.8	34.2 ± 0.9	34.5 ± 0.9	0.633
	Minimum	33.6 ± 1.1	33.6 ± 1.2	34.1 ± 1.1	0.559
	Average	33.9 ± 0.9	34.0 ± 1.1	34.3 ± 1.0	0.622
R15	Maximum	34.0 ± 0.8	34.3 ± 0.8	34.4 ± 0.9	0.495
	Minimum	33.6 ± 1.0	33.8 ± 1.1	34.1 ± 1.0	0.567
	Average	33.8 ± 0.9	34.0 ± 1.0	34.3 ± 1.0	0.570
R1 vs. R2 Difference	Maximum	0.03 ± 0.72	−0.09 ± 0.22	0.26 ± 0.43	0.494
	Minimum	0.55 ± 1.45	−0.59 ± 0.95	0.62 ± 1.38	0.307
	Average	0.14 ± 0.95	−0.33 ± 0.41	0.33 ± 0.54	0.321
R3 vs. R4 Difference	Maximum	0.22 ± 0.37	0.06 ± 0.17	0.17 ± 0.39	0.754
	Minimum	0.44 ± 0.61	0.46 ± 0.68	0.53 ± 1.31	0.977
	Average	0.27 ± 0.45	0.27 ± 0.39	0.20 ± 0.53	0.949
R5 vs. R6 Difference	Maximum	−0.36 ± 0.46	0.12 ± 0.49	0.05 ± 0.42	0.089
	Minimum	−0.34 ± 0.39 [a]	0.27 ± 0.53 [b]	0.11 ± 0.31 [b]	0.015
	Average	−0.38 ± 0.44 [a]	0.20 ± 0.51 [ab]	0.09 ± 0.34 [b]	0.026
R7 vs. R8 Difference	Maximum	0.21 ± 0.30	0.16 ± 0.76	−0.19 ± 0.48	0.163
	Minimum	0.36 ± 0.42	0.05 ± 0.52	−0.14 ± 0.52	0.088
	Average	0.28 ± 0.33	0.09 ± 0.69	−0.23 ± 0.49	0.072
R10 vs. R11 Difference	Maximum	−0.31 ± 0.61	0.04 ± 0.31	−0.01 ± 0.42	0.333
	Minimum	−0.25 ± 1.15	−0.15 ± 0.74	−0.02 ± 0.40	0.842
	Average	−0.33 ± 0.67	0.10 ± 0.66	0.05 ± 0.39	0.252
R12 vs. R13 Difference	Maximum	−0.08 ± 0.38	0.02 ± 0.25	−0.12 ± 0.34	0.533
	Minimum	−0.06 ± 0.51	0.06 ± 0.48	−0.07 ± 0.43	0.885
	Average	−0.04 ± 0.43	0.01 ± 0.29	−0.14 ± 0.33	0.740
R14 vs. R15 Difference	Maximum	0.09 ± 0.11	−0.04 ± 0.18	0.02 ± 0.14	0.293
	Minimum	−0.03 ± 0.22	−0.25 ± 0.24	−0.04 ± 0.19	0.183
	Average	0.02 ± 0.13	−0.05 ± 0.07	−0.01 ± 0.13	0.593

Legend: R1—right medial palpebral corner, R2—left medial palpebral corner, R3—right lateral palpebral corner, R4—left lateral palpebral corner, R5—right frontal, R6—left frontal, R7—right temporal, R8—left temporal, R9—nasal tip, R10—right nasolabial, R11—left nasolabial, R12—right lateral commissure, R13—left lateral commissure, R14—right infralabial, and R15—left infralabial. [a,b] Equal letters do not differ according to the Tukey test at 5% significance.

There was a significant difference between the predominant sides only in the difference between R5 vs. R6 in the minimum ($p = 0.015$) and average ($p = 0.026$) values. Patients complaining of pain on the right showed greater differences between the two temperatures in this region (lower temperatures on the right side than on the left) when compared to participants complaining of pain on the left side and bilateral (on average, those with predominance on the right side did not differ significantly from those with predominance on the left side, only from those with bilateral).

There was no statistically significant difference between the predominant sides regarding the variables presented in Table 8.

Table 8. Comparative Analysis of Aura, VAS, PAS, DHI, and WHOQOL—groups with unilateral right-sided pain (n = 10), unilateral left-sided pain (n = 4), and bilateral pain (n = 10).

Variables	Predominant Side			p
	Right (n = 10)	Left (n = 4)	Bilateral (n = 10)	
	Median (Min–Max)	Median (Min–Max)	Median (Min–Max)	
Presence of Aura—n (%)	9 (90.0)	2 (50.0)	5 (50.0)	0.122
VAS	7 (0–8)	7 (7–8)	7 (6–8)	0.626
PAS	5.5 (1–27)	3.5 (0–14)	2 (0–40)	0.515
DHI	50 (0–70)	12 (2–74)	24 (0–60)	0.298
WHOQOL—mean ± SD	13.0 ± 3.8	13.8 ± 3.1	13.9 ± 2.5	0.791

The associations of temperature differences between regions (considering the average) and the VAS, PAS, DHI, and WHOQOL measurements are presented in Table 9. There was a statistically significant inverse association between the differences in R1 vs. R2 and DHI scores in patients with predominantly bilateral sides; that is, the greater the negative difference (with lower values on the right side), the higher the DHI score, as can be seen in Figure 2. In the group with a predominance of the right side, there was a statistically significant inverse association between the differences in R14 vs. R15 and the VAS scores; that is, the greater the negative difference (with lower values on the right side), the higher the VAS score, as can be seen in Figure 3. Finally, there was a statistically significant positive association between the differences in R14 vs. R15 and the DHI scores in the group with bilateral predominance; that is, the greater the positive difference (with higher values on the right side), the higher the DHI score, according to can be seen in Figure 4.

Table 9. Association between temperature differences between regions (considering the average) and VAS, PAS, DHI, and WHOQOL measurements using Spearman and Pearson correlation coefficients on the predominant right and bilateral sides.

Variables	VAS	PAS	DHI	WHOQOL
	r_s (p)	r_s (p)	r_s (p)	r (p)
R1 vs. R2 Difference				
Right predominant side	−0.03 (0.945)	0.02 (0.960)	0.35 (0.328)	−0.43 (0.212)
Bilateral predominant side	0.18 (0.623)	−0.31 (0.390)	−0.86 (0.001)	0.22 (0.535)
R3 vs. R4 Difference				
Right predominant side	−0.04 (0.918)	−0.46 (0.179)	−0.56 (0.090)	0.41 (0.235)
Bilateral predominant side	−0.15 (0.676)	−0.27 (0.452)	0.47 (0.171)	0.31 (0.380)
R5 vs. R6 Difference				
Right predominant side	0.48 (0.160)	−0.32 (0.374)	0.15 (0.676)	0.08 (0.818)
Bilateral predominant side	0.45 (0.188)	0.48 (0.157)	−0.40 (0.249)	−0.41 (0.245)
R7 vs. R8 Difference				
Right predominant side	0.17 (0.642)	0.21 (0.567)	0.10 (0.777)	−0.43 (0.213)
Bilateral predominant side	−0.05 (0.885)	−0.62 (0.054)	−0.59 (0.075)	0.57 (0.085)
R10 vs. R11 Difference				
Right predominant side	0.14 (0.706)	0.12 (0.738)	0.18 (0.627)	0.10 (0.778)
Bilateral predominant side	0.17 (0.637)	0.27 (0.452)	0.18 (0.613)	−0.59 (0.075)

Table 9. *Cont.*

Variables	VAS	PAS	DHI	WHOQOL
	r_s (*p*)	r_s (*p*)	r_s (*p*)	r (*p*)
R12 vs. R13 Difference				
Right predominant side	0.14 (0.706)	0.37 (0.300)	0.20 (0.580)	−0.03 (0.934)
Bilateral predominant side	0.47 (0.167)	0.38 (0.280)	0.09 (0.802)	−0.46 (0.183)
R14 vs. R15 Difference				
Right predominant side	−0.64 (0.048)	−0.46 (0.185)	−0.08 (0.829)	0.45 (0.192)
Bilateral predominant side	−0.16 (0.650)	0.25 (0.485)	0.66 (0.038)	−0.19 (0.603)

r_s = Spearman correlation coefficient; r = Pearson correlation coefficient.

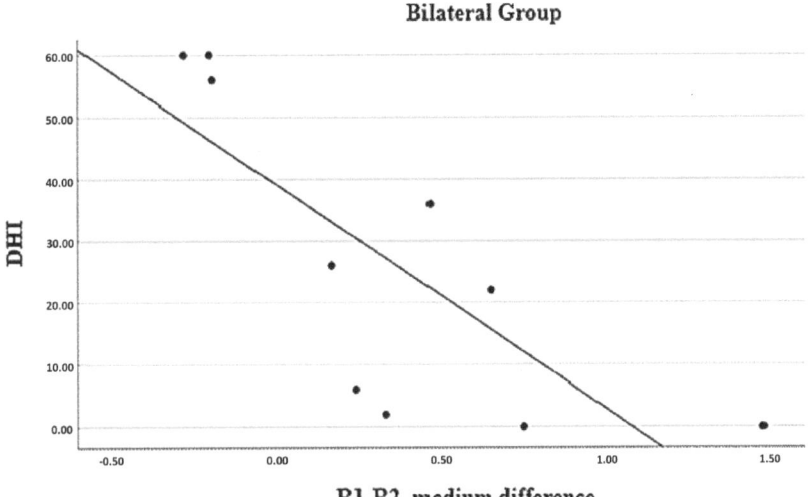

Figure 2. Relationship between mean difference of R1 vs. R2 with DHI in bilateral pain group. (Region of interests R1—right medial palpebral corner; R2—left medial palpebral corner).

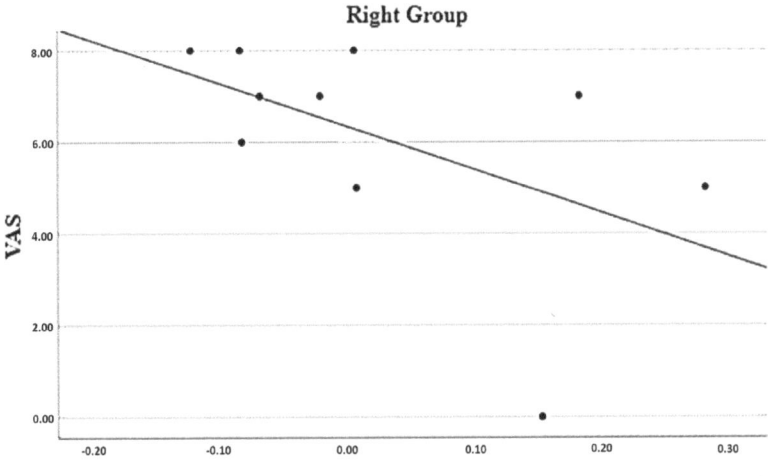

Figure 3. Relationship between mean difference of R14 vs. R15 with VAS in right pain group. (Region of interests R14—right infralabial; R15—left infralabial).

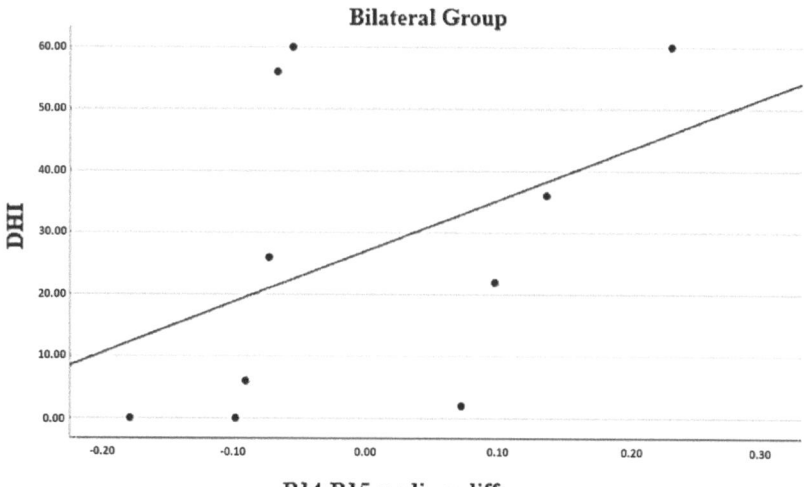

Figure 4. Relationship between mean difference of R14 vs. R15 with DHI in bilateral pain group. (Region of interests R14—right infralabial; R15—left infralabial).

For the group with predominantly right-sided pain, patients with aura showed significantly smaller R1 vs. R2 differences than those without aura (however, it is worth remembering that we have nine patients with aura and only one without aura in this group).

The difference between the frontal sides (R5 vs. R6) was 0.38 °C ± 0.07 °C, while the difference between the temporal sides (R7 vs. R8) was 0.28 °C ± 0.05 °C. Combining results from both regions, the average temperature difference was approximately 0.33 °C ± 0.06 °C. These findings indicate that participants with right-sided unilateral pain had significant temperature differences, with the right frontal region cooler and the right temporal region thermally more intense.

From the Receiver Operating Characteristic (ROC) curve, it was possible to determine the best cutoff point for differences between temperatures only between R5 vs. R6 and R7 vs. R8, as shown in Table 10.

Table 10. Variability in Sensitivity and Specificity in the Comparison of Thermoanatomic Points in Participants with Right and Bilateral Complaints.

Variables			Predominant Side (Right vs. Bilateral)		
	AUC (95% CI)	p	Cutoff	Sensitivity	Specificity
R5 vs. R6 Difference Average	0.79 (0.58–1.00)	0.007	−0.11	80.0%	80.0%
R7 vs. R8 Difference Average	0.81 (0.60–1.02)	0.003	0.001	90.0%	80.0%
Variables			Right	Bilateral	p
			n (%)	n (%)	
Difference average R5 vs. R6 ≥ −0.111			2 (20.0)	8 (80.0)	0.025
Difference average R7 vs. R8 ≥ 0.001			9 (90.0)	2 (20.0)	0.005

Legend: R5—right frontal, R6—left frontal, R7—right temporal, R8—left temporal.

It can be noted that instances of migraines with pain on the right side differ from cases with bilateral pain, displaying an average temperature difference of R7 < 0.001 °C compared to R8 (with a sensitivity of 90% and specificity of 80%). It is also possible to notice that in cases of migraine with bilateral pain with complaints of pain on the right, R5 presents a temperature <0.11 °C about R6 (with sensitivity and specificity of 80%). It was not possible to make comparisons with cases complaining of pain on the left due to the small sample size. Figure 5 illustrates a detailed visual comparison among the three clinical scenarios, emphasizing cutaneous perfusion, particularly in the frontal region.

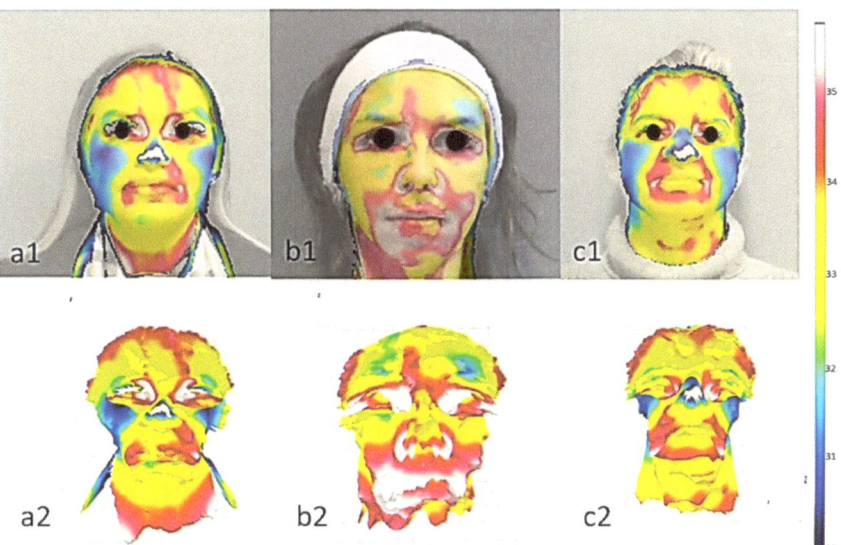

Figure 5. Illustrating the distinctions among the studied groups, this figure begins by exploring groups (**a**) Right-sided pain, (**b**) Left-sided pain, and (**c**) Bilateral pain. The top row (1) showcases thermal images overlaid with visual information, while the bottom row (2) features 3D thermal images, both captured through infrared POC thermography. Note the hypointensity and reduced frontal perfusion, highlighted in blue, in cases (**a1,a2**) with right-sided pain, and (**b1,b2**) with left-sided pain.

4. Discussion

This study aimed to characterize the facial thermographic profile of women with chronic migraine by quantifying temperature differences in 15 regions of interest at thermoanatomical points on the face. The authors observed that women with right unilateral headaches exhibited significant differences in facial thermographic data compared to women with left unilateral headaches or bilateral headaches, particularly in the right frontal and temporal regions. These findings can contribute to our understanding of the thermoregulatory aspects of migraine.

The most prominent finding in this study was the temperature asymmetry observed in participants with right unilateral headache, where the right frontal region showed cooler temperatures, while the right temporal region exhibited hyperperfusion, as indicated by statistically significant differences when compared to the left side in women with migraine outside of the crisis phase. Participants with right-sided pain demonstrated a bilateral difference in the pattern of distribution in the frontal and temporal regions. The thermal profile comprised a 0.33 °C discrepancy in the frontal and temporal regions ($p < 0.05$). Women with chronic migraine exhibited facial temperatures in the analyzed regions of interest, ranging from T = 28.06 °C at the tip of the nose (minimum value) to T = 36.45 °C in the left temporal region (maximum value).

Dalla Volta et al. [16] suggested that patients should receive tDCS therapy on the same side where lower frontal skin temperature is observed. While some of the literature supports the presence of thermal asymmetry in the frontal region during migraine, it remains a matter of debate, as some authors argue that the location of the cold area is not consistently related to the side of the pain [29]. This discrepancy may be attributed to variations in temperature during a migraine attack or differences in headache lateralization within individuals (unilateral or bilateral), as proposed by Drummond and Lance [30].

As Shevel [31] highlighted, vasodilation is considered a source of pain in migraine, but this dilation primarily involves extracranial rather than intracranial vessels. Our findings of temperature disparities in the frontotemporal region suggest that there may be variations in neural control and vasomotor activity between different facial areas. Specifically, the temporal area receives its primary blood supply from the superficial temporal artery, which branches from the external carotid artery and is primarily under sympathetic neural influence, which can potentially lead to neurogenic inflammation or inhibition and subsequent vasodilation. In contrast, the frontal area is vascularized by supra-orbital arteries, which are branches of the ophthalmic artery, themselves derived from the internal carotid artery, regulated by a more complex interplay of sympathetic and parasympathetic neural mechanisms, leading to variable effects under different conditions. The nasal region receives blood supply from the supra-orbital arteries, which anastomose with branches of the angular artery from the facial artery, stemming from the external carotid artery, potentially contributing to temperature variations. This vascular anatomy explanation aligns with the recent literature [32].

Jensen [33] also suggested that both extracranial arteries and myofascial structures receive innervation from unmyelinated trigeminal sensory nerve fibers containing various neuropeptides, which are released during migraine attacks. The observed tenderness during migraine attacks may be attributed to axonal reflexes between extracranial arteries and neighboring myofascial tissues, along with referred pain mechanisms.

The thermal discrepancy in the frontotemporal region observed in our study is consistent with the findings of Antonaci et al. [17]. They suggested that this discrepancy could represent a neurochemical imbalance in facial microcirculation between the two sides in migraine patients, reflecting vasoconstriction within the carotid territory because of autonomic-trigeminovascular system interactions. In a previous study, Ford and Ford [34] observed that 85.4% of participants with migraine without aura exhibited thermal changes in the frontal region, while 89.1% of those with migraine with aura displayed such manifestations. This thermal behavior may be reversible in 85.3% of patients with prophylactic treatments such as beta-blockers or calcium channel blockers, challenging the notion of fixed thermal changes in migraine patients [35]. This is in contrast to the perspective of Swerdlow and Dieter [29], who considered the thermal changes in migraine patients as fixed clinical and geographic entities.

It is worth noting that the dilation of the middle meningeal artery, another branch of the external carotid artery originating from the maxillary artery, has been linked to the onset of migraine attacks [5]. Khan et al. [5] observed that the initiation of a migraine attack was linked to an increase in the circumference of the middle meningeal artery on the side of the headache, suggesting the activation of perivascular dural nociceptors. The increase in temperature observed in the region supplied by the superficial temporal artery on the right side of participants with right-sided headaches suggests a possible relationship, as both the superficial temporal and middle meningeal arteries originate from the external carotid artery.

We utilized thermoanatomical points proposed by Haddad et al. [26] for our analysis, demonstrating high inter-rater agreement. This approach provided reliable results and allowed for a point-by-point comparison of temperature differences. Our findings support the notion that specific thermographic points may be more dependable for detecting thermal asymmetry in headache patients compared to assessing temperature across an entire area. Specifically, the authors reported the following average temperatures (T=) for various points: the medial palpebral commissure had an average temperature of T = 35.38 °C ± 0.41 (compared to T = 34.48 °C ± 0.91 in our study), the labial commissure had an average temperature of T = 34.84 °C ± 0.61 (matching T = 34.84 °C ± 0.61 in our study), the temporal region exhibited T = 34.8 °C ± 0.48 (compared to T = 33.84 °C ± 0.67 in our study), the frontal region displayed T = 34.5 °C ± 0.57 (in contrast to T = 33.85 °C ± 0.72 in our study), the lower lip presented T = 34.3 °C ± 0.80 (as opposed to T = 33.84 °C ± 0.89 in our study), the lateral palpebral commissure showed T = 34.27 °C ± 0.55 (versus T = 33.55 °C ± 0.97 in our study), and the nasolabial region registered T = 34.1 °C ± 0.92 (compared to T = 33.24 °C ± 0.85 in our study) [26]. In the study conducted by Antonaci et al. [17], researchers also chose to perform point-by-point temperature measurements rather than assessing temperature across an entire area due to observed differences in results between patient and control groups. While patients with headaches exhibited a colder area in the frontal region, healthy controls did not display this characteristic, rendering the area-based assessment unreliable and non-reproducible. Consequently, the researchers opted to evaluate temperature at specific and symmetrical points on the face to ensure more consistent outcomes. The data suggest that this approach may be more dependable for detecting the location of the cold area in headache patients when conducting this kind of thermal research.

Migraine with left-sided pain is generally associated with a lower quality of life, anxiety, bipolar disorder, post-traumatic stress disorder, reduced sympathetic activity, and increased parasympathetic activity. Conversely, migraine with right-sided pain is associated with poorer performance in various cognitive tests, a higher degree of anisocoria (unequal pupil size), alterations in skin temperature, higher diastolic blood pressure, changes in blood flow in the middle and basilar cerebral arteries, and alterations in electroencephalograms [15]. More specifically, Blum et al. [15], when considering the topography of the complaint, propose that headaches manifesting on the right side are associated with changes in cutaneous temperature, while those on the left are related to increased parasympathetic activity.

Supporting our findings, Iversen et al. [36] measured the diameter of frontal branches of the superficial temporal artery with high-resolution ultrasound during a spontaneous migraine attack and concluded that it was increased on the side of the reported pain, with no diameter increase compared to the pain-free state. Amin et al. [37] using magnetic resonance angiography reported bilateral increases in the circumference of the middle cerebral artery and the cavernous portion of the internal carotid artery during a migraine attack compared to a day without an attack. Although extracranial arteries did not dilate during the migraine attack in their study, the authors did not rule out the possibility of dilation of dural branches of the middle meningeal artery, as these are small arterial branches that are difficult to visualize using the technique employed in their study.

In this study we did not compare the findings with a sample of women without migraine. However, in a study conducted by Haddad et al. [26], thermoanatomical points were described on the faces of healthy individuals and the authors did not report any statistically significant differences between corresponding hemifaces. The average temperature of the labial commissure was similar to that found in our study. However, the average temperatures for other points on the face, including the medial palpebral commissure, temporal region, frontal region, lower lip, lateral palpebral commissure, and nasolabial region, exhibited higher values than those presented by the women in this study. Our findings suggest that thermographic points in patients with chronic migraine exhibit distinct temperature patterns compared to those observed in healthy individuals. In our study, individuals with migraine displayed bilateral differences between termoanatomical points and cooler facial temperatures in six specific thermoanatomical points that ranged from −0.49 °C in the lower lip region to −0.96 °C in the temporal region.

Interestingly, our study did not identify thermal pattern discrepancies in participants with complaints of bilateral pain, contrary to some of the existing literature. This observation raises questions about potential diagnostic errors or differences in the neurophysiopathological mechanisms underlying bilateral migraine presentations. Given the predominantly clinical nature of migraine diagnosis and the lack of universally accepted diagnostic markers, our research highlights the importance of further investigations into facial temperature patterns to improve diagnostic accuracy. This inference gains substantial support when considering that the diagnosis of migraine remains predominantly clinical and lacks universally accepted markers or laboratory tests for confirmation [38]. These cases could be categorized as 'probable migraine,' which is defined as migraine-like episodes lacking one of the necessary features to fulfill all diagnostic criteria [2].

The examination of the nasal tip (R9) temperature revealed significant variation at this thermoanatomical point. Previous studies have also reported lower nasal temperatures in migraineurs [27], potentially associated with negative emotions and pain [39]. This could be attributed to differences in vasomotor control mechanisms, with vasoconstrictor tone dominating in the nose and active vasodilation in the forehead [40]. Our findings align with these observations, as participants with right-sided pain exhibited lower nasal temperatures compared to those with left-sided pain or bilateral pain. Zaproudina et al. [27,41] noted that individuals with a family history of migraine who developed headaches after sublingual nitroglycerin had lower nasal temperatures than control subjects. The skin temperature values in individuals with migraine were below 30 °C in the nose in 58% of cases, compared to 31% in the control group, which were 0.8 °C lower than the malar region. This behavior aligns with our study, where participants with right-sided pain exhibited an average temperature of 29.5 ± 1.63 °C, those with left-sided pain had 31.45 °C ± 2.69, and those with bilateral pain had 30.81 ± 2.59 °C.

To advance our understanding of this intriguing phenomenon, further research is needed. Future studies should include larger and more diverse samples to enhance the generalizability of our findings to broader populations. Additionally, the limited number of participants with left-sided pain hindered a comprehensive analysis of thermal differences in this subgroup. Moreover, our study's cross-sectional design provides information from a specific moment, preventing causal inferences regarding the relationship between chronic migraine and facial thermographic changes. Future longitudinal investigations could provide insights into the dynamic nature of facial thermographic patterns in migraine patients, potentially unravelling the complex interplay between neural control and vasomotor activity. Finally, the absence of a control group limits our ability to conclude whether the observed thermographic changes are specific to women with chronic migraine. Including a control group in future research would allow for a more comprehensive comparison.

While we provide cautious conclusions firmly rooted in our data, the path forward involves continued research to validate and expand upon our observations. Our findings may be of interest to clinicians and researchers in the field of headache disorders, as they offer a novel perspective on migraine pathophysiology. Understanding the thermal patterns associated with migraine can aid in refining diagnostic criteria and potentially inform treatment strategies. Facial point-of-care thermography may serve as a potential adjunctive tool for understanding and diagnosing chronic migraine, particularly in cases of right unilateral headache. However, the clinical implications of our findings should be approached with caution, given the relatively small sample size, the absence of a control group with healthy women, and the absence of the evaluation of women during ongoing attacks. Therefore, we suggest future research to contribute to our findings and validate our observations. This journey holds promise for improving the diagnosis and management of chronic migraine, ultimately enhancing the quality of life for affected individuals.

In considering the potential clinical application of facial POC thermography in the management of chronic migraine, the authors envision a precise and targeted approach. Building upon the observed temperature disparities in the frontotemporal region, a tailored therapeutic strategy could be developed. For instance, the authors propose that patients with right unilateral headaches, displaying cooler temperatures in the right frontal region, may benefit from targeted interventions aimed at modulating neural and vasomotor activity in this specific area. This could involve the application of transcranial direct current stimulation (tDCS) on the same side as the lower frontal skin temperature, as suggested by Dalla Volta et al. [16]. This targeted approach aligns with the notion that thermoregulatory aspects play a role in migraine pathophysiology [33,41–43]. Moreover, the authors highlight the potential of facial POC thermography in guiding prophylactic treatments, such as beta-blockers or calcium channel blockers, particularly given the observed reversibility of thermal changes in a significant percentage of patients. The integration of facial thermography into clinical practice could enhance diagnostic precision and contribute to individualized treatment plans, ultimately improving the quality of life of individuals affected by chronic migraine [16,33]. However, the authors emphasize the need for cautious interpretation, given the study's limitations, and advocate for further research to validate and refine these potential applications in clinical settings.

5. Conclusions

In summary, our study contributes valuable insights into the facial thermographic profile of women with chronic migraine. We observed temperature asymmetry in the frontotemporal region, suggesting variations in neural control, and vasomotor activity. While our findings align with some of the existing literature, further research is needed to confirm and expand upon these observations. Our study highlights the potential utility of facial thermography as an adjunctive tool in migraine diagnosis and understanding the neurophysiological underpinnings of this complex condition.

Author Contributions: Conceptualization, B.V.F. and T.M.; methodology, B.V.F., M.L.B. and T.M.; software, M.L.B.; validation B.V.F. and T.M.; formal analysis, B.V.F., M.L.B. and T.M.; investigation, B.V.F. and R.B.C.; resources, M.L.B., B.V.F. and T.M.; data curation, B.V.F., M.L.B. and T.M.; writing—original draft preparation, B.V.F., M.L.B. and T.M.; writing—review and editing, B.V.F., M.L.B. and T.M.; visualization; supervision, M.L.B. and T.M.; project administration, T.M.; funding acquisition, M.L.B. and B.V.F. All authors have read and agreed to the published version of the manuscript.

Funding: This study was financed in part by the Coordenação de Aperfeiçoamento de Pessoal de Nível Superior—Brazil (CAPES)—Finance Code 001.

Institutional Review Board Statement: This research received approval from the Ethics and Research Committee of the Regional University of Alto Uruguai and Missions through CAAE (Certificate of Presentation for Ethical Appreciation) number 35901320.6.0000.5351, approval date 6 November 2020.

Informed Consent Statement: Informed consent was obtained from all subjects involved in the study.

Data Availability Statement: The analyzed data can be accessed through the following link: https://docs.google.com/spreadsheets/d/1tDiGkRjv9RMbCH3AdIoFKNgV3QR-XWY9TU6UbzeTzas/edit?usp=drive_link (accessed on 30 October 2023).

Acknowledgments: We appreciate the voluntary participation of all research participants.

Conflicts of Interest: The authors declare no conflict of interest. The funders had no role in the design of the study; in the collection, analysis, or interpretation of the data; in the writing of the manuscript; or in the decision to publish the results.

References

1. Malta, D.C.; Bernal, R.T.I.; Lima, M.G.; Araújo, S.S.C.; Silva, M.M.A.; Freitas, M.I.F.; Barros, M.B.A. Noncommunicable diseases and the use of health services: Analysis of the National Health Survey in Brazil. *Rev. Saúde Pública* **2017**, *51*, 4s. [CrossRef]
2. HIS. Headache Classification Committee of the International Headache Society. The International Classification of Headache Disorders, 3rd edition. *Cephalalgia Int. J. Headache* **2018**, *38*, 1–211. [CrossRef] [PubMed]
3. Ashina, M.; Katsarava, Z.; Do, T.P.; Buse, D.C.; Pozo-Rosich, P.; Özge, A.; Krymchantowski, A.; Lebedeva, E.R.; Ravishankar, K.; Yu, S.; et al. Migraine: Epidemiology and systems of care. *Lancet* **2021**, *397*, 1485–1495. [CrossRef] [PubMed]
4. Vos, T.; Lim, S.S.; Abbafati, C.; Abbas, K.M.; Abbasi, M.; Abbasifard, M.; Abbasi-Kangevari, M.; Abbastabar, H.; Abd-Allah, F.; Abdelalim, A.; et al. Global Burden of 369 Diseases and Injuries in 204 Countries and Territories, 1990–2019: A Systematic Analysis for the Global Burden of Disease Study 2019. *Lancet* **2020**, *396*, 1204–1222. [CrossRef]
5. Khan, S.; Amin, F.S.; Christensen, C.E.; Ghanizada, H.; Younis, S.; Olinger, A.C.R.; Koning, P.J.H.; Larsson, H.B.W.; Ashina, M. Meningeal contribution to migraine pain: A magnetic resonance angiography study. *Brain* **2019**, *142*, 93–102. [CrossRef] [PubMed]
6. Vicente, B.N.; Oliveira, R.; Martins, I.P.; Gil-Gouveia, R. Cranial Autonomic Symptoms and Neck Pain in Differential Diagnosis of Migraine. *Diagnostics* **2023**, *13*, 590. [CrossRef] [PubMed]
7. Buse, D.C.; Greisman, J.D.; Baigi, K.; Lipton, R.B. Migraine progression: A systematic review. *Headache* **2019**, *59*, 306–338. [CrossRef] [PubMed]

8. Karsan, N.; Goadsby, P.J. Migraine Is More Than Just Headache: Is the Link to Chronic Fatigue and Mood Disorders Simply Due to Shared Biological Systems? *Front. Hum. Neurosci.* **2021**, *15*, 646692. [CrossRef]
9. Togha, M.; Jafari, E.; Moosavian, A.; Farbod, A.; Ariyanfar, S.; Farham, F. Sintomas autonômicos cranianos em enxaqueca episódica e crônica: Um estudo transversal no Irã. *BMC Neurol.* **2021**, *21*, 493.
10. Goadsby, P.J.; Holland, P.R.; Martins-Oliveira, M.; Hoffmann, J.; Schankin, C.; Akerman, S. Pathophysiology of migraine: A disorder of sensory processing. *Physiol. Rev.* **2017**, *97*, 553–622. [CrossRef]
11. Do, T.P.; Hougaard, A.; Dussor, G.; Brennan, K.C.; Amin, F.M. Migraine attacks are of peripheral origin: The debate goes on. *J. Headache Pain* **2023**, *24*, 3. [CrossRef] [PubMed]
12. Vincent, M.B. Fisiopatologia da enxaqueca. *Arq. Neuro-Psiquiatr.* **1998**, *56*, 841–851. [CrossRef] [PubMed]
13. Waschek, J.A.; Baca, S.M.; Akerman, S. PACAP and migraine headache: Immunomodulation of neural circuits in autonomic ganglia and brain parenchyma. *J. Headache Pain* **2018**, *19*, 23. [CrossRef] [PubMed]
14. Fraser, C.L.; Hepschke, J.L.; Jenkins, B.; Prasad, S. Migraine aura: Pathophysiology, mimics, and treatment options. *Semin. Neurol.* **2019**, *39*, 739–748. [CrossRef] [PubMed]
15. Blum, A.S.S.; Riggins, N.Y.; Hersey, D.P.; Atwood, G.S.; Littenberg, B. Left-vs right-sided migraine: A scoping review. *J. Neurol.* **2023**, *270*, 2938–2949. [CrossRef] [PubMed]
16. Dalla Volta, G.; Marceglia, S.; Zavarise, P.; Antonaci, F. Cathodal tDCS guided by thermography as adjunctive therapy in chronic migraine patients: A sham-controlled pilot study. *Front. Neurol.* **2020**, *11*, 121. [CrossRef]
17. Antonaci, F.; Rossi, E.; Voiticovschi-Iosob, C.; Dalla Volta, G.; Marceglia, S. Frontal infrared thermography in healthy individuals and chronic migraine patients: Reliability of the method. *Cephalalgia* **2019**, *39*, 489–496. [CrossRef] [PubMed]
18. Dalla Volta, G.; Griffini, S.; Pezzini, A. Influence of sumatriptan on the autonomic system during migraine attacks. *J. Headache Pain* **2006**, *7*, 116. [CrossRef]
19. Rosier, E.M.; Iadarola, M.J.; Coghill, R.C. Reproducibility of pain measurement and pain perception. *Pain* **2002**, *98*, 205–216. [CrossRef]
20. Castro, A.S.; Gazzola, J.M.; Natour, J.; Ganança, F.F. Versão brasileira do dizziness handicap inventory. *Pro-Fono* **2007**, *19*, 97–104. [CrossRef]
21. Karapolat, H.; Eyigor, S.; Kirazlı, Y.; Celebisoy, N.; Bilgen, C.; Kirazlı, T. Reliability, validity and sensitivity to change of Turkish Dizziness Handicap Inventory (DHI) in patients with unilateral peripheral vestibular disease. *J. Int. Adv. Otol.* **2009**, *5*, 237–245.
22. Ito, L.M.; Ramos, R.T. Escalas de avaliação clínica: Transtorno de pânico. *Rev. Psychiatr. Clin.* **1998**, *25*, 294–302.
23. Shear, M.K.; Frank, E.; Rucci, P.; Fagiolini, D.A.; Grochocinski, V.J.; Houck, P.; Cassano, G.B.; Kupfer, D.J.; Endicott, J.; Maser, J.D.; et al. Panic-agoraphobic spectrum: Reliability and validity of assessment instruments. *J. Psychiatr. Res.* **2001**, *35*, 59–66. [CrossRef] [PubMed]
24. Kluthcovsky, A.C.G.; Kluthcovsky, F.A. O WHOQOL-bref, um instrumento para avaliar qualidade de vida: Uma revisão sistemática. *Rev. Psiquiatr. Rio Gd. Sul* **2009**, *31*, a07s1. [CrossRef]
25. Schwartz, R.G.; Getson, P.; O'Young, B.; Campbell, J.S. Guidelines for dental-oral and systemic health infrared thermography. *Pan Am. J. Med. Thermol.* **2015**, *2*, 44–53. [CrossRef]
26. Haddad, D.S.; Brioschi, M.L.; Baladi, M.G.; Arita, E.S. A new evaluation of heat distribution on facial skin surface by infrared thermography. *Dentomaxillofac. Radiol.* **2016**, *45*, 20150264. [CrossRef]
27. Zaproudina, N.; Teplov, V.; Nippolainen, E.; Lipponen, J.A.; Kamshilin, A.A.; Närhi, M.; Karjalainn, P.A.; Giniatullin, R. Asynchronicity of facial blood perfusion in migraine. *PLoS ONE* **2013**, *8*, e80189. [CrossRef]
28. Terwee, C.B.; Bot, S.D.; Boer, M.R.; van der Windt, D.A.W.M.; Knol, D.L.; Dekker, J.; Bouter, L.M.; Vet, H.C.W. Quality criteria were proposed for the measurement properties of health status questionnaires. *J. Clin. Epidemiol.* **2007**, *60*, 34–42. [CrossRef]
29. Swerdlow, B.; Dieter, J.N. The vascular 'cold patch' is not a prognostic index for headache. *Headache* **1989**, *29*, 562–568. [CrossRef]
30. Drummond, P.D.; Lance, J.W. Thermographic changes in cluster headache. *Neurology* **1984**, *34*, 1292–1298. [CrossRef]
31. Shevel, E. The extracranial vascular theory of migraine—A great story confirmed by the facts. *Headache* **2011**, *51*, 409–417. [CrossRef] [PubMed]
32. Drake, R.; Vogl, A.W.; Mitchell, A.W. *Dorland's/Gray's Pocket Atlas of Anatomy E-Book*; Elsevier Health Sciences: Amsterdam, The Netherlands, 2008.
33. Jensen, K. Extracranial blood flow, pain and tenderness in migraine. Clinical and experimental studies. *Acta Neurol. Scand.* **1993**, *147*, 1–27.
34. Ford, R.G.; Ford, K.T. Thermography in the diagnosis of headache. *Semin. Neurol.* **1997**, *17*, 343–349. [CrossRef] [PubMed]
35. Dalla Volta, G.; Anzola, G.P.; Dimonda, V. The disappearance of the "cold patch" in recovered migraine patients: Thermographic findings. *Headache* **1991**, *31*, 305–309. [CrossRef] [PubMed]
36. Iversen, H.K.; Nielsen, T.H.; Olesen, J.; Tfelt-Hansen, P. Arterial responses during migraine headache. *Lancet* **1990**, *336*, 837–839. [CrossRef] [PubMed]
37. Amin, F.M.; Asghar, M.S.; Hougaard, A.; Hansen, A.E.; Larsen, V.A.; de Koning, P.J.; Larsson, H.B.; Olesen, J.; Ashina, M. Magnetic resonance angiography of intracranial and extracranial arteries in patients with spontaneous migraine without aura: A cross-sectional study. *Lancet Neurol.* **2013**, *12*, 454–461. [CrossRef] [PubMed]
38. Marcelino, M.T.M.C. Revisão Atualizada da Enxaqueca e do Seu Tratamento. Master's Thesis, Universidade Beira Interior, Covilhã, Portugal, 2022.

39. Miyaji, A.; Hayashi, S.; Hayashi, N. Diferenças regionais nas respostas do fluxo sanguíneo da pele facial à estimulação térmica. *Eur. J. Appl. Physiol.* **2019**, *119*, 1195–1201. [CrossRef] [PubMed]
40. Kashima, H.; Ikemura, T.; Hayashi, N. Regional differences in facial skin blood flow responses to the cold pressor and static handgrip tests. *Eur. J. Appl. Physiol.* **2019**, *113*, 1035–1041. [CrossRef]
41. Zaproudina, N.; Lipponen, J.A.; Karjalainen, P.A.; Kamshilin, A.A.; Giniatullin, R.; Närhi, M. Acral coldness in migraineurs. *Auton. Neurosci.* **2014**, *180*, 70–73. [CrossRef]
42. Drummond, P.D.; Lance, J.W. Extracranial vascular changes and the source of pain in migraine headache. *Ann. Neurol.* **1983**, *13*, 32–37. [CrossRef]
43. Lin, P.H.; Echeverria, A.; Poi, M.J. Infrared thermography in the diagnosis and management of vasculitis. *J. Vasc. Surg. Cases Innov. Tech.* **2017**, *14*, 112–114. [CrossRef] [PubMed]

Disclaimer/Publisher's Note: The statements, opinions and data contained in all publications are solely those of the individual author(s) and contributor(s) and not of MDPI and/or the editor(s). MDPI and/or the editor(s) disclaim responsibility for any injury to people or property resulting from any ideas, methods, instructions or products referred to in the content.

Article

Improved Outcomes and Therapy Longevity after Salvage Using a Novel Spinal Cord Stimulation System for Chronic Pain: Multicenter, Observational, European Case Series

Philippe Rigoard [1,*], Maxime Billot [1], Renaud Bougeard [2], Jose Emilio Llopis [3], Sylvie Raoul [4], Georgios Matis [5], Jan Vesper [6] and Hayat Belaïd [7]

1. PRISMATICS Lab, Poitiers University Hospital, 86021 Poitiers, France; maxime.billot@chu-poitiers.fr
2. Clinique de la Sauvegarde, 69009 Lyon, France; dr.bougeard@renaudbougeard.fr
3. Hospital Universitario de la Ribera, 46600 Alzira, Valencia, Spain; llopis_joscal@gva.es
4. CHU de Nantes-Hopital Laennec, 44800 Saint-Herblain, France; sylvie.raoul@chu-nantes.fr
5. Uniklinik Köln, 50937 Köln, Germany; georgios.matis@uk-koeln.de
6. Universitaetsklinikum Dusseldorf, 40225 Dusseldorf, Germany; jan.vesper@med.uni-duesseldorf.de
7. Fondation Adolphe de Rothschild, 75019 Paris, France; hbelaid@for.paris
* Correspondence: philippe.rigoard@chu-poitiers.fr

Abstract: Spinal cord stimulation (SCS) is proven to effectively relieve chronic neuropathic pain. However, some implanted patients may face loss of efficacy (LoE) over time, and conversion to more recent devices may rescue SCS therapy. Recent SCS systems offer novel stimulation capabilities, such as temporal modulation and spatial neural targeting, and can be used to replace previous neurostimulators without changing existing leads. Our multicenter, observational, consecutive case series investigated real-world clinical outcomes in previously implanted SCS patients who were converted to a new implantable pulse generator. Data from 58 patients in seven European centers were analyzed (total follow-up 7.0 years, including 1.4 years after conversion). In the Rescue (LoE) subgroup (n = 51), the responder rate was 58.5% at the last follow-up, and overall pain scores (numerical rating scale) had decreased from 7.3 ± 1.7 with the previous SCS system to 3.5 ± 2.5 ($p < 0.0001$). Patients who converted for improved battery longevity (n = 7) had their pain scores sustained below 3/10 with their new neurostimulator. Waveform preferences were diverse and patient dependent (34.4% standard rate; 44.8% sub-perception modalities; 20.7% combination therapy). Our results suggest that patients who experience LoE over time may benefit from upgrading to a more versatile SCS system.

Keywords: chronic pain; spinal cord stimulation; system conversion; waveform therapy

1. Introduction

Chronic pain is a distressing condition, thought to affect around one-quarter of people worldwide [1], and is a leading cause of disability and disease burden. Low back pain is one of the top 10 contributors to years lived with disability in adults [2], impacting psychological and social conditions [3–5]. Since its first application in the late 1960s [6], spinal cord stimulation (SCS) using conventional paresthesia-based stimulation has proven to be an effective and efficient therapy for chronic low back and/or leg pain [7–10]. New SCS paradigms have been developed over the last 15 years, introducing neural-targeting algorithms, sub-perception therapies, and waveform combination capabilities supported by substantial clinical evidence [11–20].

While significant benefits from SCS therapy are sustained in the long term in most patients, some may become suboptimal over time and face loss of efficacy (LoE) [21–24]. LoE can occur when pain coverage is lost (i.e., with new onset pain or when stimulation is no longer perceived in the previous area [21,25]) or when patients have suboptimal pain relief despite no loss of coverage, implying stimulation tolerance that can affect up to one-third of patients in the long term [22,23]. The pathophysiology of stimulation tolerance is not yet fully understood but may include neural plasticity or fibrosis around the lead [21].

Once all of the potential device-related causes of LoE (e.g., lead migration, lead fracture, battery depletion, etc.) have been excluded and/or managed accordingly, several rescue strategies can be implemented. The objective of rescue therapy is to regain and sustain clinically significant pain relief and thus expand the durability of SCS therapy and avoid the need for explanting the SCS system [26–28]. If the implanted device is capable of delivering at least one alternative SCS modality, non-invasive reprogramming strategies can be useful to rescue LoE [16,29–32] and should be conducted first. However, the lack of programming capabilities in previous generations of implantable pulse generators (IPG) able to deliver only one stimulation modality may limit the possibilities for sustained pain relief.

Yet, it is possible to use a more versatile SCS device with advanced programming capabilities that provide full access to a wide range of therapeutic options. These modalities include supra- and sub-perception stimulation therapies that can be used either in isolation or in combination and enable the use of advanced temporal and spatial neural-targeting algorithms (e.g., customized field shapes using multiple independent current control, MICC) [14–18,20,33,34]. Simple, minimally invasive replacement of the IPG, using an adapter or not, can be performed, enabling access to multiple programmable solutions that allow stimulation to be tailored and adjusted over time. This ability could potentially overcome tolerance and avoid the need for explantation [34]. Several monocentric clinical studies have reported promising results after LoE patients were offered IPG conversion procedures, resulting in improvements in pain intensity, functional disability, and quality of life [34], as well as successful rescue of 78% of patients who then sustained significant benefits for up to one year after conversion [35].

Besides LoE, other patients with older-generation SCS devices may face suboptimal battery longevity and/or charging inconvenience. These patients may also benefit from an upgrade to more recent battery technology, which could expand the IPG's longevity and simplify their charging experience.

Our objective in this multicenter, European study was to investigate real-world clinical outcomes in previously implanted SCS patients who converted to a multimodal SCS IPG offering multiple waveform options. We hypothesized that patients who converted to a newer system would report an improvement in overall pain scores that would be sustained in the long term.

2. Materials and Methods

2.1. Study Design

These are the initial results from a retrospective review of data obtained from de-identified patient records from a consecutive case series performed in seven centers throughout Europe. Ethics Committee approval was obtained from each site, and the study was conducted in accordance with Good Clinical Practice (ISO14155) guidelines and the Declaration of Helsinki. All patients provided written, informed consent, as required per local regulatory authorities.

2.2. Study Setting and Participants

Consecutive chronic pain patients (aged $\geq$ 18 years) who had been converted, via a direct lead connection or with the use of an adapter to a new SCS device (Boston Scientific Neuromodulation, Valencia, CA, USA) after they had received SCS therapy with a previously implanted system (any manufacturer, apart from Boston Scientific) were included. IPG conversion procedures were conducted between April 2016 and June 2022.

Each center applied its standard practice to decide whether to convert the patient's existing IPG. The reasons for replacing the previous IPG with a different technology varied. In most cases, decisions to convert the previous device were motivated by suboptimal pain relief (patients experiencing moderate to severe pain and/or <50% pain relief with the previous device), reprogramming limitations (no alternative waveforms with the previous device), and/or longevity or charging issues. Two subgroups were further defined to differentiate patients who had a conversion procedure to restore the efficacy of SCS therapy ("Rescue" group) from those who were converted to a new IPG for a better experience with device longevity and/or charging ("Sustain" group).

There were no exclusion criteria, as per the study protocol. All patients eligible for SCS whose indications were compliant with the new device's "directions for use" labeling and with local regulations were included in the study.

Data collection was organized by the center and consisted of reporting documented outcomes from patients' medical files as they had been evaluated per standard of care. As a result, the type of clinical evaluations and the number and timing of follow-up visits could vary across sites and patients.

2.3. IPG Conversion

Patients who were previously implanted with SCS systems from multiple manufacturers had their IPG replaced with a multimodal Boston Scientific IPG (Spectra Wavewriter, Precision Spectra, Wavewriter Alpha, Precision Montage, Precision Novi, or Precision Plus) using an implantable adapter if needed (Precision M8 for Medtronic leads, Precision S8 for Abbott leads). For Nevro leads, a direct connection to the new IPG was possible and performed without using any adapter. In all patients, SCS leads from the previously implanted SCS system were kept in place. The conversion procedure consisted of performing a cutaneous incision at the level of the IPG pocket to remove the previous neurostimulator and connecting the new one to the implanted lead or extension.

The multiple independent current control (MICC) technology and customized algorithms embedded in the new SCS system were used to tailor stimulation programming, including adapting the shape of the electrical field to optimize spatial neural targeting and adjusting the temporal resolution of the signal using one or several waveform(s). The programming capabilities offered by the new IPG included one or more of the following SCS modalities:

- MICC-tonic SCS: supra-perception, paresthesia-based SCS modality that uses MICC technology and the Illumina 3D™ programming algorithm (Boston Scientific). Illumina 3D™ is a proprietary, neural-targeting algorithm that takes into account the 3D anatomical environment around the SCS leads to compute the electrical field that will best engage specific dorsal column fibers and cover the desired pain areas.
- Customized burst SCS (Burst 3D or MicroBurst 3D, Boston Scientific): sub-perception SCS modality delivering packets of burst stimuli in a regular manner. Burst stimulation leverages the Illumina 3D™ algorithm to target the stimulation area and offers various settings (e.g., intra-burst frequency, inter-burst frequency, pulse width, number of pulses, etc.) that help to personalize the waveform to each patient.
- High-frequency/dorsal horn modulation (DHM) SCS: sub-perception SCS modality using high-frequency (≤ 1.2 kHz) stimulation and MICC and/or the Illumina 3D algorithm. High-frequency SCS can either use a focal target or a broad uniform field of stimulation using the Contour algorithm (Boston Scientific). High-frequency SCS has been shown to significantly reduce the wide dynamic range output [36], and the Contour algorithm implements a stimulation field designed to preferentially modulate the dorsal horn inhibitory interneurons [18,37].
- Fast-acting sub-perception SCS therapy (FAST) enables rapid onset of analgesia that combines precise placement of the stimulating electric field and precise dosing of a biphasic symmetric waveform at low frequency in a manner intended to engage surround inhibition for pain relief [38,39]. FAST therapy is programmed with the proprietary Illumina 3D™ algorithm and uses a 90 Hz active recharge waveform to achieve 100% coverage before reducing the amplitude to a sub-perception level.
- Combination SCS therapy allows multiple waveforms to be layered in a simultaneous or sequential manner to engage various modalities and mechanisms of action.

For example, MICC-tonic SCS could be simultaneously delivered with Contour SCS to produce both dorsal column activation and dorsal horn modulation to optimize pain relief.

2.4. Outcome Measures

All data were collected by the sites and their medical staff, as per standard practice and without sponsor involvement. Patient assessments were made before any SCS system was implanted, as well as prior to (pre-conversion) and immediately after implantation of the new SCS system (immediate post-conversion follow-up), and at the latest available follow-up (last follow-up). Demographic information was recorded, along with pain location, surgical history, and reason for conversion. Pain intensity was evaluated using the numerical rating scale (NRS, scored from 0 = no pain to 10 = worst pain; a score ≤3 corresponds to mild pain, 4–6 to moderate pain, and ≥7 to severe pain [40]). Patient preference for a programming modality was also recorded. The Oswestry Disability Index (ODI; 0 = no disability to 100 = highest level of disability) for assessing functional disability and responder rates (number of patients with at least 50% reduction in pain scores) were calculated for the "Rescue" subgroup.

Due to the retrospective design of this study, study outcomes reflect the clinical evaluations that were documented by the sites, as per their standard practice, and the available data were analyzed from only those patients who had completed follow-up at the time of the data snapshot. As such, the number of patients assessed fluctuated over time.

2.5. Statistical Analysis

A Kolmogorov–Smirnov test was performed to confirm the normality of the change in NRS score. For demographic data and NRS scores, means and standard deviations were determined for the Overall group of patients, as well as for the "Rescue" and "Sustain" subgroups. Descriptive analysis was used for the responder rates, which were calculated based on individual NRS pain scores before and after IPG conversion. A paired t-test with a two-sided 0.05 significance level was used to calculate whether the mean reduction in pre-conversion baseline pain was greater than 0. For the statistical procedure measuring overall NRS changes over time in both the Overall group and the Rescue subgroup, the Mixed Effect Model was used with three time points (baseline, post-conversion immediate follow-up, and last follow-up). Continuous variables are presented as mean ± standard deviation, while categorical variables are presented by frequency and percentage. All statistical analyses were performed using SAS System Version 9.3 software or above (SAS Institute Inc., Cary, NC, USA). The missing data were not imputed.

3. Results

3.1. Patient Population

Fifty-eight eligible patients (mean age 58.3 ± 9.5 years, 46.5% females) were included in the analysis. Patients suffered from pain in their low back and/or legs (Table 1). Prior to any SCS implant, the mean overall pain score (NRS) was 7.8 ± 1.9. At the time of conversion, patients had been treated with spinal cord stimulation for a mean of 5.6 ± 4.1 years.

Treatment goals and expectations differed depending on the motivations for converting to a different IPG. The most frequent reasons patients chose to convert to a new SCS system were to improve pain relief (71%), to obtain access to multiple stimulation modalities (34%), for coverage of new pain areas (33%), and/or for better battery longevity (12%). Some patients reported multiple reasons (Figure 1).

Table 1. Patient characteristics (n = 58).

Characteristics	Patients
Sex—female, n (%)	27 (46.5)
Age (years), mean ± SD	58.3 ± 9.5, n = 52
Pain location prior to IPG conversion, n (%)	Low back/legs, 33 (57.0)
(multiple locations may be reported)	Lower limbs, 25 (43.1)
Pain prior to any SCS implant, mean ± SD	7.8 ± 1.9, n = 47
Pain prior to IPG conversion, mean ± SD	
ALL patients	6.6 ± 2.5, n = 56
Rescue group	7.3 ± 1.7, n = 49
Sustain group	1.5 ± 1.2, n = 7
Follow-up duration (years), mean ± SD [range in years]	
With previous IPG	5.6 ± 4.1 [0.02–8.25], n = 58
With new IPG	1.4 ± 1.4 [0.04–18.98], n = 50
Waveform used priori conversion	
Paresthesia-based	n = 39
Paresthesia-free	n = 15

IPG, implantable pulse generator; SCS, spinal cord stimulation; SD, standard deviation.

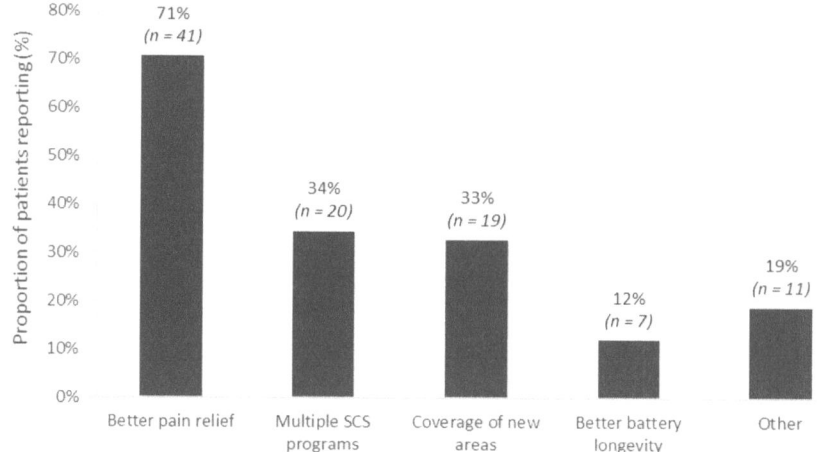

Figure 1. Reasons for converting to the new spinal cord stimulation implantable pulse generator (N = 58). Multiple reasons could be selected by each patient.

Two subgroups were further defined to delineate the outcomes in converted patients based on their pre-conversion pain scores and reasons for conversion:

- Rescue of LoE (Rescue group): patients who had moderate to severe pain based on pre-conversion overall pain scores (NRS $\geq$ 4/10) or those who chose to convert for any one of the following reasons: better pain relief, access to multiple stimulation modalities, or coverage of new pain areas (n = 51).
- Sustain group: patients who had mild pain based on their pre-conversion overall pain score (NRS $\leq$ 3/10) or who chose to convert for better battery longevity (n = 7).

The overall average pre-conversion pain score (NRS) was 7.3 ± 1.7 in the Rescue group (n = 49) and 1.5 ± 1.2 in the Sustain group (n = 7).

3.2. Conversion Procedure

In all patients, SCS leads/extensions from the previous implanted system remained in place. In all patients but five (8.6%), adaptors were used to connect the leads/extensions to the new IPG (Table 2). Spectra Wavewriter was implanted in the majority of patients (n = 29, 50.0%), followed by Wavewriter Alpha (n = 12, 20.7%).

Table 2. Device-related information (N = 58).

Device-Related Information	Patients
Patients prior to conversion, type of adaptors used n (%)	
M8/M1 adaptor	44 (75.9)
S8 adaptor	9 (15.5)
No adaptor	5 (8.6)
Patients after conversion, type of IPG implanted, n (%)	
Spectra Wavewriter	29 (50.0)
Wavewriter Alpha	12 (20.7)
Precision Spectra	11 (18.9)
Precision Montage	3 (5.2)
Precision Novi	1 (1.7)
Precision Plus	1 (1.7)
Not reported	1 (1.7)

3.3. Post-Conversion Clinical Outcomes

3.3.1. All Patients

The Overall group of patients reported an average pre-conversion pain score of 6.6 ± 2.5 ($n = 56$) with the previous system post-optimization. Following the IPG upgrade procedure, the overall NRS pain score significantly decreased to a level of 3.1 ± 2.4 ($n = 49$, $p < 0.0001$) and was sustained until the last follow-up, i.e., 1.4 years after conversion (mean NRS 3.4 ± 2.5, $n = 50$, $p < 0.0001$) (Figure 2). With their new SCS therapy, patients experienced a significant and sustained reduction in their NRS score when compared to the level of their pain with the previous system.

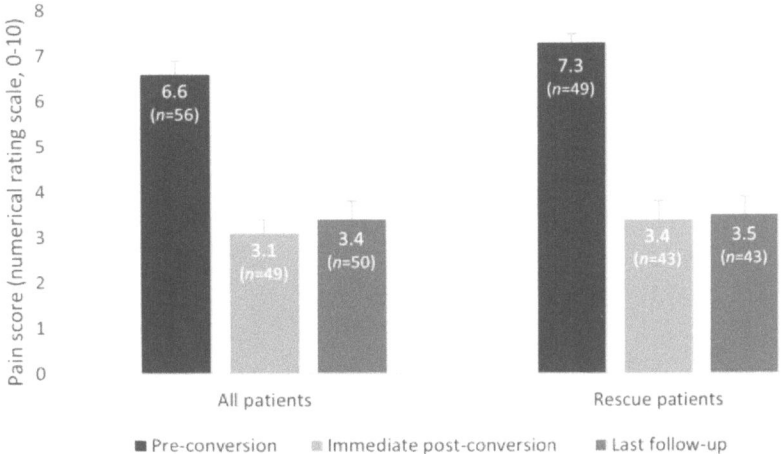

Figure 2. Overall NRS (0–10) pain scores (mean ± standard error) from the pre-conversion baseline to the immediate post-conversion and last follow-up evaluations (mean 1.4 years after new IPG implant) in the Overall and Rescue groups.

3.3.2. Rescue (LoE) Subgroup

In the Rescue (LoE) subgroup ($n = 51$), the mean pre-conversion overall pain score was 7.3 ± 1.7, despite programming optimization, and close to the level of pain reported by these patients before they started SCS therapy (7.8 ± 1.9).

After their previous device was replaced with the new IPG, patients reported a significant improvement in overall pain compared to pre-conversion (mean 4.1 ± 2.8-point reduction in the NRS score, $p < 0.0001$), with NRS pain score decreasing from 7.3 ± 1.7 before IPG was replaced to 3.4 ± 2.4 immediately after conversion ($p < 0.0001$). The improvement with the new SCS system was sustained at the last follow-up (mean NRS score 3.5 ± 2.5, *p* < 0.0001) (Figure 2).

The responder rate (proportion of patients reporting 50% pain relief or more) immediately after conversion was 78.0% (*n* = 32/41) and 58.5% (*n* = 24/41) at the last follow-up (1.4 years on average after conversion). Furthermore, 48.8% (*n* = 20/41) and 39.0% (16/41) of the Rescue patients reported ≥70% decrease in overall pain after conversion and at the last follow-up, respectively.

There was also a significant improvement in patients' disability, with a mean reduction of 18.5 points in the ODI scores when comparing the pre-conversion status (63.9 ± 14.4, *n* = 14) to the last follow-up evaluations (40.8 ± 18.8, *n* = 23) (*p* = 0.01).

3.3.3. Sustain Subgroup

In patients for whom the conversion was solely to benefit from a higher battery longevity or better charging experience (*n* = 7), the average pre-conversion pain score was 1.5 ± 1.2 and remained below 3/10 until the last follow-up (1.3 years after the new IPG was implanted).

3.3.4. Waveforms Usage

Patients reported their SCS program usage following conversion. At the last follow-up, the "MICC-paresthesia based SCS" modality was used the most, followed by combination SCS, then sub-perception therapies (burst/microburst or high-rate/DHM/FAST) (Figure 3). Patients could report the use of multiple programs and adjust their therapy as needed using their remote control.

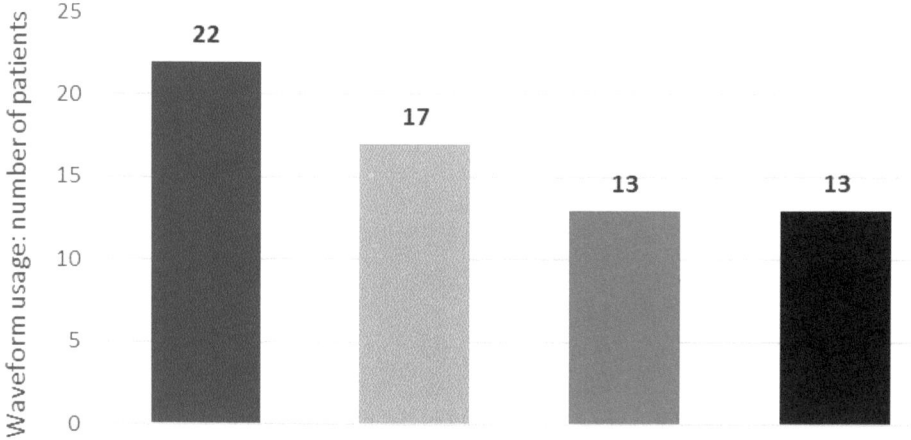

Figure 3. Waveform usage at last follow-up. Multiple waveforms may be used by each patient. DHM: dorsal horn modulation; FAST: fast-acting sub-perception; HR: high-rate SCS.

4. Discussion

Our multicenter, observational, consecutive case series demonstrated that patients who converted to a new SCS system reported a significant improvement in overall pain scores that was sustained for 1.4 years post conversion. The majority of patients (88%, *n* = 51/58) were offered an IPG conversion procedure due to the loss of efficacy they faced with their previous system despite programming optimization. These findings support our hypothesis that new IPG with the capability to deliver multiple stimulation modalities and programming options can help restore SCS efficacy and that undertaking a conversion procedure may prevent the need for future explantation.

It is now well established that some patients using SCS for chronic pain may see their therapeutic response decrease (i.e., LoE) several years after their initial implant and may become totally refractory to SCS treatment [21–24]. Multiple clinical reports have described LoE cases and shown that 12–68% of patients became refractory to their initial SCS treatment after a period of 2–4.0 years [21,23,24,41]. LoE can have serious consequences, and multiple real-world reports have demonstrated that the primary reason for explants was inadequate pain relief [26–28]. Three large patient cohorts estimated that 41–52% of SCS explants in the long term were due to LoE [26–28], while 81% of patients from a cohort of 129 patients who underwent explantation of their SCS system over a nine-year period gave LoE as the primary reason [42].

The explantation rate due to inadequate pain relief is reported to be lower when using multimodal devices (2.4% [43]) compared with traditional SCS systems (around 10% [27,44]), possibly due to the ability to easily switch programs when pain relief is no longer sufficient or when the pain condition evolves with time [31]. Most of the systems used in early studies assessing real-world, long-term outcomes in patients experiencing LoE were non-versatile and had limited reprogramming capabilities, possibly compromising their ability to rescue LoE patients with the existing IPG and thus increasing the need for explantation. In 2014, Deer et al. [22] described "stimulation tolerance" as a difficult-to-predict "biologic complication" of SCS that could occur during the course of patient follow-up. The recommendations from the Neuromodulation Appropriateness Consensus Committee (NACC) group to help prevent or alleviate stimulation tolerance included the use of more versatile IPGs, which could "offer the possibility of choosing between paresthesia and paresthesia-free stimulation and modulation capabilities" [22]. Since then, various clinical reports have documented variable rates of success in patients using standard-rate SCS who experienced LoE and were subsequently converted to a system offering different modalities such as high-density SCS [29], BurstDR stimulation [24,30], 10 kHz SCS [45,46], or system with versatile capability [34,35]. In all of these experiences, the failed therapy was conventional standard-rate SCS therapy using single-source technology; however, it has been shown that LoE can also occur with other modalities [41]. Results from the WHISPER randomized controlled trial (RCT) demonstrated that a device capable of providing multiple neurostimulation therapies provided superior long-term outcomes when subjects were able to choose the most effective therapy [47]. In the MULTIWAVE crossover RCT, the responder rate increased by up to 25% when a device capable of such versatility was used [20,33], with a responder rate of 95% considering multidimensional index assessment [48]. Our own results demonstrated that in patients with LoE who converted to a new IPG (after more than five years of successful treatment with their previous SCS system), the mean NRS pain score decreased by 4.1 points ($p < 0.0001$) compared to pre-conversion, with a treatment responder rate of 58.5% ($\geq$50% improvement in overall pain) at the last follow-up. In addition, disability also improved after conversion in these patients, as illustrated by the 18.5-point clinically significant reduction in the ODI score. Our results are consistent with previous reports of rescue experiences using similar devices [34,35], which have found that 12 months after conversion, pain scores were reduced by 4.4 points and 4.6 points, respectively, and ODI improved by 13.7 points [34]. The "sustain" subgroup of patients, although limited in size ($n = 7$), maintained the efficacy of SCS with their new device for up to 1.3 years after conversion. Previous studies had reported that SCS efficacy can be sustained over time after replacing the IPG, and that pain relief after replacement did not differ when compared to de novo implants [49,50].

Interestingly, we found that a significant number of patients (N = 22) used the MICC-tonic SCS modality as part of their rescue therapy, suggesting that spatial neural targeting may be an important factor to consider when optimizing standard-rate SCS and may play a role in overcoming lead fibrosis issues. Indeed, a study in chronic low back pain has demonstrated that SCS using 3D neural targeting led to better long-term pain relief over two years compared to conventional SCS, regardless of pain location [14]. Another finding derived from our evaluation was that the improvement in efficacy observed following conversion, in contrast to the use of monotherapy that precipitated the subsequent LoE, did not appear to be dependent on a particular preference for a specific rescue waveform. After conversion, 37.9% of patients used standard-rate paresthesia-based MICC SCS therapy, 44.8% used one of the various sub-perception modalities now available on their device, while 29.3% used combination SCS therapy. These results suggest that device versatility and programming capabilities are likely important for achieving optimal and personalized responses within the highly diverse cohort of patients who experience LoE and are consistent with the findings of Andrade et al. [35] and Rigoard et al. [34]. Furthermore, sustaining the efficacy of SCS therapy for years after implantation is important for relieving the level of burden on patients and healthcare systems. In our study, LoE patients had already experienced 5.6 years of successful therapy with their initial SCS system. The IPG conversion procedure enabled them to regain that efficacy and prolong the benefits of therapy for an additional mean of 1.4 years to date, resulting in almost 7 years of significant pain relief when using SCS therapy. In fact, the cumulative, real-world data collected over such a long time period in consecutive patients are a strength of our multicenter, international study and confirm that adaptable SCS therapy in well-monitored patients can provide effective, long-term pain relief.

Our study does have some limitations. Due to the retrospective nature of the study, the analysis is limited to only those data points that are available based on documented medical chart review per standard of care, without protocol, constant time points, and standardized outcomes. Therefore, some data are missing, and a limited number of multidimensional assessments were reported. There was also an imbalance in the number of patients in the Rescue and Sustain subgroups. Although our findings demonstrate increased and sustained efficacy in patients who experience LoE, it is necessary to confirm these data in larger and/or controlled studies and to further analyze the impact of flexible SCS therapy in patients who have already achieved relatively good pain relief. While a 1.4-year follow-up could be considered a strength of our study, offering pain relief in LoE patients, longer follow-ups are needed to capture the potential return of LoE with the new device. Despite the positive outcomes that we observed, future research is needed to obtain a greater understanding of the causes and mechanisms of LoE and to more precisely characterize the clinical profiles of LoE patients and the evolutions in their pathology that could explain why they became refractory to SCS. More data (e.g., large samples of patients, multiple datapoints) and artificial intelligence algorithms may ultimately enable better prediction and personalization of the neurostimulative modality(-ies) utilized by patients in the context of LoE and possibly help to prevent or reduce the incidence of LoE. Finally, the characteristics between the previous and new IPGs were not collected in our study. These elements, such as MRI compatibility, should be documented to ensure, at the very least, a similar capability of the systems. Improvements in MRI conditional compatibility of such hybrid SCS systems need to be further developed in the future.

5. Conclusions

Our clinical evaluation demonstrates that a simple conversion procedure was able to salvage SCS therapy and extend therapy longevity in chronic pain patients experiencing loss of efficacy. The level of pain reduction achieved following conversion was maintained in the long term (mean 1.4 years to date). Prospective randomized controlled trials are now needed to further confirm these findings.

Author Contributions: Conceptualization: P.R. and M.B.; data collection: P.R., M.B., R.B., J.E.L., S.R., G.M., J.V. and H.B.; manuscript content review and editing: P.R., M.B., R.B., J.E.L., S.R., G.M., J.V. and H.B. All authors have read and agreed to the published version of the manuscript.

Funding: This clinical study was sponsored by Boston Scientific (Valencia, CA, USA). Study sponsor had a research agreement signed with the institution of each investigator for the reimbursement of data collection as required by the study protocol.

Institutional Review Board Statement: The study was conducted according to the guidelines of the Declaration of Helsinki, and approved by the Local Ethics Committee Hospital Universitario La Paz (protocol code PI-3250, approval date 30 April 2018); Local Ethics Committee Heinrich Heine Universitat Dusseldorf (protocol code 2019085218, approval date 5 March 2020); Local Ethics Committee Hospital Universitario de la Ribera (protocol code A7005, approval date 10 September 2020) and Local Ethics Committee CNIL (protocol code 2214468 v 0, approval date 19 July 2019).

Informed Consent Statement: All patients provided written, informed consent as per local regulatory requirements.

Data Availability Statement: The data, analytic methods, and study materials for this clinical study will be made available to other researchers in accordance with the Boston Scientific Data Sharing Policy: https://www.bostonscientific.com (accessed on 5 February 2024).

Acknowledgments: The authors wish to express their great appreciation to Deborah Nock (Medical WriteAway, Norwich, U.K.) for drafting the initial version of this published manuscript. Contributors to this published manuscript who reported employment with Boston Scientific during the conduct of this work are acknowledged at the request of the primary author.

Conflicts of Interest: P.R. reports a consulting agreement with Boston Scientific and grants and personal fees from Medtronic and Abbott outside the submitted work. S.R. and G.M. report consulting agreements with Boston Scientific. J.V. reports a consulting agreement with Boston Scientific, Medtronic, Abbott, and uniQure and has received grants from the German Research Council and Medtronic, outside the submitted work, and speaker honoraria from Abbott, outside the submitted work. All other authors report no conflicts.

References

1. Mansfield, K.E.; Sim, J.; Jordan, J.L.; Jordan, K.P. A systematic review and meta-analysis of the prevalence of chronic widespread pain in the general population. *Pain* **2016**, *157*, 55–64. [CrossRef]
2. Vos, T.; Lim, S.S.; Abbafati, C.; Abbas, K.M.; Abbasi, M.; Abbasifard, M.; Abbasi-Kangevari, M.; Abbastabar, H.; Abd-Allah, F.; Abdelalim, A.; et al. Global burden of 369 diseases and injuries in 204 countries and territories, 1990–2019: A systematic analysis for the Global Burden of Disease Study 2019. *Lancet* **2020**, *396*, 1204–1222. [CrossRef]
3. Cohen, S.P.; Vase, L.; Hooten, W.M. Chronic pain: An update on burden, best practices, and new advances. *Lancet* **2021**, *397*, 2082–2097. [CrossRef]
4. Naiditch, N.; Billot, M.; Moens, M.; Goudman, L.; Cornet, P.; Le Breton, D.; Roulaud, M.; Ounajim, A.; Page, P.; Lorgeoux, B.; et al. Persistent Spinal Pain Syndrome Type 2 (PSPS-T2), a Social Pain? Advocacy for a Social Gradient of Health Approach to Chronic Pain. *J. Clin. Med.* **2021**, *10*, 2817. [CrossRef] [PubMed]
5. Naiditch, N.; Billot, M.; Goudman, L.; Cornet, P.; Roulaud, M.; Ounajim, A.; Page, P.; Lorgeoux, B.; Baron, S.; Nivole, K.; et al. Professional Status of Persistent Spinal Pain Syndrome Patients after Spinal Surgery (PSPS-T2): What Really Matters? A Prospective Study Introducing the Concept of "Adapted Professional Activity" Inferred from Clinical, Psychological and Social Influence. *J. Clin. Med.* **2021**, *10*, 5055. [CrossRef] [PubMed]
6. Shealy, C.N.; Mortimer, J.T.; Reswick, J.B. Electrical inhibition of pain by stimulation of the dorsal columns: Preliminary clinical report. *Anesth. Analg.* **1967**, *46*, 489–491. [CrossRef] [PubMed]
7. Kumar, K.; Taylor, R.S.; Jacques, L.; Eldabe, S.; Meglio, M.; Molet, J.; Thomson, S.; O'Callaghan, J.; Eisenberg, E.; Milbouw, G.; et al. Spinal cord stimulation versus conventional medical management for neuropathic pain: A multicentre randomised controlled trial in patients with failed back surgery syndrome. *Pain* **2007**, *132*, 179–188. [CrossRef]
8. Kumar, K.; Rizvi, S. Cost-effectiveness of spinal cord stimulation therapy in management of chronic pain. *Pain Med.* **2013**, *14*, 1631–1649. [CrossRef]
9. Vallejo, R.; Gupta, A.; Cedeno, D.L.; Vallejo, A.; Smith, W.J.; Thomas, S.M.; Benyamin, R.; Kaye, A.D.; Manchikanti, L. Clinical Effectiveness and Mechanism of Action of Spinal Cord Stimulation for Treating Chronic Low Back and Lower Extremity Pain: A Systematic Review. *Curr. Pain Headache Rep.* **2020**, *24*, 70. [CrossRef]
10. Eckermann, J.M.; Pilitsis, J.G.; Vannaboutathong, C.; Wagner, B.J.; Province-Azalde, R.; Bendel, M.A. Systematic Literature Review of Spinal Cord Stimulation in Patients With Chronic Back Pain Without Prior Spine Surgery. *Neuromodulation* **2021**, *25*, 648–656. [CrossRef]
11. Chakravarthy, K.; Malayil, R.; Kirketeig, T.; Deer, T. Burst Spinal Cord Stimulation: A Systematic Review and Pooled Analysis of Real-World Evidence and Outcomes Data. *Pain Med.* **2019**, *20*, S47–S57. [CrossRef] [PubMed]
12. Baranidharan, G.; Edgar, D.; Bretherton, B.; Crowther, T.; Lalkhen, A.G.; Fritz, A.K.; Vajramani, G. Efficacy and Safety of 10 kHz Spinal Cord Stimulation for the Treatment of Chronic Pain: A Systematic Review and Narrative Synthesis of Real-World Retrospective Studies. *Biomedicines* **2021**, *9*, 180. [CrossRef]

13. Rigoard, P.; Billot, M.; Ingrand, P.; Durand-Zaleski, I.; Roulaud, M.; Peruzzi, P.; Dam Hieu, P.; Voirin, J.; Raoul, S.; Page, P.; et al. How Should we Use Multicolumn Spinal Cord Stimulation to Optimize Back Pain Spatial Neural Targeting? A Prospective, Multicenter, Randomized, Double-Blind, Controlled Trial (ESTIMET Study). *Neuromodulation* **2021**, *24*, 86–101. [CrossRef]
14. Veizi, E.; Hayek, S.M.; North, J.; Brent Chafin, T.; Yearwood, T.L.; Raso, L.; Frey, R.; Cairns, K.; Berg, A.; Brendel, J.; et al. Spinal Cord Stimulation (SCS) with Anatomically Guided (3D) Neural Targeting Shows Superior Chronic Axial Low Back Pain Relief Compared to Traditional SCS-LUMINA Study. *Pain Med.* **2017**, *18*, 1534–1548. [CrossRef] [PubMed]
15. Kallewaard, J.W.; Paz-Solís, J.F.; De Negri, P.; Canós-Verdecho, M.A.; Belaid, H.; Thomson, S.J.; Abejón, D.; Vesper, J.; Mehta, V.; Rigoard, P.; et al. Real-World Outcomes Using a Spinal Cord Stimulation Device Capable of Combination Therapy for Chronic Pain: A European, Multicenter Experience. *J. Clin. Med.* **2021**, *10*, 4085. [CrossRef] [PubMed]
16. Metzger, C.S.; Hammond, M.B.; Pyles, S.T.; Washabaugh, E.P., 3rd; Waghmarae, R.; Berg, A.P.; North, J.M.; Pei, Y.; Jain, R. Pain relief outcomes using an SCS device capable of delivering combination therapy with advanced waveforms and field shapes. *Expert. Rev. Med. Devices* **2020**, *17*, 951–957. [CrossRef]
17. Thomson, S.J.; Tavakkolizadeh, M.; Love-Jones, S.; Patel, N.K.; Gu, J.W.; Bains, A.; Doan, Q.; Moffitt, M. Effects of Rate on Analgesia in Kilohertz Frequency Spinal Cord Stimulation: Results of the PROCO Randomized Controlled Trial. *Neuromodulation* **2018**, *21*, 67–76. [CrossRef]
18. Paz-Solís, J.; Thomson, S.; Jain, R.; Chen, L.; Huertas, I.; Doan, Q. Exploration of High- and Low-Frequency Options for Subperception Spinal Cord Stimulation Using Neural Dosing Parameter Relationships: The HALO Study. *Neuromodulation* **2022**, *25*, 94–102. [CrossRef]
19. Head, J.; Mazza, J.; Sabourin, V.; Turpin, J.; Hoelscher, C.; Wu, C.; Sharan, A. Waves of Pain Relief: A Systematic Review of Clinical Trials in Spinal Cord Stimulation Waveforms for the Treatment of Chronic Neuropathic Low Back and Leg Pain. *World Neurosurg.* **2019**, *131*, 264–274.e263. [CrossRef]
20. Rigoard, P.; Ounajim, A.; Moens, M.; Goudman, L.; Roulaud, M.; Lorgeoux, B.; Baron, S.; Nivole, K.; Many, M.; Lampert, L.; et al. Should we Oppose or Combine Waveforms for Spinal Cord Stimulation in PSPS-T2 Patients? A Prospective Randomized Crossover Trial (MULTIWAVE Study). *J. Pain* **2023**, *24*, 2319–2339. [CrossRef]
21. Kumar, K.; Hunter, G.; Demeria, D. Spinal cord stimulation in treatment of chronic benign pain: Challenges in treatment planning and present status, a 22-year experience. *Neurosurgery* **2006**, *58*, 481–496. [CrossRef]
22. Deer, T.R.; Mekhail, N.; Provenzano, D.; Pope, J.; Krames, E.; Thomson, S.; Raso, L.; Burton, A.; DeAndres, J.; Buchser, E.; et al. The appropriate use of neurostimulation: Avoidance and treatment of complications of neurostimulation therapies for the treatment of chronic pain. Neuromodulation Appropriateness Consensus Committee. *Neuromodulation* **2014**, *17*, 571–597, discussion 597–578. [CrossRef] [PubMed]
23. Aiudi, C.M.; Dunn, R.Y.; Burns, S.M.; Roth, S.A.; Opalacz, A.; Zhang, Y.; Chen, L.; Mao, J.; Ahmed, S.U. Loss of Efficacy to Spinal Cord Stimulator Therapy: Clinical Evidence and Possible Causes. *Pain Physician* **2017**, *20*, E1073–E1080. [CrossRef]
24. Hunter, C.W.; Carlson, J.; Yang, A.; Patterson, D.; Lowry, B.; Mehta, P.; Rowe, J.; Deer, T. BURST(able): A Retrospective, Multicenter Study Examining the Impact of Spinal Cord Stimulation with Burst on Pain and Opioid Consumption in the Setting of Salvage Treatment and "Upgrade". *Pain Physician* **2020**, *23*, E643–E658.
25. Rigoard, P.; Nivole, K.; Blouin, P.; Monlezun, O.; Roulaud, M.; Lorgeoux, B.; Bataille, B.; Guetarni, F. A novel, objective, quantitative method of evaluation of the back pain component using comparative computerized multi-parametric tactile mapping before/after spinal cord stimulation and database analysis: The "Neuro-Pain't" software. *Neurochirurgie* **2015**, *61* (Suppl. 1), S99–S108. [CrossRef]
26. Hayek, S.M.; Veizi, E.; Hanes, M. Treatment-Limiting Complications of Percutaneous Spinal Cord Stimulator Implants: A Review of Eight Years of Experience From an Academic Center Database. *Neuromodulation* **2015**, *18*, 603–608, discussion 608–609. [CrossRef]
27. Van Buyten, J.P.; Wille, F.; Smet, I.; Wensing, C.; Breel, J.; Karst, E.; Devos, M.; Pöggel-Krämer, K.; Vesper, J. Therapy-Related Explants After Spinal Cord Stimulation: Results of an International Retrospective Chart Review Study. *Neuromodulation* **2017**, *20*, 642–649. [CrossRef] [PubMed]
28. Pope, J.E.; Deer, T.R.; Falowski, S.; Provenzano, D.; Hanes, M.; Hayek, S.M.; Amrani, J.; Carlson, J.; Skaribas, I.; Parchuri, K.; et al. Multicenter Retrospective Study of Neurostimulation With Exit of Therapy by Explant. *Neuromodulation* **2017**, *20*, 543–552. [CrossRef] [PubMed]
29. De Jaeger, M.; Goudman, L.; Putman, K.; De Smedt, A.; Rigoard, P.; Geens, W.; Moens, M. The Added Value of High Dose Spinal Cord Stimulation in Patients with Failed Back Surgery Syndrome after Conversion from Standard Spinal Cord Stimulation. *J. Clin. Med.* **2020**, *9*, 3126. [CrossRef]
30. Courtney, P.; Espinet, A.; Mitchell, B.; Russo, M.; Muir, A.; Verrills, P.; Davis, K. Improved Pain Relief With Burst Spinal Cord Stimulation for Two Weeks in Patients Using Tonic Stimulation: Results From a Small Clinical Study. *Neuromodulation* **2015**, *18*, 361–366. [CrossRef]
31. Sammak, S.E.; Mualem, W.; Michalopoulos, G.D.; Romero, J.M.; Ha, C.T.; Hunt, C.L.; Bydon, M. Rescue therapy with novel waveform spinal cord stimulation for patients with failed back surgery syndrome refractory to conventional stimulation: A systematic review and meta-analysis. *J. Neurosurg. Spine* **2022**, *37*, 670–679. [CrossRef]

32. Haider, N.; Ligham, D.; Quave, B.; Harum, K.E.; Garcia, E.A.; Gilmore, C.A.; Miller, N.; Moore, G.A.; Bains, A.; Lechleiter, K.; et al. Spinal Cord Stimulation (SCS) Trial Outcomes After Conversion to a Multiple Waveform SCS System. *Neuromodulation* **2018**, *21*, 504–507. [CrossRef]
33. Billot, M.; Naiditch, N.; Brandet, C.; Lorgeoux, B.; Baron, S.; Ounajim, A.; Roulaud, M.; Roy-Moreau, A.; de Montgazon, G.; Charrier, E.; et al. Comparison of conventional, burst and high-frequency spinal cord stimulation on pain relief in refractory failed back surgery syndrome patients: Study protocol for a prospective randomized double-blinded cross-over trial (MULTIWAVE study). *Trials* **2020**, *21*, 696. [CrossRef] [PubMed]
34. Rigoard, P.; Ounajim, A.; Goudman, L.; Banor, T.; Héroux, F.; Roulaud, M.; Babin, E.; Bouche, B.; Page, P.; Lorgeoux, B.; et al. The Challenge of Converting "Failed Spinal Cord Stimulation Syndrome" Back to Clinical Success, Using SCS Reprogramming as Salvage Therapy, through Neurostimulation Adapters Combined with 3D-Computerized Pain Mapping Assessment: A Real Life Retrospective Study. *J. Clin. Med.* **2022**, *11*, 272. [CrossRef] [PubMed]
35. Andrade, P.; Heiden, P.; Visser-Vandewalle, V.; Matis, G. 1.2 kHz High-Frequency Stimulation as a Rescue Therapy in Patients With Chronic Pain Refractory to Conventional Spinal Cord Stimulation. *Neuromodulation* **2021**, *24*, 540–545. [CrossRef] [PubMed]
36. Li, S.; Farber, J.P.; Linderoth, B.; Chen, J.; Foreman, R.D. Spinal Cord Stimulation with "Conventional Clinical" and Higher Frequencies on Activity and Responses of Spinal Neurons to Noxious Stimuli: An Animal Study. *Neuromodulation* **2018**, *21*, 440–447. [CrossRef] [PubMed]
37. Rubinstein, J.T. Axon termination conditions for electrical stimulation. *IEEE Trans. Biomed. Eng.* **1993**, *40*, 654–663. [CrossRef] [PubMed]
38. Metzger, C.S.; Hammond, M.B.; Paz-Solis, J.F.; Newton, W.J.; Thomson, S.J.; Pei, Y.; Jain, R.; Moffitt, M.; Annecchino, L.; Doan, Q. A novel fast-acting sub-perception spinal cord stimulation therapy enables rapid onset of analgesia in patients with chronic pain. *Expert. Rev. Med. Devices* **2021**, *18*, 299–306. [CrossRef] [PubMed]
39. Gilbert, J.E.; Titus, N.; Zhang, T.; Esteller, R.; Grill, W.M. Surround Inhibition Mediates Pain Relief by Low Amplitude Spinal Cord Stimulation: Modeling and Measurement. *Eneuro* **2022**, *9*, ENEURO.0058-22.2022. [CrossRef] [PubMed]
40. Boonstra, A.M.; Stewart, R.E.; Köke, A.J.; Oosterwijk, R.F.; Swaan, J.L.; Schreurs, K.M.; Schiphorst Preuper, H.R. Cut-Off Points for Mild, Moderate, and Severe Pain on the Numeric Rating Scale for Pain in Patients with Chronic Musculoskeletal Pain: Variability and Influence of Sex and Catastrophizing. *Front. Psychol.* **2016**, *7*, 1466. [CrossRef]
41. D'Souza, R.S.; Her, Y.F. Stimulation holiday rescues analgesia after habituation and loss of efficacy from 10-kilohertz dorsal column spinal cord stimulation. *Reg. Anesth. Pain. Med.* **2022**, *47*, 722–727. [CrossRef]
42. Patel, S.K.; Gozal, Y.M.; Saleh, M.S.; Gibson, J.L.; Karsy, M.; Mandybur, G.T. Spinal cord stimulation failure: Evaluation of factors underlying hardware explantation. *J. Neurosurg. Spine* **2019**, *32*, 133–138. [CrossRef]
43. Love-Jones, S.; Thomson, S.; Rauck, R.; Group, R.; Woon, R.; Jain, R. ESRA19-0159 A prospective global registry of real-world outcomes using spinal cord stimulation systems for chronic pain. *Reg. Anesth. Pain Med.* **2019**, *44*, A77. [CrossRef]
44. Deer, T.; Skaribas, I.; McJunkin, T.; Nelson, C.; Salmon, J.; Darnule, A.; Braswell, J.; Russo, M.; Fernando Gomezese, O. Results From the Partnership for Advancement in Neuromodulation Registry: A 24-Month Follow-Up. *Neuromodulation* **2016**, *19*, 179–187. [CrossRef]
45. Kapural, L.; Sayed, D.; Kim, B.; Harstroem, C.; Deering, J. Retrospective Assessment of Salvage to 10 kHz Spinal Cord Stimulation (SCS) in Patients Who Failed Traditional SCS Therapy: RESCUE Study. *J. Pain. Res.* **2020**, *13*, 2861–2867. [CrossRef] [PubMed]
46. Cordero Tous, N.; Sánchez Corral, C.; Ortiz García, I.M.; Jover Vidal, A.; Gálvez Mateos, R.; Olivares Granados, G. High-frequency spinal cord stimulation as rescue therapy for chronic pain patients with failure of conventional spinal cord stimulation. *Eur. J. Pain* **2021**, *25*, 1603–1611. [CrossRef] [PubMed]
47. North, J.; Loudermilk, E.; Lee, A.; Sachdeva, H.; Kaiafas, D.; Washabaugh, E.; Sheth, S.; Scowcroft, J.; Mekhail, N.; Lampert, B.; et al. Outcomes of a Multicenter, Prospective, Crossover, Randomized Controlled Trial Evaluating Subperception Spinal Cord Stimulation at ≤1.2 kHz in Previously Implanted Subjects. *Neuromodulation* **2020**, *23*, 102–108. [CrossRef] [PubMed]
48. Rigoard, P.; Ounajim, A.; Goudman, L.; Louis, P.Y.; Slaoui, Y.; Roulaud, M.; Naiditch, N.; Bouche, B.; Page, P.; Lorgeoux, B.; et al. A Novel Multi-Dimensional Clinical Response Index Dedicated to Improving Global Assessment of Pain in Patients with Persistent Spinal Pain Syndrome after Spinal Surgery, Based on a Real-Life Prospective Multicentric Study (PREDIBACK) and Machine Learning Techniques. *J. Clin. Med.* **2021**, *10*, 4910. [CrossRef] [PubMed]
49. Goudman, L.; Rigoard, P.; Billot, M.; De Smedt, A.; Roulaud, M.; Consortium, D.; Moens, M. Spinal Cord Stimulation–Naïve Patients vs. Patients with Failed Previous Experiences with Standard Spinal Cord Stimulation: Two Distinct Entities or One Population? *Neuromodulation* **2023**, *26*, 157–163. [CrossRef] [PubMed]
50. Leplus, A.; Voirin, J.; Cuny, E.; Onno, M.; Billot, M.; Rigoard, P.; Fontaine, D. Is Spinal Cord Stimulation Still Effective After One or More Surgical Revisions? *Neuromodulation* **2023**, *26*, 1102–1108. [CrossRef] [PubMed]

Disclaimer/Publisher's Note: The statements, opinions and data contained in all publications are solely those of the individual author(s) and contributor(s) and not of MDPI and/or the editor(s). MDPI and/or the editor(s) disclaim responsibility for any injury to people or property resulting from any ideas, methods, instructions or products referred to in the content.

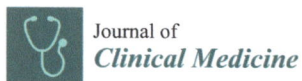 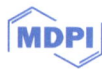

Article

Medial or Lateral, That Is the Question: A Retrospective Study to Compare Two Injection Techniques in the Treatment of Knee Osteoarthritis Pain with Hyaluronic Acid

Giacomo Farì [1,2,*], Rachele Mancini [1], Laura Dell'Anna [1], Vincenzo Ricci [3], Simone Della Tommasa [4], Francesco Paolo Bianchi [5], Ilaria Ladisa [1], Carlo De Serio [1], Silvia Fiore [6], Danilo Donati [7], Maurizio Ranieri [1], Andrea Bernetti [2] and Marisa Megna [1]

1. Department of Translational Biomedicine and Neuroscience, Aldo Moro University, 70121 Bari, Italy; maurizio.ranieri@uniba.it (M.R.)
2. Department of Biological and Environmental Science and Technologies, University of Salento, 73100 Lecce, Italy
3. Physical and Rehabilitation Medicine Unit, Luigi Sacco University Hospital, 20121 Milano, Italy
4. Department for Horses, University of Leipzig, 04103 Leipzig, Germany
5. Interdisciplinary Department of Medicine, University of Bari, 70124 Bari, Italy
6. School of Specialization in Rheumatology, Fondazione Polclinico Universitario Agostino Gemelli IRCCS, 00168 Roma, Italy
7. Clinical and Experimental Medicine PhD Program, University of Modena and Reggio Emilia, 41121 Modena, Italy
* Correspondence: giacomo.fari@unisalento.it; Tel.: +39-083-675-410

Abstract: **Background**: Mild-to-moderate knee osteoarthritis (KOA) can be successfully treated using intra-articular hyaluronic acid (IA-HA). The medial infrapatellar (MIP) approach and lateral infrapatellar (LIP) approach are two of the most used techniques for performing IA-HA, but it is still not clear which one is preferable. **Objectives**: The study aims to find the best knee injection technique between MIP and LIP approaches. Methods: In total, 161 patients were enrolled, divided into two groups (MIP or LIP). Each technique was performed once a week for three weeks. Patients were evaluated using the Numeric Rating Scale (NRS), Knee Injury and Osteoarthritis Outcome Score (KOOS) and Roles and Maudsley Score (RMS) at T0 (before the first injection), T1 (one week after the third injection) and T2 (six months after). **Results**: NRS, KOOS and RMS showed a statistically significant improvement in both groups at all the detection times, without significant differences. No differences were detected between the groups in terms of systemic effect effusions, while the MIP group presented a mildly higher number of bruises in comparison with the LIP group ($p = 0.034$). **Conclusions**: Both the IA-HA techniques are equally effective in measured outcomes. The MIP approach seems to produce some local and transient side effects. So, the choice of the LIP or MIP approach depends on the operator's skill and experience.

Keywords: knee osteoarthritis; hyaluronic acid; intra-articular hyaluronic acid; medial infrapatellar approach; lateral infrapatellar approach; rehabilitation

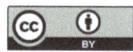

1. Introduction

Osteoarthritis (OA) is a chronic degenerative articular disease [1–3]. Knee osteoarthritis (KOA) is the most frequent since the knee joint is particularly exposed to mechanical overloads [4], causing chronic pain and severe motor impairments, which lead to disability and loss of independence in carrying out the activities of daily living [5].

There are many therapies for KOA treatment, from drugs and new nutraceutical products to relieve pain [6,7] to prosthetic surgery during the most severe stages [8].

Hyaluronic acid (HA) is a glycosaminoglycan that occurs naturally in the knee synovial fluid. In KOA, due to decreased HA production, degradation and increased clearance, synovial fluid HA concentration is lower than in healthy knees. The aim of HA intra-articular injections (IA-HA) is the restoration of its viscoelastic properties, preventing cartilage degradation, promoting its regeneration and reducing chronic pain [9]. IA-HA represents a valid and effective option for mild-to-moderate KOA management, as well as for severe non-surgical management [10].

There are many approaches to performing knee IA-HA injections. Maricar et al. identified eight different knee injection sites for the palpation-guided technique. Nevertheless, physician experience largely influences the accuracy of injections. A high parapatellar approach is preferred for fluid evacuation, while two of the most used are the lateral infrapatellar (LIP) approach and the medial infrapatellar (MIP) one [11]. In both cases, the IA-HA injection is performed with the knee flexed at 90°, accessing the knee joint by passing next to the patella and the related tendon with the medial or lateral patellofemoral approach.

KOA most often affects the medial tibiofemoral compartment. As a consequence, patients frequently report pain located in the medial compartment of the knee [12]. Consequently, among patients, it is commonly thought that the MIP approach could be more effective due to the needle placement nearer the pain site.

Although previous studies have been conducted to evaluate the most effective needle placement into the knee intra-articular space, to our knowledge, none of the previous investigations compared these two approaches in terms of effectiveness and local side effects.

Since there is still no evidence available that the medial approach grants better outcomes or whether one of the two techniques is more valid than the other, a retrospective study was carried out to compare the effectiveness of these two techniques in terms of clinical outcomes and local side effects for treating KOA with HA injections.

2. Materials and Methods

This study is an observational retrospective one. It was carried out according to the Declaration of Helsinki Principles, and it received the approval of the human ethical committee of the General Hospital of Bari, Italy, protocol number 1402/CEL, 13 December 2023.

The written informed consent of each enrolled subject was originally collected as an express acceptance to undergo the injection treatments and to allow the use of the data for scientific research purposes.

2.1. Study Population

We retrospectively enrolled 161 patients (74 men and 87 women) affected by KOA who attended the Physical Medicine and Rehabilitation outpatient service of the Bari General Hospital from January 2019 to March 2023.

The inclusion criteria were as follows:
- Diagnosis of KOA confirmed by a clinical medical evaluation and by an X-ray taken within the previous 12 months;
- Kellgren–Lawrence (KL) REF grade 2–3;
- Age between 55 and 75 years;
- Monolateral Knee Pain (NRS > 3) lasting for at least 3 months or longer.

The exclusion criteria were as follows:
- Previous knee surgery;
- Diagnosis of other musculoskeletal or neurological or rheumatological disorders affecting the lower limbs;
- Any KOA local and systemic treatment in the previous 6 months (therapeutic exercises, physical therapy, other injections, NSAIDs, etc.);
- Pharmacological therapies or systemic diseases which contraindicate injection treatments (e.g., anticoagulant drugs, coagulopathies).

The patients were retrospectively divided into two different groups according to the injection site. Group A consisted of 79 KOA patients treated once a week for three consecutive weeks with three HA MIP injections; group B consisted of 82 KOA patients treated with three HA LIP injections once a week for three consecutive weeks. All injections were performed by an expert physiatrist who had 5 years of experience in knee IA injections.

2.2. Intervention

The patient was positioned supine with the hip flexed at approximately 45° and the knee flexed at approximately 45°. Before each injection, a meticulous skin disinfection was performed using sterile gauzes soaked in povidone iodine solution. The same high-molecular-weight (>1500 kDalton) HA was used for each injection using a 2.0 in (5.1 cm) 21-gauge needle. Each vial contained 30 mg of HA in 2 mL. The performed injection techniques were the standard LIP and MIP techniques delivered in an ultrasound-assisted way (Figure 1).

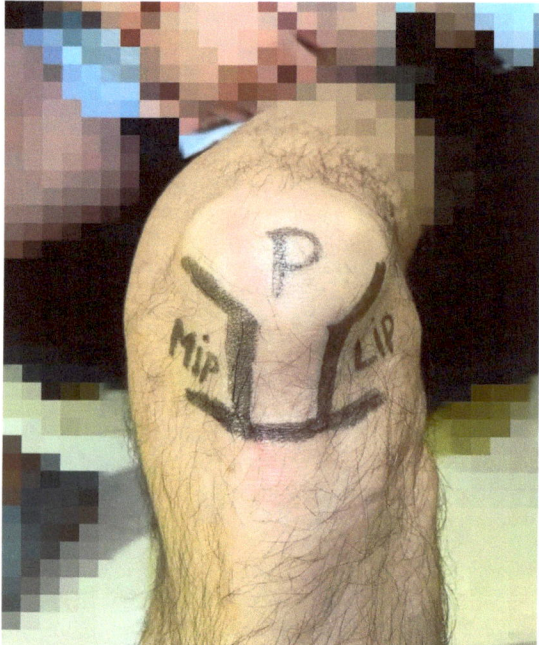

Figure 1. MIP and LIP knee joint injection access (left knee).

The preliminary ultrasound assessment is useful for evaluating the anatomical structures and for establishing the correct needle direction [13]. In the LIP technique, the needle is inserted about 1 cm below and 1 cm lateral to the inferior lateral margin of the patella, and then it is directed diagonally, going from the lateral side behind the patella (Figure 2).

In the MIP technique, the needle is inserted about 1 cm below and 1 cm medially to the inferior medial aspect of the patella, and then it is directed obliquely, going from the medial side behind the patella (Figure 3).

2.3. Timing

All the involved patients were evaluated by three different physiatrists at the following detection times:

- T0: at the enrolment, which overlapped with the date of the first injection;
- T1: one week after completing the IA-HA cycle, three weeks after the first injection;
- T2: six months after the first IA-HA injection.

The first injection was administered at T0, the second one a week after the first and the third one a week after the second.

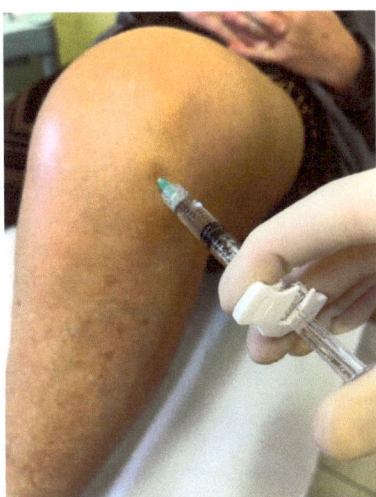

Figure 2. LIP technique performed in the left knee.

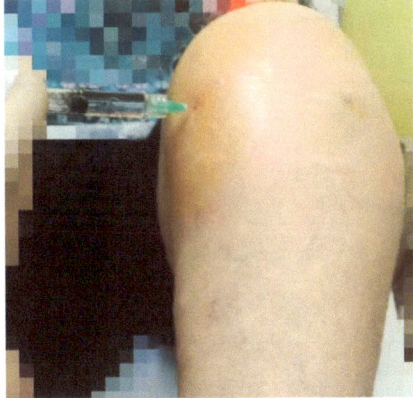

Figure 3. MIP technique performed in the left knee.

2.4. Outcome Measures

The aim of this study was to assess the best clinical knee injection approach between MIP and LIP techniques in terms of knee pain and functional improvement and local side effects. At T0, T1 and T2, after a medical and ultrasound evaluation of the treated knee, each patient was evaluated with the Numeric Rating Scale (NRS) and Knee Injury and Osteoarthritis Outcome Score (KOOS). The NRS is a validated pain scale with a score ranging from 0 (no pain) to 10 (maximum pain) [14]. The KOOS is a 42-item questionnaire useful for assessing self-reported progress in knee functions [15]. At T1 and T2, the Roles and Maudsley Score (RMS) was also collected for each patient. The RMS is a subjective patient assessment of pain, and it was used as an instrument to evaluate the satisfaction with the treatment in terms of effectiveness, discomfort related to the execution and the procedure's side effects. At T1 and T2, for each patient, the examining physiatrist filled out a diary with all the local effects reported after the injections. The side effects were recorded after an inspection and palpatory examination to highlight bruises, hematomas and sites of pain; then, they were further investigated with an ultrasound evaluation.

2.5. Statistical Analysis

Data were analyzed using Stata MP18 software. We expressed continuous variables as mean ± standard deviation (SD) and range; categorical data were expressed as proportions. The Skewness and Kurtosis test was used to compare normal distribution of continuous data, and, whenever possible, we created a normal model for those data not normally distributed. For parametric data, a Student's *t*-test was used to compare continuous variables between the two groups. The continuous variables were compared between the two groups using the Student's *t*-test for independent data or using the Wilcoxon signed-rank test for non-parametric data. An ANOVA test was used for repetitive measures, comparing different timing. The Chi-squared test was used to compare categorical variables between groups. A multivariate linear regression was used for the analysis of the relationship between the NRS and KOOS outcomes at T0 and T2, and between sex, age, BMI and groups. Confidence interval was set at 95%, while a *p*-value was considered statistically significant if <0.05.

3. Results

The study sample was made up of 161 (74 men and 87 women) patients suffering from KOA, divided into group A, composed of 79 people (49.1%), and group B, composed of 82 subjects (59.9%). The average age was 66 ± 4.3 years (range 56–75). The groups were homogenous regarding age, gender and BMI. The sample's characteristics are resumed in Table 1.

Table 1. Characteristics of the sample divided per group.

Parameter	Group A	Group B	Total	*p*-Value
Age (years); mean ± SD (range)	65.8 ± 4.3 (56–73)	66.3 ± 4.4 (57–75)	66.0 ± 4.3 (56–75)	0.481
Male; *n* (%)	35 (44.3)	39 (47.6)	74 (46.0)	0.678
BMI (kg/m^2); mean ± SD (range)	27.5 ± 2.6 (22–35)	27.2 ± 2.5 (23–36)	27.4 ± 2.5 (22–36)	0.249
Side; *n* (%) left right	35 (44.3) 44 (55.7)	31 (37.8) 51 (62.2)	66 (41.0) 95 (59.0)	0.402
Doppler activity; *n* (%)	6 (7.6)	9 (11.0)	15 (9.3)	0.461

BMI = body mass index; SD = standard deviation.

The outcome variables, by group and detection time, are described in Table 2. The NRS showed a statistically significant reduction in subsequent time points in both groups (group A: T1 6.6 ± 1.0 (4–8), T2 2.5 ± 0.8 (1–5), T3 2.2 ± 0.7 (0–4); group B: T1 6.7 ± 1.0 (4–8), T2 2.2 ± 0.7 (0–4), T3 2.0 ± 0.7 (0–4)). In all the KOOS scale's sections, values increased between T0 and T1 and T2 in group A as well as in group B in a statistically significant way ($p < 0.0001$). All these findings are fully described in Table 2.

The ANOVA test for repeated measurements showed a statistically significant difference for all the aforementioned outcome measures in the comparison between times. The Roles and Maudsley Score, assessing procedure satisfaction as a self-reported outcome, showed a minimum decrement between T1 and T2 and a difference between groups ($p = 0.042$), both not statistically relevant. Every single outcome is also visually represented as line graphs in Figures 4 and 5, showing the evolution over time for each scale. Figure 6 displays the Roles and Maudsley Score at each evaluation time. The figure underlines the difference between the two groups, but, as outlined in Table 2, the *p*-value is >0.05; therefore, it is not statistically significant.

Table 2. Average ± SD and range of outcomes per time and group.

	T0	T1	T2	Group Comparison	Time Comparison	Time and Group Interaction
			NRS			
Group A	6.6 ± 1.0 (4–8)	2.5 ± 0.8 (1–5)	2.2 ± 0.7 (0–4)	0.283	<0.0001	0.117
Group B	6.7 ± 1.0 (4–8)	2.2 ± 0.7 (0–4)	2.0 ± 0.7 (0–4)			
Total	6.6 ± 1.0 (4–8)	2.4 ± 0.8 (0–5)	2.1 ± 0.7 (0–4)			
			KOOS—Symptoms			
Group A	60.8 ± 5.6 (50.1–71.0)	73.0 ± 6.9 (54.6–89.0)	76.4 ± 5.8 (64.7–91.0)	0.348	<0.0001	0.770
Group B	61.8 ± 5.0 (52.4–72.0)	73.9 ± 7.5 (57.0–88.0)	76.7 ± 6.9 (60.4–90.0)			
Total	61.3 ± 5.3 (50.1–72.0)	73.5 ± 7.2 (54.6–89.0)	76.5 ± 6.4 (60.4–91.0)			
			KOOS—Pain			
Group A	55.6 ± 6.2 (40–72)	69.7 ± 7.5 (53–88)	74.6 ± 7.8 (60–94)	0.528	<0.0001	0.756
Group B	55.6 ± 7.3 (39–73)	70.5 ± 6.5 (54–84)	75.3 ± 5.0 (60–92)			
Total	55.6 ± 6.8 (39–73)	70.1 ± 7.0 (53–88)	75.0 ± 6.5 (60–94)			
			KOOS—Activity of Daily Life			
Group A	66.8 ± 7.4 (46.5–83.4)	78.8 ± 6.3 (61.0–95.0)	79.1 ± 6.7 (65.0–90.2)	0.628	<0.0001	0.398
Group B	67.1 ± 5.4 (48.8–87.3)	77.7 ± 6.2 (63.6–95.0)	78.8 ± 5.4 (64.0–90.0)			
Total	66.9 ± 6.4 (46.5–87.3)	78.3 ± 6.2 (61.0–95.0)	79.0 ± 6.1 (64.0–90.2)			
			KOOS—Sport			
Group A	32.1 ± 6.0 (16–50)	42.2 ± 5.7 (22.0–52.0)	43.0 ± 5.4 (28–51)	0.354	<0.0001	0.633
Group B	32.4 ± 5.0 (17–48)	43.1 ± 5.4 (26–51)	43.9 ± 5.4 (28–54)			
Total	32.3 ± 5.5 (16–50)	42.7 ± 5.6 (22–52)	43.4 ± 5.4 (28–54)			
			KOOS—Quality of Life			
Group A	33.3 ± 5.0 (18–48)	45.9 ± 5.7 (25–65)	46.8 ± 5.0 (25–66)	0.852	<0.0001	0.854
Group B	33.1 ± 4.9 (17–48)	46.2 ± 5.8 (25–66)	47.0 ± 4.6 (40–65)			
Total	33.2 ± 4.9 (17–48)	46.1 ± 5.7 (25–66)	46.9 ± 4.8 (25–66)			
			Roles and Maudsley Score			
Group A	-	1.9 ± 0.5 (1–3)	1.8 ± 0.5 (1–3)	0.051	0.042	0.849
Group B	-	1.8 ± 0.5 (1–3)	1.6 ± 0.5 (1–3)			
Total	-	1.8 ± 0.5 (1–3)	1.7 ± 0.5 (1–3)			

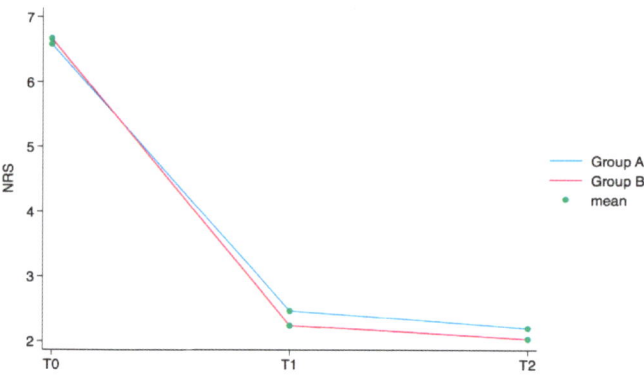

Figure 4. NRS by group and detection time.

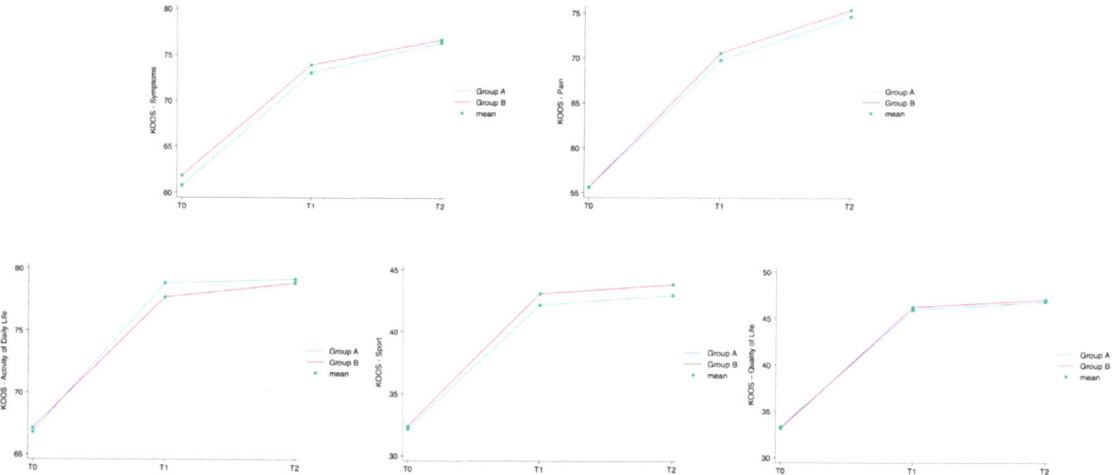

Figure 5. KOOS scale—Symptoms, Pain, Activity of Daily Life, Sport, Quality of Life—by group.

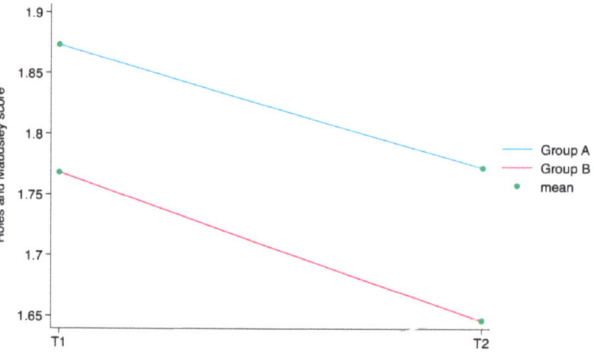

Figure 6. Roles and Maudsley Score, by group.

Tables 3–8 describe the multivariate linear regression analyses by single outcome. Sex, age, BMI and knee side were identified as potential confounders and included in the multivariate linear regression analysis to investigate any influence on every single outcome measure.

Table 3. A multivariate linear regression model to analyze the NRS variations between T2 and T0.

Variable	Coef.	95%CI	p-Value
Group (B vs. A)	−0.20	−0.52–0.13	0.238
Age (years)	−0.02	−0.06–0.16	0.248
Sex (male vs. female)	−0.38	−0.71–−0.05	0.024
BMI (kg/m^2)	0.01	−0.05–0.08	0.658
Side (right vs. left)	−0.42	−0.76–0.09	0.014

BMI = body mass index; Coef. = coefficient; CI = confidence interval.

Table 4. A multivariate linear regression model to analyze the KOOS variations in Symptoms between T2 and T0.

Variable	Coef.	95%CI	p-Value
Group (B vs. A)	−0.72	−2.93–1.49	0.520
Age (years)	0.18	−0.07–0.44	0.157
Sex (male vs. female)	1.42	−0.79–3.64	0.206
BMI (kg/m^2)	0.51	0.06–0.96	0.025
Side (right vs. left)	1.00	−1.26–3.26	0.386

BMI = body mass index; Coef. = coefficient; CI = confidence interval.

Table 5. A multivariate linear regression model to analyze the KOOS variations in Pain between T2 and T0.

Variable	Coef.	95%CI	p-Value
Group (B vs. A)	0.74	−1.89–3.38	0.578
Age (years)	0.24	−0.07–0.54	0.123
Sex (male vs. female)	0.41	−2.22–3.05	0.758
BMI (kg/m^2)	0.25	−0.28–0.78	0.362
Side (right vs. left)	−0.34	−3.02–2.35	0.805

BMI = body mass index; Coef. = coefficient; CI = confidence interval.

Table 6. A multivariate linear regression model to analyze the KOOS variations in Activity of Daily Life between T2 and T0.

Variable	Coef.	95%CI	p-Value
Group (B vs. A)	−0.78	−3.27–1.71	0.536
Age (years)	−0.13	−0.42–0.15	0.363
Sex (male vs. female)	0.41	−2.08–2.90	0.747
BMI (kg/m^2)	−0.30	−0.80–0.20	0.239
Side (right vs. left)	1.07	−1.47–3.60	0.408

BMI = body mass index; Coef. = coefficient; CI = confidence interval.

Table 7. A multivariate linear regression model to analyze KOOS variations in Sport between T2 and T0.

Variable	Coef.	95%CI	p-Value
Group (B vs. A)	0.69	−1.20–2.58	0.474
Age (years)	−0.01	−0.23–0.21	0.933
Sex (male vs. female)	0.99	−0.91–2.88	0.304

Table 7. Cont.

Variable	Coef.	95%CI	p-Value
BMI (kg/m^2)	0.22	−0.17–0.60	0.266
Side (right vs. left)	0.28	−1.64–2.21	0.774

BMI = body mass index; Coef. = coefficient; CI = confidence interval.

Table 8. A multivariate linear regression model to analyze KOOS variations in Quality of Life between T2 and T0.

Variable	Coef.	95%CI	p-Value
Group (B vs. A)	0.29	−1.73–2.31	0.778
Age (years)	0.13	−0.11–0.36	0.287
Sex (male vs. female)	0.38	−1.64–2.40	0.711
BMI (kg/m^2)	−0.10	−0.50–0.31	0.641
Side (right vs. left)	−0.22	−2.28–1.83	0.834

BMI = body mass index; Coef. = coefficient; CI = confidence interval.

In Table 9, the side effect prevalence is explained. No systemic adverse events and no allergic reactions (skin rash, hives) were reported. Only local adverse events were recorded, such as bruises and effusions. The presence of bruises was observed in 23 subjects (14.3%), and there was a statistically significant difference between groups (group A: 16, 20.3% vs. group B: 7, 8.5%; p-value = 0.034). For 23 (14.3%) patients, there was effusion, without statistically significant differences between the groups (group A: 15, 19.0% vs. group B: 8, 9.8%; p-value = 0.094).

Table 9. Side effect prevalence ("bruise" and "effusion") per group.

Variable	Group A (n = 79)	Group B (n = 82)	Total (n = 161)	p-Value
Effusion; n (%)	15 (19.0)	8 (9.8)	23 (14.3)	0.094
Bruise; n (%)	16 (20.3)	7 (8.5)	23 (14.3)	0.034

4. Discussion

The efficacy of IA-HA injections for treating KOA is already well known [16]. In fact, it represents a simple and safe procedure which grants short- and medium-term pain relief with a positive effect on joint functionality. Currently, there is weak evidence in the literature about the long-term effects of IA-HA for pain relief, but some studies demonstrated that IA-HA can delay knee arthroplasty surgery [17].

The best approach for knee injection is still uncertain; the procedure choice is often based only on the physician's experience. The goal is to deliver an adequate quote of medication in the IA space, to improve the technique accuracy and to reduce the risk that, during the injection, the needle may engage with the medial knee plica or the fat pad.

Our findings demonstrated the efficacy of IA-HA. In fact, both groups significantly improved between T0 and T2 both in terms of pain reduction according to NRS scores ($p < 0.0001$) and in terms of joint function, according to KOOS ($p < 0.0001$).

Particularly, the NRS decreased by approximately four points in both groups. These results are in line with the current scientific literature, which states the effectiveness of IA-HA injections in relieving knee pain during up to 6 months of follow up [18]. Similarly, KOOS values improved in both groups and for each scale section. Also, these results are in line with the available evidence of IA-HA injections' effectiveness [19,20].

The multivariate linear regression analysis ruled out that these results were influenced by the determinants described in Table 1, except for two aspects. Particularly, sex seemed to slightly affect the NRS scores ($p = 0.024$) so that females seemed to have a better response to IA-HA. This gap may be due to a different experience of pain between men and women. NRS values slightly differ among people. Furthermore, women experience pain more frequently due to the role of sex and gender; this aspect could refer to many causes, ranging from factors related to biological sex to those related to psychosocial gender. Moreover, to our knowledge, the previous literature never reported or investigated gender differences in IA-HA effects, and it would be desirable for this aspect to be explored in future studies. The other apparently significant determinant is the BMI with respect to the trend of the KOOS Symptoms score ($p = 0.025$). In this case, an explanation could be the fact that people with a higher BMI usually have a lower KOOS Symptoms rate at baseline, and, therefore, they obtain a more marked increase in KOOS Symptoms rate between T0 and T2 due to the benefits derived from IA-HA.

No weight-related difference was found in pain scale between the two groups. Partially in contrast with our results, a study conducted by D'Alessandro et al. compared the accuracy of other injection techniques in overweight patients (BMI > 25) affected by KOA. They found no variation of injection-related pain in IA-HA between anterolateral and superolateral access. According to their research, an increase in BMI seems to be indicative of greater pain during anterolateral access. They explained this evidence as a consequence of a greater local production of adipocytokines, due to the augmented subcutaneous tissue in overweight patients, rather than to Hoffa's fat pad, whose volume seems to not be related to weight [21].

Most importantly for our research, there were no significant differences between the two groups according to NRS and KOOS. Based on our results, MIP and LIP approaches are equally effective as minimally invasive KOA treatments so neither approach is preferable to the other.

In the available scientific literature, data are lacking in the specific comparison between MIP and LIP approaches. A comparison study by Toda et al. [22] deepened the accuracy rates of three different knee IA approaches, namely, LIP and MIP approaches with the patient in a seated position and the modified Waddell approach, an anteromedial approach with manipulative ankle traction at 30 degrees of knee flexion. Although the number of patients was small, no significant differences were detected between the three techniques for KL 2 and 3 patients ($p > 0.05$), in line with our results.

The anterolateral approach, both medial and lateral, seems to be more accurate and effective than the traditional superolateral one [23]. In fact, the MIP and LIP techniques are useful when the knee is dry, without joint effusions, with no anatomical variations, and when the knee cannot be fully extended [24]. Moreover, these approaches are easy to perform also with a palpatory landmark guide in the absence of an ultrasound guide [25].

Regarding RMS, at each detection time, both groups had a high satisfaction with the received injection treatment. Even though there was no statistically significant difference between the groups, we observed an interesting trend in favor of the LIP approach ($p = 0.051$). Although this is only a trend, this can probably be justified by the fact that the LIP technique seems to be more accurate when the knee is dry; therefore, with the same effectiveness, it can be less painful for patients as it allows for a more accurate infiltration [26]. In fact, a study by Jackson et al. compared different IA knee injections using real-time fluoroscopic imaging with contrast material and affirmed that a lateral midpatellar injection (an injection into the patellofemoral joint) was the most precise one since it was intra-articular in 93% of cases [27]. This finding is also validated in a paper by Park et al. that investigated the injection accuracy rate in three different knee sites with an ultrasound-guided approach. They stated that, in KOA, ultrasound-guided IA-HA injections in the mediolateral or superolateral space were more accurate than those through the medial space [28].

This reasoning could be extended also to the analysis of the findings regarding the local side effects. In fact, there were no systemic adverse effects, while the results obtained for bruises and joint effusions were different in statistical terms. No differences were detected between the groups in terms of effusions, while the MIP group (group A) presented a significantly higher number of bruises in comparison with the LIP group ($p = 0.034$). The higher frequency of bruises could be due to the fact that, in the MIP approach, there is a higher risk of crossing subcutaneous small veins. Our results are in line with a previous study published by Lussier et al. [29] that confirms that both techniques are safe, but the LIP one seems to be more accurate, making even minimal injection-related discomforts less frequent.

In conclusion, MIP and LIP techniques appear to be totally equivalent in terms of effectiveness. This evidence is far from obvious or without usefulness. On the contrary, it allows us to choose the approach based on the skills of the operator performing the injections or based on the clinical contingency. Sometimes, KOA determines an alteration of the joint anatomy and a deformity such as to force access from one side rather than another [30,31]. Particularly, the medial knee compartment is more frequently altered by KOA, and the bone reshaping could be an obstacle to a correct and easy injection using the MIP technique [32,33]. In these cases, the LIP approach could be preferred, as well as in cases where there is an increased risk of bleeding and bruising caused by the infiltration itself (for example, in patients taking anticoagulants). Similarly, when there are no preferences due to the physician's expertise or due to specific anatomical contingencies, the LIP technique could be more advantageous due to a lower risk of even minimal side effects.

The current study presents some limitations. First of all, pain is a difficult parameter to assess in an objective way. In fact, pain outcomes were self-reported, but it was a mandatory condition to evaluate it. Then, in the literature, various knee entry sites are described for injecting HA, but, as we said above, we chose the two most used techniques. Therefore, further studies are needed to investigate the best injective way, including also other techniques and different operators. We established a relatively long-term follow up (6 months); however, it would be interesting to better understand long-term efficacy to investigate the differences in terms of injection frequency between the two techniques in a perspective study.

5. Conclusions

MIP and LIP techniques seem to be equally effective and safe as IA-HA injection procedures for patients suffering from chronic pain related to KOA. Therefore, the choice of the technique to be performed can be based on the operators' practical experience, thus reducing the risk of side effects.

Anatomical variations and specific risk factors, such as coagulopathies, may make the execution of the LIP technique more suitable, just as the degree of patient satisfaction may require switching to one approach rather than another during the same injection cycle.

Further studies are needed to deepen these aspects and to continuously refine knee infiltration techniques in order to increase the patients' satisfaction and compliance with therapies.

Author Contributions: Conceptualization, G.F. and M.M.; methodology, G.F.; software, F.P.B.; validation, M.R., A.B. and D.D.; formal analysis, F.P.B.; investigation, R.M.; resources, C.D.S.; data curation, F.P.B.; writing—original draft preparation, R.M.; writing—review and editing, L.D.; visualization, I.L. and S.F.; supervision, S.D.T.; project administration, V.R.; funding acquisition, G.F. All authors have read and agreed to the published version of the manuscript.

Funding: This research was funded by the University of Bari.

Institutional Review Board Statement: The study was conducted in accordance with the Declaration of Helsinki and approved by the Institutional Ethics Committee (human ethical committee) of the General Hospital of Bari, Italy (protocol number 1402/CEL 13/12/2023).

Informed Consent Statement: Informed consent was obtained from all subjects involved in the study.

Data Availability Statement: The datasets used and/or analyzed during the current study will be made available upon reasonable request to the corresponding author (G.F.).

Conflicts of Interest: The authors declare no conflicts of interest.

References

1. Dainese, P.; Wyngaert, K.V.; De Mits, S.; Wittoek, R.; Van Ginckel, A.; Calders, P. Association between knee inflammation and knee pain in patients with knee osteoarthritis: A systematic review. *Osteoarthr. Cartil.* **2022**, *30*, 516–534. [CrossRef]
2. Di Nicola, V. Degenerative osteoarthritis a reversible chronic disease. *Regen. Ther.* **2020**, *15*, 149–160. [CrossRef]
3. Iaconisi, G.N.; Gallo, N.; Caforio, L.; Ricci, V.; Fiermonte, G.; Della Tommasa, S.; Bernetti, A.; Dolce, V.; Farì, G.; Capobianco, L. Clinical and Biochemical Implications of Hyaluronic Acid in Musculoskeletal Rehabilitation: A Comprehensive Review. *J. Pers. Med.* **2023**, *13*, 1647. [CrossRef]
4. Primorac, D.; Molnar, V.; Rod, E.; Jeleč, Ž.; Čukelj, F.; Matišić, V.; Vrdoljak, T.; Hudetz, D.; Hajsok, H.; Borić, I. Knee Osteoarthritis: A Review of Pathogenesis and State-Of-The-Art Non-Operative Therapeutic Considerations. *Genes* **2020**, *1*, 1854. [CrossRef]
5. Litwic, A.; Edwards, M.H.; Dennison, E.M.; Cooper, C. Epidemiology and burden of osteoarthritis. *Br. Med. Bull.* **2013**, *105*, 185–199. [CrossRef] [PubMed]
6. Farì, G.; Megna, M.; Scacco, S.; Ranieri, M.; Raele, M.V.; Noya, E.C.; Macchiarola, D.; Bianchi, F.P.; Carati, D.; Gnoni, A.; et al. Effects of Terpenes on the Osteoarthritis Cytokine Profile by Modulation of IL-6: Double Face versus Dark Knight? *Biology* **2023**, *12*, 1061. [CrossRef]
7. Farì, G.; Megna, M.; Scacco, S.; Ranieri, M.; Raele, M.V.; Chiaia Noya, E.; Macchiarola, D.; Bianchi, F.P.; Carati, D.; Panico, S.; et al. Hemp Seed Oil in Association with β-Caryophyllene, Myrcene and Ginger Extract as a Nutraceutical Integration in Knee Osteoarthritis: A Double-Blind Prospective Case-Control Study. *Medicina* **2023**, *59*, 191. [CrossRef]
8. Singh, J.A.; Tugwell, P.; Zanoli, G.; Wells, G.A. Total joint replacement surgery for knee osteoarthritis and other non-traumatic diseases: A network meta-analysis. *Cochrane Database Syst. Rev.* **2019**, *9*, CD011765. [CrossRef]
9. Migliore, A.; Procopio, S. Effectiveness and utility of hyaluronic acid in osteoarthritis. *Clin. Cases Min. Bone Metab.* **2015**, *12*, 31–33. [CrossRef] [PubMed]
10. Bhandari, M.; Bannuru, R.R.; Babins, E.M.; Martel-Pelletier, J.; Khan, M.; Raynauld, J.P.; Frankovich, R.; Mcleod, D.; Devji, T.; Phillips, M.; et al. Intra-articular hyaluronic acid in the treatment of knee osteoarthritis: A Canadian evidence-based perspective. *Ther. Adv. Musculoskeleton Dis.* **2017**, *9*, 231–246. [CrossRef] [PubMed]
11. Maricar, N.; Parkes, M.J.; Callaghan, M.J.; Ferson, D.T.; O'Neill, T.W. Where and how to inject the knee—A systematic review. *Semin. Arthritis Rheum.* **2013**, *43*, 195–203.
12. Stoddart, J.C.; Dandridge, O.; Garner, A.; Cobb, J.; van Arkel, R.J. The compartmental distribution of knee osteoarthritis—A systematic review and meta-analysis. *Osteoarthr. Cartil.* **2021**, *29*, 445–455. [CrossRef]
13. Lueders, D.R.; Smith, J.; Sellon, J.L. Ultrasound-Guided Knee Procedures. *Phys. Med. Rehabil. Clin. N. Am.* **2016**, *27*, 631–648. [CrossRef]
14. Karcioglu, O.; Topacoglu, H.; Dikme, O.; Dikme, O. A systematic review of the pain scales in adults: Which to use? *Am. J. Emerg. Med.* **2018**, *36*, 707–714. [CrossRef]
15. Monticone, M.; Ferrante, S.; Salvaderi, S.; Rocca, B.; Totti, V.; Foti, C.; Roi, G.S. Development of the Italian version of the knee injury and osteoarthritis outcome score for patients with knee injuries: Cross-cultural adaptation, dimensionality, reliability, and validity. *Osteoarthr. Cartil.* **2012**, *20*, 330–335. [CrossRef] [PubMed]
16. Tenti, S.; Mondanelli, N.; Bernetti, A.; Mangone, M.; Agostini, F.; Capassoni, M.; Cheleschi, S.; De Chiara, R.; Farì, G.; Frizziero, A.; et al. Impact of COVID-19 pandemic on injection-based practice: Report from an italian multicenter and multidisciplinary survey. *Ann. Ig. Med. Prev. Comunita* **2022**, *34*, 501–514.
17. Ong, K.L.; Runa, M.; Lau, E.; Altman, R. Is Intra-Articular Injection of Synvisc Associated with a Delay to Knee Arthroplasty in Patients with Knee Osteoarthritis? *Cartilage* **2019**, *10*, 423–431. [CrossRef] [PubMed]
18. Trueba Davalillo, C.Á.; Trueba Vasavilbaso, C.; Navarrete Álvarez, J.M.; Coronel Granado, P.; García Jiménez, O.A.; Gimeno Del Sol, M.; Gil Orbezo, F. Clinical efficacy of intra-articular injections in knee osteoarthritis: A prospective randomized study comparing hyaluronic acid and betamethasone. *Open Access Rheumatol. Res. Rev.* **2015**, *7*, 9–18.
19. Askari, A.; Gholami, T.; NaghiZadeh, M.M.; Farjam, M.; Kouhpayeh, S.A.; Shahabfard, Z. Hyaluronic acid compared with corticosteroid injections for the treatment of osteoarthritis of the knee: A randomized control trail. *SpringerPlus* **2016**, *5*, 1–6. [CrossRef] [PubMed]
20. Tang, J.Z.; Nie, M.J.; Zhao, J.Z.; Zhang, G.C.; Zhang, Q.; Wang, B. Platelet-rich plasma versus hyaluronic acid in the treatment of knee osteoarthritis: A meta-analysis. *J. Orthop. Surg. Res.* **2020**, *15*, 403. [CrossRef] [PubMed]
21. D'Alessandro, R.; Falsetti, P.; Conticini, E.; Al Khayyat, S.G.; Bardelli, M.; Baldi, C.; Gentileschi, S.; Cantarini, L.; Frediani, B. Difference in pain and accuracy of two hyaluronic acid injection techniques for symptomatic knee osteoarthritis in overweight patients. *Reumatology* **2021**, *59*, 23–26. [CrossRef] [PubMed]
22. Toda, Y.; Tsukimura, N. A comparison of intra-articular hyaluronan injection accuracy rates between three approaches based on radiographic severity of knee osteoarthritis. *Osteoarthr. Cartil.* **2008**, *16*, 980–985. [CrossRef] [PubMed]
23. Chernchujit, B.; Tharakulphan, S.; Apivatgaroon, A.; Prasetia, R. Accuracy comparisons of intra-articular knee injection between the new modified anterolateral Approach and superolateral approach in patients with symptomatic knee osteoarthritis without effusion. *Asia-Pac. J. Sports Med. Arthrosc. Rehabil. Technol.* **2019**, *17*, 1–4. [CrossRef] [PubMed]
24. Moser, T.; Moussaoui, A.; Dupuis, M.; Douzal, V.; Dosch, J.C. Anterior approach for knee arthrography: Tolerance evaluation and comparison of two routes. *Radiology* **2008**, *246*, 193–197. [CrossRef] [PubMed]

25. Hunter, C.W.; Deer, T.R.; Jones, M.R.; Chang Chien, G.C.; D'Souza, R.S.; Davis, T.; Eldon, E.R.; Esposito, M.F.; Goree, J.H.; Hewan-Lowe, L.; et al. Consensus Guidelines on Interventional Therapies for Knee Pain (STEP Guidelines) from the American Society of Pain and Neuroscience. *J. Pain. Res.* **2022**, *15*, 2683–2745. [CrossRef] [PubMed]
26. Telikicherla, M.; Kamath, S.U. Accuracy of Needle Placement into the Intra-Articular Space of the Knee in Osteoarthritis Patients for Viscosupplementation. *J. Clin. Diagn. Res.* **2016**, *10*, RC15. [CrossRef]
27. Jackson, D.W.; Evans, N.A.; Thomas, B.M. Accuracy of needle placement into the intra-articular space of the knee. *J. Bone Jt. Surg. Am. Vol.* **2002**, *84*, 1522–1527. [CrossRef]
28. Park, Y.; Lee, S.C.; Nam, H.S.; Lee, J.; Nam, S.H. Comparison of sonographically guided intra-articular injections at 3 different sites of the knee. *J. Ultrasound Med.* **2011**, *30*, 1669–1676. [CrossRef]
29. Lussier, A.; Cividino, A.A.; McFarlane, C.A.; Olszynski, W.P.; Potashner, W.J.; De Médicis, R. Viscosupplementation with hylan for the treatment of osteoarthritis: Findings from clinical practice in Canada. *J. Rheumatol.* **1996**, *23*, 1579–1585.
30. Khajehsaeid, H.; Abdollahpour, Z. Progressive deformation-induced degradation of knee articular cartilage and osteoarthritis. *J. Biomech.* **2020**, *111*, 109995. [CrossRef] [PubMed]
31. Geng, R.; Li, J.; Yu, C.; Zhang, C.; Chen, F.; Chen, J.; Ni, H.; Wang, J.; Kang, K.; Wei, Z.; et al. Knee osteoarthritis: Current status and research progress in treatment (Review). *Exp. Ther. Med.* **2023**, *26*, 481. [CrossRef] [PubMed]
32. Chavda, S.; Rabbani, S.A.; Wadhwa, T. Role and Effectiveness of Intra-articular Injection of Hyaluronic Acid in the Treatment of Knee Osteoarthritis: A Systematic Review. *Cureus* **2022**, *14*, e24503. [CrossRef] [PubMed]
33. Briem, K.; Axe, M.J.; Snyder-Mackler, L. Medial knee joint loading increases in those who respond to hyaluronan injection for medial knee osteoarthritis. *J. Orthop. Res.* **2009**, *27*, 1420–1425. [CrossRef] [PubMed]

Disclaimer/Publisher's Note: The statements, opinions and data contained in all publications are solely those of the individual author(s) and contributor(s) and not of MDPI and/or the editor(s). MDPI and/or the editor(s) disclaim responsibility for any injury to people or property resulting from any ideas, methods, instructions or products referred to in the content.

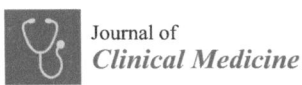 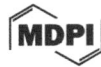

Review

Clinical Patient-Relevant Outcome Domains for Persistent Spinal Pain Syndrome—A Scoping Review and Expert Panels

Ferdinand Bastiaens [1,2,3,*], Jessica T. Wegener [3], Raymond W. J. G. Ostelo [4,5], Bert-Kristian W. P. van Roosendaal [2], Kris C. P. Vissers [2,3] and Miranda L. van Hooff [1,6]

1. Department of Research, Sint Maartenskliniek, 9500 GM Nijmegen, The Netherlands
2. Department of Anesthesiology, Pain, and Palliative Medicine, Radboud University Medical Center, Geert Grooteplein Zuid 10, 6525 GA Nijmegen, The Netherlands
3. Department of Anesthesiology and Pain Medicine, Sint Maartenskliniek, 9500 GM Nijmegen, The Netherlands
4. Department of Health Sciences, Faculty of Science and Amsterdam Movement Science Research Institute, Vrije Universiteit, Van der Boechorststraat 7, 1081 BT Amsterdam, The Netherlands
5. Department of Epidemiology and Data Science, Amsterdam University Medical Centre, Vrije Universiteit, Meibergdreef 9, 1105 AZ Amsterdam, The Netherlands
6. Department of Orthopedics, Radboud University Medical Center, Geert Grooteplein Zuid 10, 6525 GA Nijmegen, The Netherlands
* Correspondence: f.bastiaens@maartenskliniek.nl

Abstract: Large variation exists in the monitoring of clinical outcome domains in patients with persistent spinal pain syndrome (PSPS). Furthermore, it is unclear which outcome domains are important from the PSPS patient's perspective. The study objectives were to identify patient-relevant outcome domains for PSPS and to establish a PSPS outcomes framework. PubMed, CINAHL, Cochrane, and EMBASE were searched to identify studies reporting views or preferences of PSPS patients on outcome domains. The Arksey and O'Malley framework was followed to identify outcome domains. An expert panel rated the domains based on the importance for PSPS patients they have treated. A framework of relevant outcome domains was established using the selected outcome domains by the expert panel. No studies were found for PSPS type 1. Five studies with 77 PSPS type 2 patients were included for further analysis. Fourteen outcome domains were identified. An expert panel, including 27 clinical experts, reached consensus on the domains pain, daily activities, perspective of life, social participation, mobility, mood, self-reliance, and sleep. Eleven domains were included in the PSPS type 2 outcomes framework. This framework is illustrative of a more holistic perspective and should be used to improve the evaluation of care for PSPS type 2 patients. Further research is needed on the prioritization of relevant outcome domains.

Keywords: persistent spinal pain syndrome; scoping review; outcome domains; patient participation; expert panel

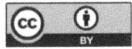

1. Introduction

Persistent spinal pain syndrome (PSPS) encompasses a diversity of clinical symptoms. These include chronic or recurrent pain of spinal origin, paresthesia, numbness, stiffness, muscle spasms, and weakness, most commonly situated in the lumbosacral region [1–4]. Spinal surgery may have occurred (PSPS type 2, formerly known as failed back surgery syndrome (FBSS)) or not (PSPS type 1) [4]. PSPS patients commonly suffer from severe complaints [5], impacting their ability to work [6] and diminishing their quality of life [7]. A multitude of interventions are frequently offered to PSPS patients in primary care and dedicated pain centers, ranging from conservative therapy to invasive pain treatments [8–10].

Clinical outcome domains are defined as concepts to be measured in terms of a further specification of an aspect of health [11]. Ideally, there should be a consensus-based set of outcomes that can be monitored over time, reported in research trials, and in daily clinical practice of a specific clinical area [12]. Although PSPS patients often share epidemiological, demographic, and phenotypical characteristics, a large variation exists in the monitoring of clinical outcome domains [13]. This is partly because of the possible refractory character of this syndrome and the various clinical approaches and care pathways provided by different medical specialties who are involved in the management of PSPS patients. Furthermore, the tools used to measure the properties of these outcome domains vary largely [14–16]. These inconsistencies impede large-scale evaluations and the ability to make informed decisions about healthcare [17].

A standardized set of outcomes that focuses on biomedical, psychosocial, and behavioral domains is needed to map the health status of chronic pain patients [18]. In general, classification models such as the International Classification of Diseases (ICD-11) and the International Classification of Functioning, Disability and Health (ICF) aim to identify the right patient populations and emphasize a broader view on health, where health encompasses more than the absence of a disease [19,20]. In addition, conversational tools such as the Positive Health Model focus on the multidimensional exploration of patient preferences in the clinical setting [21].

There are also initiatives that recommend multidimensional outcome domains for (non-specific) low back pain [22,23]. However, due to the chronic and multi-dimensional nature of PSPS, these recommendations may not be appropriate for PSPS patients [10,24]. In addition, there are recommendations on outcome domains in chronic pain trials, as well as a consensus statement on outcome domains for PSPS type 2 patients utilizing a multidisciplinary team approach [15,25]. However, these recommendations are treatment related and based on the perspectives of clinical and scientific experts. Overall, it is important that the patient's perspective on outcome domains is more involved in these clinical outcome sets to ensure the clinical relevance [26].

The clinical relevance of measured outcome domains is important in addressing the healthcare needs of patients and facilitate the process of shared decision making [27–31]. Due to the chronic nature of PSPS and multidimensional limitations in daily life for PSPS patients, it is important to consider the value of different domains from a patient's perspective. Hence, a more multidimensional evaluation is necessary to determine which outcome domains are deemed important from the perspective of PSPS patients. The primary objective of this study is to identify outcome domains from the perspective of patients with PSPS (patient-relevant outcome domains). Additionally, we aim to link the identified outcome domains to items of the ICF model.

2. Materials and Methods

This study is the first part of a research project to identify a shortlist of patient-relevant outcome domains. The research project follows an iterative design in accordance with the core outcome set process described in the COMET Handbook [17]. A scoping review of the literature is performed to identify existing evidence, followed by a consensus process with a panel of clinical and research experts to elicit views about the outcome domains. In a subsequent study, focus groups will be held with PSPS patients to weigh and prioritize (and possibly expand the list of) the identified outcome domains of the current publication.

In this study, a scoping literature review was performed to explore the perspectives and preferences of PSPS patients on important outcome domains. The framework of Arksey and O'Malley was followed [26]. This framework provides a comprehensive foundation for scoping review methodology comprising five stages: (1) identifying the research question; (2) identifying relevant studies; (3) study selection; (4) charting the data; and (5) collating, summarizing, and reporting the results. The list of outcome domains was evaluated by

(6) consulting expert panels to determine a framework of relevant outcome domains. The study is performed and reported according to the Preferred Reporting Items for Systematic Reviews and Meta-Analysis (PRISMA) statement for scoping reviews [32].

2.1. Identifying the Research Question

The aim of the scoping review was to identify patient-relevant outcome domains for PSPS patients that could be used by PSPS patients to weigh and prioritize the identified domains. The following research questions were formulated: 1. Which outcome domains are deemed relevant for the general health of PSPS patients? 2. Can the identified outcome domains be linked to the items of the ICF model and used to create a PSPS outcome-framework.

2.2. Identifying Relevant Studies

The literature search using PubMed, CINAHL, Embase, and Cochrane Library was performed in November 2023. The search strategy was set up with the aid of an information specialist and consisted of keywords, subject headings, and free-text words. The search string was built upon a combination of the patient populations (e.g., chronic pain), possible interventions (e.g., pain management), and outcomes (e.g., patient participation). The complete search string is shown in Supplementary Materials Section S1. Studies found through the search results were imported and managed in Rayyan QCRI [33].

2.3. Study Selection

Studies focusing on PSPS patients encompassing a diversity of clinical symptoms were eligible for inclusion. These include chronic or recurrent pain of spinal origin, paresthesia, numbness, stiffness, muscle spasms, and weakness, most commonly situated in the lumbosacral region and [1–4]. Spinal surgery may have occurred (PSPS type 2, including previous diagnoses such as FBSS and post-laminectomy syndrome) or not (PSPS type 1) [4]. Furthermore, studies had to contain views or preferences of PSPS patients on outcome domains. Both qualitative and quantitative studies were eligible for inclusion. Case reports, animal studies, in vitro studies, biomechanical studies, simulation studies, and literature reviews were excluded. Non-English language studies, conference abstracts, and study protocols were excluded as well. In Table 1, an overview is presented of the selection criteria following the participants/population, intervention, comparator and outcome model (PICO).

Table 1. PICO for the scoping review.

Category	Selection Criteria
Participants/population	Adult (≥18 years) PSPS patients who present back and/or leg pain and irrespective of whether they have undergone prior back surgery or not. This includes study samples with an FBSS diagnosis.
Intervention	Not applicable
Comparator	Not applicable
Outcome	Views or preferences of PSPS patients on outcome domains.

After checking for duplicates, all the studies of the initial search were screened based on title and abstract. Included studies were checked on full text-availability. All full-text studies were then subjugated to full-text screening. Both screening processes were conducted separately by two reviewers (F.B. and B.R.). In case of disagreements, the reviewers discussed the study until consensus was reached.

2.4. Charting the Data and Collating, Summarizing and Reporting the Results

The following categories of information were extracted from included studies: author(s), year of publication, objective(s), study design, setting, country, study population, and sample size. In quantitative studies, identified outcome domains and their rationale were charted and compiled into a list. Qualitative studies were analyzed through theoretical thematic analysis [34,35]. The first step was familiarization of the collected data. Secondly, all key themes were identified in order to further develop the framework. Thirdly, data were indexed in textual form by coding the relevant information from the studies. Fourthly, data were linked to the relevant part of the thematic framework in concordance with the ICF rules [19,36,37]. Outcome domains recurring in multiple studies were considered as patient-relevant outcome domains and included for further evaluation by the expert panels in order to establish a PSPS outcomes framework.

2.5. Expert Panel Consultation

The list of outcome domains linked to the ICF models was presented to an expert panel. The expert panel consultation consisted of a two-round online questionnaire, followed by a consensus meeting. The experts were medical specialists experienced in treating PSPS patients and were recruited from the Orthopedics and Chronic Pain departments of the Sint Maartenskliniek Nijmegen and Radboud University Medical Center Nijmegen. The expert panel was asked to complete a questionnaire in which they were asked to rate the domains based on the importance for PSPS patients they have treated. In the first round, experts were asked to rate each outcome domain using the Grading of Recommendations Assessment, Development and Evaluation (GRADE) scale, a nine-point scale that is commonly divided into three categories for Core Outcome Set projects: not important (1–3), important but not critical (4–6), and critically important (7–9) [38]. A free-text option was also included to add comments or suggestions for additional outcomes. After the first round, the results of the first round were discussed in a consensus meeting by participating experts. Descriptive statistics (e.g., median and interquartile range (IQR)) were used to analyze the results of both rounds.

In the first round, 18 experts from the chronic pain department (chronic pain expert panel) and nine experts from the orthopedic department (orthopedic expert panel) participated. In total, 11 experts from the chronic pain department also participated in the second round. The chronic pain expert panel consisted of seven anesthesiologists, six neurosurgeons, and five nursing specialists, whereas the orthopedic panel consisted of four orthopedic spinal surgeons, four general orthopedists, and one spine orthopedist.

Defining consensus for inclusion of an outcome in the shortlist was based on the systematic review on consensus in Delphi studies by Diamond et al. (2014) [39]. Consensus was defined a priori as $\geq 75\%$ of the participants in all stakeholder groups rating the outcome as critically important (GRADE score = 7–9) [39]. Consensus for exclusion of an outcome from the shortlist was defined as 50% or less of respondents in all stakeholder groups rating the outcome as critically important [40]. Added suggestions were reviewed by the research team and, if appropriate, included as an outcome domain in the second round.

Prior to the second round, an overview of the included and excluded domains from the first round was shown and discussed with the experts. The experts were asked to give a new GRADE rating. Inclusion/exclusion of outcome domains was based on the aforementioned consensus measures. After the second round, outcome domains that did not meet either measure were assessed by the research team. A framework of relevant outcome domains was established using the ICF model, in which the outcome domains selected by the two rounds of experts were linked to items of the ICF classification [19,36,37]. The outcome domains were linked to the most precise ICF level of classification (or category). The ICF categories 'other specified' and 'unspecified' were avoided in the linking process. The main researcher (FB) performed the initial linking process, which was discussed the main research team (JW, MH, JV, and KV) in order to reach consensus for the final linkage decisions. Outcome domains that could not be classified in the ICF were labeled as "not covered", and those that were not precise enough were labeled as "not definable", apart from outcome domains that were considered as personal factors.

3. Results

3.1. Study Selection

The databases yielded 3405 potentially relevant published studies, of which 2398 studies remained after the duplication check. After screening the titles and abstracts, 18 studies remained. During the full-text availability check, 4 studies could not be retrieved. Of the 14 studies that underwent a full-text screening, 9 were excluded due to wrong populations (e.g., non-specific low-back pain, spinal cord injury, fibromyalgia, diabetes, etc.) and/or absence of reported patient perspectives on outcome domains [41–49]. A final number of 5 studies were included for further analysis. The screening process is shown in the study flow diagram (Figure 1).

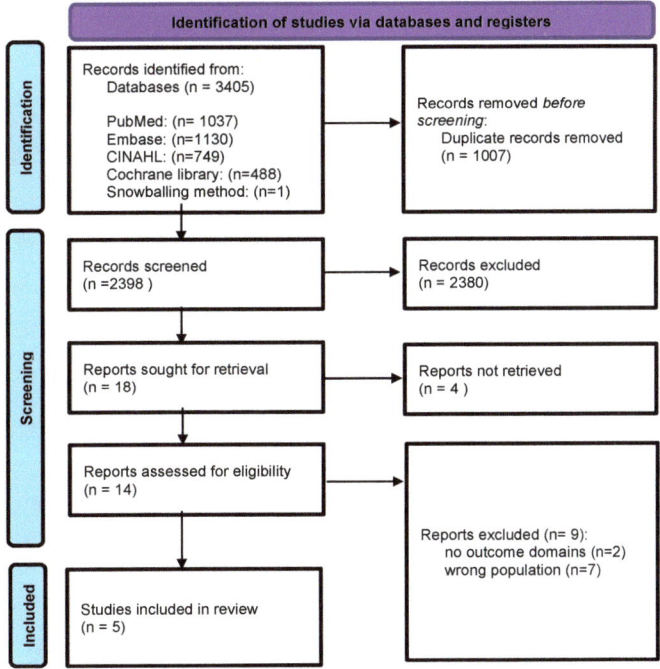

Figure 1. PRISMA flowchart of the study selection and eligibility process.

3.2. Study Characteristics

Included studies were conducted in four different European countries. All studies were qualitative single-center studies conducted in a hospital setting. Sample sizes in the studies ranged from 12 to 20 participants, with 77 participants in total. All the included study populations are classified as PSPS type 2. Specifically, four of the included studies focused on spinal cord stimulation (SCS) in PSPS type 2 patients either treated with SCS or being considered candidates for SCS treatment. Three studies reported to have no conflicts of interest, and one study lacked a report on conflicts of interest. One study was funded by a medical company, while another study was supported by a medical company. An overview of the characteristics is shown in Table 2.

Table 2. Study characteristics of the included studies.

Author (Year)	Objective(s)	Design	Country (Setting)	Study Population	Sample Size	Conflict of Interest & Funding
Abbot et al. (2011) [50]	To describe within the context of the ICF, patients' experiences post-lumber fusion regarding back problems, recovery, and expectations of rehabilitation.	(Semi-structured) interview study	Sweden (Hospital: Orthopedic department)	CLBP patients post lumbar-fusion (PSPS type 2)	20	No conflicts of interest statement. This study was funded by a research grant obtained from the Health Care Sciences Postgraduate School, Karolinska Institute.
Goudman et al. (2020) [51]	Explore if applying goal setting, as a form of patient empowerment, in potential candidates for SCS may further improve the outcome of SCS.	(Semi-structured) interview study	Belgium (Hospital: Neurosurgery department)	SCS candidates with FBSS or FNSS (PSPS type 2)	15	Authors have no conflicts of interest to declare. Study was supported by Medtronic.
Hamm-Faber et al. (2020) [52]	To explore perspectives on personal health and quality of life in FBSS patients concerning their physical, psychological and spiritual well-being prior to receiving an SCS system.	(Semi-structured) interview study	Netherlands (Hospital: Pain medicine department)	SCS candidates with FBSS (PSPS type 2)	17	No competing interests. Study received no external funding.
Ryan et al. (2019) [53]	To explore the experience of SCS for patients with FBSS.	(Semi-structured) interview study	United Kingdom (Hospital: Pain clinic)	SCS patients with FBSS (PSPS type 2)	12	Dr. Cormac G Ryan and Professor Denis J. Martin are named inventors on a patent application for a novel device that delivers sensory discrimination training. The device could be used in the treatment of people with chronic pain. The remaining authors have no conflicts of interest to declare. Funded by Medtronic.
Witkam et al. (2021) [54]	To qualitatively and quantitatively map the FBSS patients' experiences with SCS and the effects of SCS on low back pain caused by FBSS.	Qualitatively driven mixed method analysis	Netherlands (Hospital: Anaesthesiology department)	SCS patients with FBSS (PSPS type 2)	13	The authors reported no conflict of interest. No financial support.

CLBP: chronic low back pain

3.3. Patient-Relevant Outcome Domains

Based on the data chart, fourteen patient-relevant outcome domains were identified. The outcome domains pain and mobility were identified in all the included studies, whereas pain medication, daily activities, work, social participation, leisure activities, and mood were identified in four studies. In three studies, the outcome domains coping strategy, sleep, and energy were reported. The outcome domains of acceptance, perspective of life, and self-reliance were noted twice in the included studies. An overview of the characteristics is shown in Table 3. Thirteen outcome domains were identified in only a single study and therefore not included. A qualitative overview of the identified outcome domains can be seen in Supplementary Materials Section S2.

Table 3. Included outcome domains.

		Abbot et al. (2011) [50]	Goudman et al. (2020) [51]	Hamm-Faber et al. (2020) [52]	Ryan et al. (2019) [53]	Witkam (2021) [54]
1.	Pain	X	X	X	X	X
2.	Mobility	X	X	X	X	X
3.	Work	X	X	X		X
4.	Social participation	X	X	X		X
5.	Mood	X	X		X	X
6.	Pain medication use	X		X	X	X
7.	Daily activities	X		X	X	X
8.	Leisure activities/hobbies	X	X	X		X
9.	Coping strategy	X		X		X
10.	Energy	X		X		X
11.	Sleep			X	X	X
12.	Acceptance			X		X
13.	Perspective of life			X		X
14.	Self-reliance			X		X

X indicates that the outcome domain is described in the specific study.

3.4. Expert Panel Consultation

3.4.1. First Consensus Round

After the first round, the following domains reached consensus for inclusion: pain, sleep, daily activities, perspective of life, social participation, mood, and self-reliance. The domains coping strategy, work, and acceptance were excluded from the framework. While discussing the results of the first round, the participating experts noted that coping strategy and acceptance were relevant domains for patients, but only at a later stage in their care journey. In addition, work was considered less relevant due to the relatively large proportion of PSPS patients who are retired or about to retire or are on long-term disability. A complete overview of the results from the first round is shown in Table 4.

Table 4. GRADE results from the first round of expert panels.

Outcome Domain	Score 7–9 (n Panelists)	Score 4–6 (n Panelists)	Score 1–3 (n Panelists)	Median (IQR) *	Consensus #
Pain	26	0	1	8 (8–9)	≥75%
Coping Strategy	8	18	1	6 (5–7)	<50%
Pain Medication Use	19	8	0	7 (6–8)	50–75%
Sleep	21	6	0	8 (7–8)	≥75%
Daily Activities	22	5	0	8 (7–8)	≥75%
Mobility	20	7	0	7 (6.5–8)	50–75%
Work	11	16	0	6 (5–7)	<50%
Acceptance	10	13	4	6 (4.5–7)	<50%
Perspective of life	23	4	0	7 (7–8)	≥75%
Social participation	24	3	0	7 (7–8)	≥75%
Mood	21	6	0	7 (7–8)	≥75%
Self-Reliance	21	6	0	7 (6–8)	≥75%
Leisure Activities	19	8	0	7 (7–8)	50–75%
Energy	16	10	1	7 (6–8)	50–75%

* IQR interquartile range; #: <50% = excluded, 50–75% = subject to further discussion, ≥75% = included.

3.4.2. Second Consensus Round

The outcomes suggested by panelists secondary gain and external perception were included in the second round. However, both were subsequently excluded. A complete overview of suggested outcomes is shown in Supplementary Materials Section S3. The outcome domain mobility was included based on consensus. An overview of the results from the second round is shown in Table 5.

Table 5. GRADE results from the second round of expert panels.

Outcome Domain	Score 7–9 (n Panelists)	Score 4–6 (n Panelists)	Score 1–3 (n Panelists)	Median (IQR) *	Consensus [#]
Pain Medication Use	6	5	0	7 (6–7.5)	50–75%
Mobility	10	1	0	7 (7–8)	≥75%
Leisure Activities	8	3	0	7 (6.5–7.5)	50–75%
Energy	7	4	0	7 (6–7)	50–75%
External Perception	4	6	1	6 (5–7)	<50%
Secondary gain	1	5	5	4 (2.5–5)	<50%

* IQR interquartile range; [#]: <50% = excluded, 50–75% = subject to further discussion, ≥75% = included.

The remaining outcome domains (pain medication use, leisure activities and energy) were included in the final framework after a discussion among the research team, alongside the previously included domains from the first round. A complete overview of the results of the second round is shown in Table 5. The final framework, the PSPS type 2 outcomes framework, was determined by linking the included outcome domains to items of the ICF model (Figure 2).

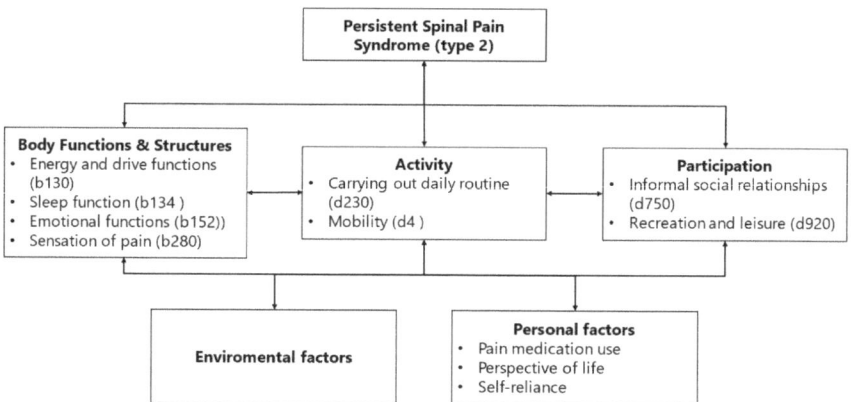

Figure 2. The PSPS type 2 outcomes framework of patient-relevant outcome domains for PSPS type 2 with ICF classifications.

4. Discussion

With this scoping review, we aimed to identify relevant outcome domains for PSPS from the patient perspective (patient-relevant outcome domains). Five studies (77 patients) were included in this scoping review. Out of these studies, 14 patient-relevant outcome domains were identified. In two expert panel rounds, consisting of 27 experts, the outcome domains were rated on their importance until consensus was reached. The following 11 outcome domains reached consensus and were included in the PSPS type 2 outcomes framework and based on the ICF classification: pain, daily activities, perspective of life, social participation, sleep, mobility, mood, pain medication, leisure activities, energy, and self-reliance (Figure 2).

4.1. Comparison with Other Studies

The identified outcome domains in the PSPS type 2 outcomes framework comprise an expansive set, illustrative of a holistic perspective on PSPS. Several outcome sets for chronic (low back) pain exist. For example, the International Consortium for Health Outcomes Measurement (ICHOM) has developed a set of Patient-Centered Outcome Measures for Low Back Pain [22]. Additionally, the Initiative on Methods, Measurement, and Pain Assessment in Clinical Trials (IMMPACT) recommends a core set of outcome measures in chronic pain trails [14]. Comparing the ICHOM-LBP set with our framework, a notable difference is the more generalized nature of the domains (such as health-related quality of life and disability). Furthermore, the ICHOM set contains work status, while this outcome domain is excluded from the framework in the expert panels. This might be related to the relatively high percentage of retirees and work-related disability among patients with PSPS, which was mentioned in the expert panels [55].

In contrast to our developed outcomes framework, the IMMPACT core outcome set contains some intervention-related aspects, such as adverse events and treatment satisfaction. In addition to pain intensity, IMMPACT recommends emotional functioning as an outcome domain, which includes both depression and mood in general. Although patients in Goudman et al., (2020) specifically mention avoiding depression, it is not discussed in the other included studies of our scoping review [51]. This may be due to a relative lack of focus on the clinical diagnosis of depression in chronic pain patients, where more attention is paid to the impact of the complaints on their lives, such as mood and perspective of life.

Furthermore, both the recommended outcome sets of ICHOM and IMMPACT are linked to PROMs. Some PROMs, such as the Short-Form Health Survey (SF-36), have a broad and generalized character, in which multiple outcome domains are queried. However, this makes is difficult to monitor specific outcome domains, such as sleep. Moreover, ICHOM and IMMPACT recommend different PROMs for similar outcome domains, apart from the NPRS for pain. In this scoping review, we did not consider measurement instruments, such as PROMs. It is unclear which measurement instruments (e.g., PROMs) are adequate, in terms of measurement properties to coherently capture the identified patient perspectives and values. International consensus is needed on core outcome domains and corresponding outcome measures for chronic low back pain and specifically for PSPS.

4.2. Strengths and Limitations

To our knowledge, this is the first literature review focusing on the PSPS patient perspective on outcome domains. The qualitative nature of the included studies is of great added value by providing insight into the values, beliefs, and experiences of PSPS patients. It resulted in a multidimensional and clinically relevant set of outcome domains. Furthermore, the additional expert panels contributed to the existing data from the review. The experts were able to draw on their extensive experiences with a large group of PSPS patients. By including different types of healthcare disciplines involved in the diagnostic process and care for PSPS patients, we ensured the expertise on the needs of PSPS patients in different phases of their hospital care journey.

Another strength of this study is that the domains in the PSPS type 2 outcomes framework are linked to items of the ICF model. By linking the framework to the ICF, the framework consists of uniform and internationally accepted definitions. The framework is therefore very useful in various clinical settings, as well as future research, e.g., into adequate measuring instruments.

This review also has some limitations. First, a small number of relevant studies from Northern and Western Europe were included. The lack of relevant studies in the literature might be due to the specific inclusion criteria for PSPS patients, as well as the criteria for outcome domains. The relative cultural homogeneity might be of limiting influence, in particular when related to the personal factors in the PSPS type 2 framework. Second, the included studies consisted of relatively small sample sizes. This might be related to the qualitative nature of the included studies. Nonetheless, our goal is to follow up our research with a focus group study to expand and deepen the available data on this topic through an emphasis on prioritization of the relevant outcome domains. Third, the generalizability of the results seems limited due to the absence of type 1 PSPS patients. This could be explained by a recent change in terminology. While the term failed back surgery syndrome (FBSS) can be converted to PSPS type 2, it is unclear which patients can be classified as PSPS type 1. It is questionable whether the views on outcome domains of type 1 PSPS patients differ since the distinction between the two groups is based on a difference in (surgical) history rather than a difference in symptoms [56]. However, the outcome assessment of type 1 and type 2 PSPS patients will likely differ as a result of different treatment options, such as SCS.

Finally, the majority of included studies was skewed towards either PSPS patients treated with SCS or SCS candidates. In general, SCS has been the most frequently studied treatment method for type 2 PSPS patients [8,13]. However, PSPS patients treated with SCS might not be reflective of the general PSPS population. More research is needed on relevant outcome domains for PSPS patients who benefit from non-invasive and minimally invasive treatments.

4.3. Implications

The PSPS type 2 outcomes framework (Figure 2) shows a detailed and multidimensional set of relevant outcome domains for PSPS patients. It should be taken into account that the excluded domains acceptance, work, and coping strategy may also be relevant for subgroups within the PSPS population. This partly depends on the phase of the care process in which the patient is. When evaluating care, it is important that there is also room for the personal needs and goals of the patients [57].

A possible way to evaluate the multidimensional and personal picture in a clinical setting is through the Positive Health Model [21]. Although this model is used as a conversation tool for exploring patient-relevant outcome domains, one can use it to combine the complexity associated with chronic pain with setting patient-centered goals. This can also support the process of shared decision making. It should also be considered that patients themselves usually do not know in advance what to expect regarding the effect of a treatment. Therefore, it is necessary to systematically compare PROMs and patient-reported experience measures (PREMs). The expectations of the care provider about the possible effect of a treatment should also be mentioned and explored.

In summary, we recommend using the PSPS type 2 outcomes framework with patient-relevant outcome domains (Figure 2) to improve the evaluation of care for PSPS patients by evaluating healthcare multidimensionally and placing a relatively smaller focus on pain. This also applies to insurance companies and healthcare institutions that want to have high impact clinical evaluation tools to observe real, stable, and relevant long-term clinical outcomes. The framework is complementary to initiatives such as the holistic treatment response for SCS [58]. These evaluation techniques would be further substantiated with clinical outcome domains prioritized by PSPS patients.

5. Conclusions

With our scoping review and expert panels, we have identified the following 11 patient-relevant outcome domains for PSPS type 2: (1) pain, (2) sleep, (3) daily activities, (4) mobility, (5) energy, (6) mood, (7) perspective of life, (8) social participation, (9) self-reliance, (10) leisure activities, and (11) pain medication use. The outcome domains comprise an expansive set illustrative of a more holistic approach to PSPS type 2. An absence of the literature regarding the perspective of PSPS type 1 patients limited further analysis. The PSPS type 2 outcomes framework with ICF-linked domains should be used to improve the evaluation of care for PSPS type 2 patients by evaluating healthcare multidimensionally. Further research is needed on the prioritization of the relevant outcome domains for PSPS patients.

Supplementary Materials: The following supporting information can be downloaded at: https://www.mdpi.com/article/10.3390/jcm13071975/s1, Section S1: Search string (PubMed); Section S2: Qualitative overview of outcome domains from included studies.; Section S3: Expert panel suggestions and discussion (translated from Dutch).

Author Contributions: Conceptualization, F.B., J.T.W., M.L.v.H., K.C.P.V. and R.W.J.G.O.; methodology, F.B., J.T.W., M.L.v.H., K.C.P.V. and R.W.J.G.O.; validation, F.B., J.T.W., M.L.v.H. and K.C.P.V.; formal analysis, F.B. and B.-K.W.P.v.R.; investigation, F.B.; data curation, F.B. and B.-K.W.P.v.R.; writing—original draft preparation, F.B., J.T.W., M.L.v.H. and K.C.P.V.; writing—review and editing, F.B., J.T.W., M.L.v.H., K.C.P.V., B.-K.W.P.v.R. and R.W.J.G.O.; supervision, J.T.W., M.L.v.H. and K.C.P.V.; project administration, F.B. All authors have read and agreed to the published version of the manuscript.

Funding: This research received no external funding.

Institutional Review Board Statement: Not applicable.

Informed Consent Statement: Not applicable.

Data Availability Statement: The raw data supporting the conclusions of this article will be made available by the authors on request.

Acknowledgments: The authors would like to thank all participants for their time and contribution to this study.

Conflicts of Interest: The authors declare no conflicts of interest.

References

1. Merskey, H.E. Classification of chronic pain: Descriptions of chronic pain syndromes and definitions of pain terms. *Pain* **1986**, (Suppl. S3), 226.
2. Follett, K.A.; Dirks, B.A. Etiology and evaluation of the failed back surgery syndrome. *Neurosurg. Q.* **1993**, *3*, 40.
3. Leveque, J.C.; Villavicencio, A.T.; Bulsara, K.R.; Rubin, L.; Gorecki, J.P. Spinal cord stimulation for failed back surgery syndrome. *Neuromodulation* **2001**, *4*, 1–9. [CrossRef]
4. Christelis, N.; Simpson, B.; Russo, M.; Stanton-Hicks, M.; Barolat, G.; Thomson, S.; Schug, S.; Baron, R.; Buchser, E.; Carr, D.B.; et al. Persistent Spinal Pain Syndrome: A Proposal for Failed Back Surgery Syndrome and ICD-11. *Pain Med.* **2021**, *22*, 807–818. [CrossRef] [PubMed]
5. Yorimitsu, E.; Chiba, K.; Toyama, Y.; Hirabayashi, K. Long-term outcomes of standard discectomy for lumbar disc herniation: A follow-up study of more than 10 years. *Spine* **2001**, *26*, 652–657. [CrossRef] [PubMed]
6. Kumar, K.; North, R.; Taylor, R.; Sculpher, M.; Van den Abeele, C.; Gehring, M.; Jacques, L.; Eldabe, S.; Meglio, M.; Molet, J.; et al. Spinal Cord Stimulation vs. Conventional Medical Management: A Prospective, Randomized, Controlled, Multicenter Study of Patients with Failed Back Surgery Syndrome (PROCESS Study). *Neuromodulation* **2005**, *8*, 213–218. [CrossRef] [PubMed]
7. Manca, A.; Eldabe, S.; Buchser, E.; Kumar, K.; Taylor, R.S. Relationship between health-related quality of life, pain, and functional disability in neuropathic pain patients with failed back surgery syndrome. *Value Health* **2010**, *13*, 95–102. [CrossRef] [PubMed]
8. Amirdelfan, K.; Webster, L.; Poree, L.; Sukul, V.; McRoberts, P. Treatment Options for Failed back Surgery Syndrome Patients with Refractory Chronic Pain: An Evidence Based Approach. *Spine* **2017**, *42* (Suppl. S14), S41–S52. [CrossRef] [PubMed]
9. Chan, C.W.; Peng, P. Failed back surgery syndrome. *Pain Med.* **2011**, *12*, 577–606. [CrossRef]
10. Sebaaly, A.; Lahoud, M.J.; Rizkallah, M.; Kreichati, G.; Kharrat, K. Etiology, evaluation, and treatment of failed back surgery syndrome. *Asian Spine J.* **2018**, *12*, 574. [CrossRef]
11. Boers, M.; Kirwan, J.R.; Wells, G.; Beaton, D.; Gossec, L.; d'Agostino, M.A.; Conaghan, P.G.; Bingham, C.O.; Brooks, P.; Landewé, R.; et al. Developing core outcome measurement sets for clinical trials: OMERACT filter 2.0. *J. Clin. Epidemiol.* **2014**, *67*, 745–753. [CrossRef]
12. Williamson, P.R.; Altman, D.G.; Blazeby, J.M.; Clarke, M.; Devane, D.; Gargon, E.; Tugwell, P. Developing core outcome sets for clinical trials: Issues to consider. *Trials* **2012**, *13*, 132. [CrossRef]
13. Cho, J.H.; Lee, J.H.; Song, K.S.; Hong, J.Y.; Joo, Y.S.; Lee, D.H.; Hwang, C.J.; Lee, C.S. Treatment Outcomes for Patients with Failed Back Surgery. *Pain Physician* **2017**, *20*, E29–E43. [CrossRef]
14. Dworkin, R.H.; Turk, D.C.; Farrar, J.T.; Haythornthwaite, J.A.; Jensen, M.P.; Katz, N.P.; Kerns, R.D.; Stucki, G.; Allen, R.R.; Bellamy, N.; et al. Core outcome measures for chronic pain clinical trials: IMMPACT recommendations. *Pain* **2005**, *113*, 9–19. [CrossRef]
15. Rigoard, P.; Gatzinsky, K.; Deneuville, J.P.; Duyvendak, W.; Naiditch, N.; Van Buyten, J.P.; Eldabe, S. Pain Research and Management, 2019. Optimizing the management and outcomes of failed back surgery syndrome: A consensus statement on definition and outlines for patient assessment. *Pain Res. Manag.* **2019**, *2019*, 3126464. [CrossRef]

16. Clancy, C.; Quinn, A.; Wilson, F. The aetiologies of failed back surgery syndrome: A systematic review. *J. Back Musculoskelet. Rehabil.* **2017**, *30*, 395–402. [CrossRef]
17. Williamson, P.R.; Altman, D.G.; Bagley, H.; Barnes, K.L.; Blazeby, J.M.; Brookes, S.T.; Clarke, M.; Gargon, E.; Gorst, S.; Harman, N.; et al. The COMET handbook: Version 1.0. *Trials* **2017**, *18*, 280. [CrossRef]
18. Dansie, E.J.; Turk, D.C. Assessment of patients with chronic pain. *Br. J. Anaesth.* **2013**, *111*, 19–25. [CrossRef]
19. World Health Organization. *International Classification of Functioning, Disability, and Health*; World Health Organization: Geneva, Switzerland, 2001.
20. Treede, R.D.; Rief, W.; Barke, A.; Aziz, Q.; Bennett, M.I.; Benoliel, R.; Cohen, M.; Evers, S.; Finnerup, N.B.; First, M.B.; et al. Chronic pain as a symptom or a disease: The IASP classification of chronic pain for the international classification of diseases (ICD-11). *Pain* **2019**, *160*, 19–27. [CrossRef]
21. Huber, M.; van Vliet, M.; Giezenberg, M.; Winkens, B.; Heerkens, Y.; Dagnelie, P.C.; Knottnerus, J.A. Towards a 'patient-centred' operationalisation of the new dynamic concept of health: A mixed methods study. *BMJ Open* **2016**, *6*, e010091. [CrossRef]
22. Clement, R.C.; Welander, A.; Stowell, C.; Cha, T.D.; Chen, J.L.; Davies, M.; Fairbank, J.C.; Foley, K.T.; Gehrchen, M.; Hagg, O.; et al. A proposed set of metrics for standardized outcome reporting in the management of low back pain. *Acta Orthop.* **2015**, *86*, 523–533. [CrossRef]
23. Chiarotto, A.; Deyo, R.A.; Terwee, C.B.; Boers, M.; Buchbinder, R.; Corbin, T.P.; Costa, L.O.P.; Foster, N.E.; Grotle, M.; Koes, B.W.; et al. Core outcome domains for clinical trials in non-specific low back pain. *Eur. Spine J.* **2015**, *24*, 1127–1142. [CrossRef]
24. Sahin, N.; Karahan, A.Y.; Devrimsel, G.; Gezer, İ.A. Comparison among pain, depression, and quality of life in cases with failed back surgery syndrome and non-specific chronic back pain. *J. Phys. Ther. Sci.* **2017**, *29*, 891–895. [CrossRef]
25. Turk, D.C.; Dworkin, R.H.; Allen, R.R.; Bellamy, N.; Brandenburg, N.; Carr, D.B.; Cleeland, C.; Dionne, R.; Farrar, J.T.; Galer, B.S.; et al. Core outcome domains for chronic pain clinical trials: IMMPACT recommendations. *Pain* **2003**, *106*, 337–345. [CrossRef]
26. Gorst, S.L.; Young, B.; Williamson, P.R.; Wilding, J.P.; Harman, N.L. Incorporating patients' perspectives into the initial stages of core outcome set development: A rapid review of qualitative studies of type 2 diabetes. *BMJ Open Diabetes Res. Care* **2019**, *7*, e000615. [CrossRef]
27. Noonan, V.K.; Lyddiatt, A.; Ware, P.; Jaglal, S.B.; Riopelle, R.J.; Bingham, C.O., III; Figueiredo, S.; Sawatzky, R.; Santana, M.; Bartlett, S.J.; et al. Montreal Accord on Patient-Reported Outcomes (PROs) use series e Paper 3: Patient-reported outcomes can facilitate shared decision-making and guide self-management. *J. Clin. Epidemiol.* **2017**, *89*, 125–135. [CrossRef]
28. Barry, M.J.; Edgman-Levitan, S. Shared decision making—The pinnacle patient-centered care. *N. Engl. J. Med.* **2012**, *366*, 780–781. [CrossRef]
29. Epstein, R.M.; Peters, E. Beyond information: Exploring patients' preferences. *JAMA* **2009**, *302*, 195–197. [CrossRef]
30. Kramer, M.H.H.; Bauer, W.; Dicker, D.; Durusu-Tanriover, M.; Ferreira, F.; Rigby, S.P.; Roux, X.; Schumm-Draeger, P.; Weidanz, F.; van Hulsteijn, J. The changing face of internal medicine: Patient centred care. *Eur. J. Intern. Med.* **2014**, *25*, 125–127. [CrossRef]
31. Mühlbacher, A.C.; Juhnke, C. Patient preferences versus physicians' judgement: Does it make a difference in healthcare decision making? *Appl. Health Econ. Health Policy* **2013**, *11*, 163–180. [CrossRef] [PubMed]
32. Tricco, A.; Lillie, E.; Zarin, W.; O'Brien, K.K.; Colquhoun, H.; Levac, D.; Moher, D.; Peters, M.D.; Horsley, T.; Weeks, L.; et al. PRISMA extension for scoping reviews (PRISMA-ScR): Checklist and explanation. *Ann. Intern. Med.* **2018**, *169*, 467–473. [CrossRef]
33. Ouzzani, M.; Hammady, H.; Fedorowicz, Z.; Elmagarmid, A. Rayyan—A web and mobile app for systematic reviews. *Syst. Rev.* **2016**, *5*, 210. [CrossRef]
34. Braun, V.; Clarke, V. Using thematic analysis in psychology. *Qual. Res. Psychol.* **2006**, *3*, 77–101. [CrossRef]
35. Lacey, A.; Luff, D. *Qualitative Research Analysis*; The NIHR RDS for the East Midlands/Yorkshire and the Humber: Nottingham, UK, 2009; pp. 5–8.
36. Cieza, A.; Geyh, S.; Chatterji, S.; Kostanjsek, N.; Üstün, B.; Stucki, G. ICF linking rules: An update based on lessons learned. *J. Rehabil. Med.* **2005**, *37*, 212–218. [CrossRef]
37. Cieza, A.; Fayed, N.; Bickenbach, J.; Prodinger, B. Refinements of the ICF Linking Rules to strengthen their potential for establishing comparability of health information. *Disabil. Rehabil.* **2019**, *41*, 574–583. [CrossRef]
38. Guyatt, G.H.; Oxman, A.D.; Kunz, R.; Atkins, D.; Brozek, J.; Vist, G.; Alderson, P.; Glasziou, P.; Falck-Ytter, Y.; Schünemann, H.J. GRADE guidelines: 2. Framing the question and deciding on important outcomes. *J. Clin. Epidemiol.* **2011**, *64*, 395–400. [CrossRef]
39. Diamond, I.R.; Grant, R.C.; Feldman, B.M.; Pencharz, P.B.; Ling, S.C.; Moore, A.M.; Wales, P.W. Defining consensus: A systematic review recommends methodologic criteria for reporting of Delphi studies. *J. Clin. Epidemiol.* **2014**, *67*, 401–409. [CrossRef]
40. Munblit, D.; Nicholson, T.; Akrami, A.; Apfelbacher, C.; Chen, J.; De Groote, W.; Diaz, J.V.; Gorst, S.L.; Harman, N.; Kokorina, A.; et al. A core outcome set for post-COVID-19 condition in adults for use in clinical practice and research: An international Delphi consensus study. *Lancet Respir. Med.* **2022**, *10*, 715–724. [CrossRef]
41. Gardner, T.; Refshauge, K.; McAuley, J.; Goodall, S.; Hübscher, M.; Smith, L. Patient led goal setting in chronic low back pain—What goals are important to the patient and are they aligned to what we measure? *Patient Educ. Couns.* **2015**, *98*, 1035–1038. [CrossRef]
42. O'Brien, E.M.; Staud, R.M.; Hassinger, A.D.; McCulloch, R.C.; Craggs, J.G.; Atchison, J.T.W.; Price, D.D.; Robinson, M.E. Patient-centered perspective on treatment outcomes in chronic pain. *Pain Med.* **2010**, *11*, 6–15. [CrossRef]

43. Sanchez, K.; Papelard, A.; Nguyen, C.; Jousse, M.; Rannou, F.; Revel, M.; Poiraudeau, S. Patient-preference disability assessment for disabling chronic low back pain: A cross-sectional survey. *Spine* **2009**, *34*, 1052–1059. [CrossRef] [PubMed]
44. Sanchez, K.; Papelard, A.; Nguyen, C.; Bendeddouche, I.; Jousse, M.; Rannou, F.; Revel, M.; Poiraudeau, S. McMaster-Toronto Arthritis Patient Preference Disability Questionnaire sensitivity to change in low back pain: Influence of shifts in priorities. *PLoS ONE* **2011**, *6*, e20274. [CrossRef]
45. Tinetti, M.E.; Costello, D.M.; Naik, A.D.; Davenport, C.; Hernandez-Bigos, K.; Van Liew, J.R.; Esterson, J.; Kiwak, E.; Dindo, L. Outcome goals and health care preferences of older adults with multiple chronic conditions. *JAMA Netw. Open* **2021**, *4*, e211271. [CrossRef] [PubMed]
46. Moffett, J.K.; Torgerson, D.; Bell-Syer, S.; Jackson, D.; Llewlyn-Phillips, H.; Farrin, A.; Barber, J. Randomised controlled trial of exercise for low back pain: Clinical outcomes, costs, and preferences. *BMJ* **1999**, *319*, 279–283. [CrossRef]
47. Krabbe, P.F.; van Asselt, A.D.; Selivanova, A.; Jabrayilov, R.; Vermeulen, K.M. Patient-centered item selection for a new preference-based generic health status instrument: CS-Base. *Value Health* **2019**, *22*, 467–473. [CrossRef]
48. Tonkin, K.; Gustafsson, L.; Deen, M.; Broadbridge, J. Multiple-Case Study Exploration of an Occupational Perspective in a Persistent Pain Clinic. *Occup. Ther. J. Res.* **2023**, *43*, 303–312. [CrossRef] [PubMed]
49. Karran, E.L.; Fryer, C.E.; Middleton, J.T.W.; Moseley, G.L. Exploring the Social Determinants of Health Outcomes for Adults with Low Back Pain or Spinal Cord Injury and Persistent Pain: A Mixed Methods Study. *J. Pain* **2022**, *23*, 1461–1479. [CrossRef]
50. Abbott, A.D.; Hedlund, R.; Tyni-lennÉ, R. Patients' experience post-lumbar fusion regarding back problems, recovery and expectations in terms of the international classification of functioning, disability and health. *Disabil. Rehabil.* **2011**, *33*, 1399–1408. [CrossRef]
51. Goudman, L.; Bruzzo, A.; van de Sande, J.; Moens, M. Goal Identification Before Spinal Cord Stimulation: A Qualitative Exploration in Potential Candidates. *Pain Pract.* **2020**, *20*, 247–254. [CrossRef]
52. Hamm-Faber, T.E.; Engels, Y.; Vissers, K.C.P.; Henssen, D. Views of patients suffering from Failed Back Surgery Syndrome on their health and their ability to adapt to daily life and self-management: A qualitative exploration. *PLoS ONE* **2020**, *15*, e0243329. [CrossRef]
53. Ryan, C.G.; Eldabe, S.; Chadwick, R.; Jones, S.E.; Elliott-Button, H.L.; Brookes, M.; Martin, D.J. An Exploration of the Experiences and Educational Needs of Patients With Failed Back Surgery Syndrome Receiving Spinal Cord Stimulation. *Neuromodulation* **2019**, *22*, 295–301. [CrossRef]
54. Witkam, R.L.; Kurt, E.; van Dongen, R.; Arnts, I.; Steegers, M.A.H.; Vissers, K.C.P.; Henssen, D.; Engels, Y. Experiences From the Patient Perspective on Spinal Cord Stimulation for Failed Back Surgery Syndrome: A Qualitatively Driven Mixed Method Analysis. *Neuromodulation* **2021**, *24*, 112–125. [CrossRef]
55. Thomson, S.; Jacques, L. Demographic characteristics of patients with severe neuropathic pain secondary to failed back surgery syndrome. *Pain Pract.* **2009**, *9*, 206–215. [CrossRef]
56. Alves Rodrigues, T.; de Oliveira, E.J.S.G.; Morais Costa, B.; Tajra Mualem Araújo, R.L.; Batista Santos Garcia, J. Is There a Difference in Fear-Avoidance, Beliefs, Anxiety and Depression Between Post-Surgery and Non-Surgical Persistent Spinal Pain Syndrome Patients? *J. Pain Res.* **2022**, *15*, 1707–1717. [CrossRef]
57. Santana, M.J.; Manalili, K.; Jolley, R.J.; Zelinsky, S.; Quan, H.; Lu, M. How to practice person-centred care: A conceptual framework. *Health Expect.* **2018**, *21*, 429–440. [CrossRef]
58. Levy, R.M.; Mekhail, N.; Abd-Elsayed, A.; Abejón, D.; Anitescu, M.; Deer, T.R.; Eldabe, S.; Goudman, L.; Kallewaard, J.T.W.; Moens, M.; et al. Holistic Treatment Response: An International Expert Panel Definition and Criteria for a New Paradigm in the Assessment of Clinical Outcomes of Spinal Cord Stimulation. *Neuromodulation Technol. Neural Interface* **2023**, *26*, 1015–1022. [CrossRef]

Disclaimer/Publisher's Note: The statements, opinions and data contained in all publications are solely those of the individual author(s) and contributor(s) and not of MDPI and/or the editor(s). MDPI and/or the editor(s) disclaim responsibility for any injury to people or property resulting from any ideas, methods, instructions or products referred to in the content.

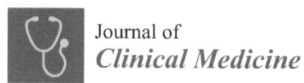 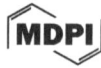

Article

YAP Ultralate Laser-Evoked Responses in Fibromyalgia: A Pilot Study in Patients with Small Fiber Pathology

Elena Ammendola [1,†], Silvia Giovanna Quitadamo [1,†], Emmanuella Ladisa [1], Giusy Tancredi [1], Adelchi Silvestri [1], Raffaella Lombardi [2], Giuseppe Lauria [2,3] and Marina de Tommaso [1,*]

[1] Neurophysiopathology Unit, DiBrain Department, Aldo Moro University, 70124 Bari, Italy; elena.ammendola@uniba.it (E.A.); sg.quitadamo@gmail.com (S.G.Q.); emmanuellemmanuellaladisa@gmail.com (E.L.); tancredi.giusy96@gmail.com (G.T.); silvestriadelchi93@gmail.com (A.S.)
[2] Neuroalgology Unit, Fondazione IRCCS Istituto Neurologico Carlo Besta, 20133 Milan, Italy; raffaella.lombardi@istituto-besta.it (R.L.); giuseppe.lauriapinter@istituto-besta.it (G.L.)
[3] Department of Medical Biotechnology and Translational Medicine, University of Milan, 20133 Milan, Italy
* Correspondence: marina.detommaso@uniba.it; Tel.: +39-334-651-2196 or +39-080-559-6739-6859 or +39-080-547-8565
† These authors contributed equally to this work.

Abstract: Background: The investigation of C-fiber-evoked ultralow-level responses (ULEPs) at somatic sites is difficult in clinical practice but may be useful in patients with small fiber neuropathy. **Aim**: The aim of the study was to investigate changes in LEPs and ULEPs in patients with fibromyalgia affected or not by abnormal intraepidermal innervation. **Methods**: We recorded LEPs and ULEPs of the hand, thigh and foot in 13 FM patients with a normal skin biopsy (NFM), 13 patients with a reduced intraepidermal nerve fiber density (IENFD) (AFM) and 13 age-matched controls. We used a YAP laser, changing the energy and spot size at the pain threshold for LEPs and at the heat threshold for ULEPs. **Results**: ULEPs occurred at a small number of sites in both the NFM and AFM groups compared to control subjects. The absence of ULEPs during foot stimulation was characteristic of AFM patients. The amplitude of LEPs and ULEPs was reduced in patients with AFM at the three stimulation sites, and a slight reduction was also observed in the NFM group. **Conclusions**: The present preliminary results confirmed the reliability of LEPs in detecting small fiber impairments. The complete absence of ULEPs in the upper and lower limbs, including the distal areas, could confirm the results of LEPs in patients with small fiber impairments. Further prospective studies in larger case series could confirm the present findings on the sensitivity of LEP amplitude and ULEP imaging in detecting small fiber impairments and the development of IENFD in FM patients.

Keywords: fibromyalgia; laser-evoked potentials; skin biopsy; small fiber neuropathy

Citation: Ammendola, E.; Quitadamo, S.G.; Ladisa, E.; Tancredi, G.; Silvestri, A.; Lombardi, R.; Lauria, G.; de Tommaso, M. YAP Ultralate Laser-Evoked Responses in Fibromyalgia: A Pilot Study in Patients with Small Fiber Pathology. *J. Clin. Med.* 2024, 13, 3078. https://doi.org/10.3390/jcm13113078

Received: 27 March 2024
Revised: 16 May 2024
Accepted: 19 May 2024
Published: 24 May 2024

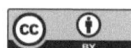

Copyright: © 2024 by the authors. Licensee MDPI, Basel, Switzerland. This article is an open access article distributed under the terms and conditions of the Creative Commons Attribution (CC BY) license (https:// creativecommons.org/licenses/by/ 4.0/).

1. Introduction

An examination of the nociceptive pathways is of crucial importance in patients with chronic pain. Laser-evoked potentials (LEPs) are a reliable tool to analyze the involvement of Aδ fibers in neuropathic pain and small fiber pathology [1], using a skin biopsy to confirm the reduction in the intraepidermal nerve fiber density (IENFD) [2]. However, the neurophysiological assessment of C-fibers is quite difficult, as the slow conduction velocity and low amplitude of evoked responses may reduce the reliability of ULEPs outside the facial area [3]. Moreover, the coactivation of Aδ fibers masks the slower C-related response, as the general principle of cortical functioning is "first come, first served". However, the use of stimulation methods capable of selectively activating C receptors could allow the detection of a late cortical response that is generally distinct from the Aδ potential [4]. In a recent article, we used a YAP laser with a thermal, non-painful intensity and a large spot, and observed an ultralate cortical response on the hand and leg in the majority of healthy volunteers [4]. Solid-state laser radiation has deeper penetration within the dermis, reducing superficial burns, with an advantage for clinical use [5].

The impairment of the small afferent fibers is often associated with fibromyalgia (FM) [6]. Recently, experienced neurologists in the field of pain have proposed the diagnostic evaluation of small fiber involvement in FM [1]. To determine the presence of small fiber impairment, it is recommended to use at least two of the following methods: heart rate variability, sympathetic skin response, Aδ-related evoked responses (LEPs), corneal confocal microscopy and skin biopsy [1].

The results of the skin biopsy are primarily based on the involvement of C-fibers. The use of laser-evoked potentials was recommended in patients with small fiber impairment [5], while the same authors stated that a single method does not completely describe the status of small afferents, so a more specific assessment of C fibers together with A delta fibers could be useful in patients with FM.

Neurophysiological studies with microneurography assessed the dysfunction of C fibers in patients with FM, which correlated with the severity of the disease [7,8]. Also, quantitative sensory testing confirmed the abnormal C-related thermal and painful sensibilities [6]. Based on previous observations, we considered conducting a pilot study to assess the function of Aδ and C fibers with the Nd:YAP laser in subgroups of fibromyalgia patients with varying degrees of cutaneous innervation in skin biopsy compared to a group of healthy subjects. The aim was to find a reliable neurophysiological signature of small fiber impairment in fibromyalgia patients.

2. Materials and Methods

2.1. Subjects

Twenty-six participants among those who had received a diagnosis of FM according to the 2016 criteria [9] agreed to undergo standard LEP and skin biopsy examination with recording of ULEPs. Two subgroups of patients were considered: fibromyalgia patients a with normal skin biopsy (FMN) and fibromyalgia patients with an altered biopsy (FMA). In addition, 13 age-matched healthy volunteers (4 men and 13 women) were included as a control group.

The study was conducted according to the rules of the Declaration of Helsinki of 1975 (https://www.wma.net/what-we-do/medical-ethics/declaration-of-helsinki/), revised in 2013. The study on skin biopsies and laser-evoked potentials was originally approved by the ethics committee of the General Hospital of Bari Policlinico in 2012. The continuation of the study was approved on December 2022. All study participants gave their informed consent, specifically reporting the possible occurrence of transitory superficial skin lesions.

2.2. Skin Biopsy

The laboratory procedure we used is described in the work of Devigili et al. [2] and in our earlier studies [10,11] (Appendix A).

The fibromyalgia patients were divided into two groups based on the results of the skin biopsy performed at two sites on the proximal and distal thigh: normal pattern (N = normal) and neuropathic pattern (A = abnormal). The groups proved to be homogeneous; each group consisted of 13 people. In the AFM group, 12 patients had non-length-dependent neuropathy and 1 patient had length-dependent neuropathy.

2.3. Laser Stimulation

For this study, we used the STIMUL 1340 system from Electronic Engineering® (El.En. S.p.A., Florence, Italy). It was equipped with two laser sources: a neodymium:yttrium aluminum perovskite laser (Nd:YAP), which emits an infrared beam, and a coaxial diode laser source, which emits a visible red beam. The stimulation procedure was similar to a previous study performed in our laboratory [4]. In this case, only the right side was stimulated to increase compliance for this type of procedure, which is known for its relatively long duration (approximately 100 min in total) and discomfort.

The parameters were set to activate the small myelinated afferents (Aδ) or the non-myelinated afferents (C).

The details of the stimulation method are described in Appendix B.

2.4. Recording

The recording methods were already described [4]. In brief, the EEG was recorded with 62 Ag–AgCl electrodes placed on the scalp with a prewired cap, according to the international 10–20 system. One electrode on the bridge of the nose served as a reference. The ground electrode was placed on the right forearm. Two electrodes placed on the upper left and lower right side of both eyes monitored eye movements and blinking. The impedance was kept below 5 kΩ.

2.5. LEP Analysis

To process the LEP data, we used the MATLAB platform and the toolboxes EEGLAB 14_1_1 and LetsWave version 7. First, we performed epoch splitting and baseline correction in the time domain (-0.1–2 s). An automatic exclusion method was set for eye movements based on EOG channels and for signals exceeding 100 μV. We applied the filters with a bandpass at 1 Hz–30 Hz; a notch filter removed the power line noise artifacts at 50 Hz (low: 48, high: 52). We visually inspected and removed bad channels and then interpolated with the neighboring electrodes. At this point, we evaluated the average of at least 21 artifact-free trials for individual responses at each stimulation site.

The latencies of LEPs N2–P2 and the ULEPs positivity wave were measured considering the maximum peak on the Cz channel.

We visually identified the main peaks in the C-related potentials. Not all patients showed C-related potentials. In cases in which an average positive response occurred at the vertex that clearly stood out from the signal noise, we determined the maximum positivity (ULEP P) considering the interval 700–2000 msec. In the present study, we did not consider those potentials that could be caused by the coactivation of Aδ fibers [4]. Therefore, the latencies of the ULEP P were measured at the maximum peak in the given interval for each subject on the Cz channel.

The amplitudes of LEPs N2–P2 and the ULEP positivity wave were evaluated on the 62 channels, considering the maximum peaks at the given intervals.

2.6. Clinical Evaluation

We tested the patients with the following scales: visual analogue scale (VAS) [12], Zung SDS and SAS [13,14], fibromyalgia-induced disability questionnaire (FIQ) [15], multidimensional assessment of fatigue (MAF) [16] and brief pain inventory (BPI) with subscales for pain severity and interference [17].

Statistical Procedure

The latencies of the Aδ-related N2–P2 complex and C-related ultralate positivity, as well as pain and heat thresholds were compared between the 3 groups using one-sided ANOVA with a post hoc Bonferroni test.

In addition, a chi-square test for independence between groups was performed to test for the presence of LEPs and ULEPs at the different stimulation sites.

The amplitude of the C-related ultralate potential and the Aδ-related components of N2 and P2 were compared between groups using the statistical package in the LetsWave vers. 7 tool. For the comparison between the controls and the AFM and FMN groups, the unpaired *t*-test with cluster-based permutation was applied at a threshold of 0.05 and 2000 permutations.

3. Results

We analyzed LEPs and ULEPs from 26 FM patients, 13 with a normal IENFD (NFM) (2 males aged 46.54 + 16.4), 13 with an abnormal skin biopsy (AFM) (2 males aged 54.62 + 9.87) and 13 age-matched controls (4 males; age 46.54 + 9.6. ANOVA F 2.47 p 0.16). In all cases, local skin burning resolved within 15 days.

We noted the pain and heat thresholds and the presence of vertex reactions of a-delta modality of the stimulation. The pain threshold for the stimulation of the Aδ fibers was similar in both groups. Perceived pain was increased in both FM groups compared to controls when the knee was stimulated (Table 1; Supplementary Table S1).

Table 1. Mean, SD and SEM of pain threshold (T) expressed in Joule (J) and pain sensation with 0–10 VAS for the sites of stimulation in Aδ fiber modality. NFM: fibromyalgia patients with normal skin biopsy. AFM: fibromyalgia patients with abnormal skin biopsy. C: controls.

Site of Stimulation	Type of Subjects	N	Mean	SD	SE	ANOVA
HAND T (J)	NFM	13	6.31	1.97	0.548	F 1.63 p 0.22
	AFM	13	6.77	3.79	1.051	
	C	13	8.54	3.93	1.090	
HAND VAS	NFM	13	74.38	15.63	4.335	F 1.88 p 0.17
	AFM	13	79.54	14.88	4.126	
	C	13	66.46	18.81	5.218	
KNEE T (J)	NFM	13	3.54	1.98	0.550	F 1.99 p 0.15
	AFM	13	5.31	2.84	0.788	
	C	13	3.54	1.85	0.514	
KNEE VAS	NFM	13	81.00	12.14	3.367	F 4.89 p 0.017 *
	AFM	13	82.54	10.85	3.010	
	C	13	64.38	18.25	5.062	
FOOT T (J)	NFM	13	6.85	2.76	0.767	F 0.277 p 0.76
	AFM	13	7.77	4.00	1.110	
	C	13	7.54	3.84	1.066	
FOOT VAS	NFM	13	76.62	13.29	3.686	F 0.777 p 0.47
	AFM	13	78.69	11.10	3.079	
	C	13	73.46	10.20	2.830	

* Post hoc Bonferroni test NFM vs. C p 0.013; AFM vs. C p 0.006.

All healthy subjects showed responses after the stimulation of the Aδ-fibers at the three stimulated sites; one patient with a normal skin biopsy had no LEPs at two stimulation sites (7.6%), 4 FM patients with abnormal skin biopsies had no LEPs at least at one site (two at two sites and two at all sites, 30.7%); (Chi-square test 9.27 p 0.15); (Supplementary Table S1, Figure 1a).

In FM patients, the absence of LEPs was consistent with the absence of ULEPs in the same stimulation region.

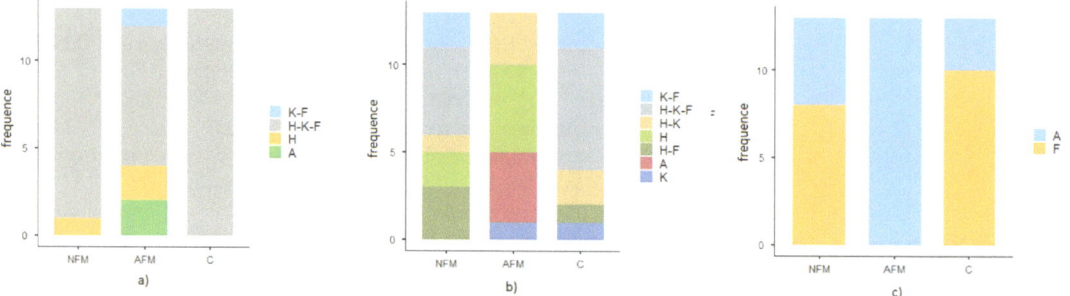

Figure 1. Presence of laser-evoked responses (LEPs) of a-delta fibers and laser-evoked responses (ULEPs) of C-fibers in 13 healthy controls (C), 13 fibromyalgia patients with normal skin biopsy (NFM) and 13 fibromyalgia patients with abnormal skin biopsy (AFM) for stimulation of the hand (H), knee (K) and foot (F). In (**a**), we showed the absence of any detectable waves and in (**b**) the presence of ULEPs. In (**c**), we showed the presence of ULEPs for foot stimulation. No patient with AFM had ULEPs during foot stimulation.

3.1. C-Modality of Stimulation

In the C modality of stimulation, the heat threshold was similar between the knee and foot stimulation groups, while the NFM group had a lower heat threshold. However, the Bonferroni test was not significant (Table 2; Supplementary Table S2).

Table 2. Warm threshold (T) expressed in Joule (J) for the three sites of stimulation in the C-fiber modality.

Site of Stimulation	Type of Subjects	N	Mean	SD	SE	ANOVA
HAND T (J)	NFM	13	6.62	3.43	0.951	F 3.63 p 0.046 *
	AFM	13	8.08	3.35	0.930	
	C	13	5.92	6.10	1.693	
KNEE T (J)	NFM	13	5.77	3.79	1.051	F 3.25 p 0.058
	AFM	13	9.62	4.25	1.180	
	C	13	6.00	5.64	1.565	
FOOT T (J)	NFM	13	11.00	2.35	0.650	F p 0.89 p 0.42
	AFM	13	12.46	3.23	0.896	
	C	13	12.00	5.07	1.405	

* Bonferroni test not significant. NFM—FM patients with normal skin biopsy AFM—patients with reduced intraepidermal nerve fiber density; C—controls.

In almost all cases, the late positivity was preceded by an early negative–positive complex. This was probably generated by the coactivation of Aδ fibers, as we had previously observed in healthy controls (see Ammendola et al., 2023) [4]. In the present study, we considered the late response attributable to C-fiber activation. In patients with a normal skin biopsy, the presence of ULEPs was 84.6% in the hand, 61.5% in the knee and 76.9% in the foot. Only five patients had ULEPs in the three stimulated sites; six patients had the ultralate potential in two sites: one in the hand and knee, two in the knee and foot and three in the hand and foot; two patients had ULEPs in the hand only (Supplementary Table S2, Figure 1b).

In the patients with an abnormal skin biopsy, the presence of ULEPs was 61.5% on the hand and 30.7% on the knee. Three patients had ULEPs on the hand and knee together, five on the hand only and one on the knee only; four had reactions at none of the stimulation sites (Figure 1b). The presence of ULEPs was different in the three groups (chi-square 27.4

p 0.007; Figure 1b). None of the thirteen patients with an abnormal skin biopsy had ULEPs at the foot level (chi-square 17.3 $p < 0.0001$; Figure 1c).

For the amplitude of the parietal waves, at the hand level, we found a slight reduction in the Aδ-related N2 amplitude in FMN patients compared to controls, which was restricted to the central regions, whereas AFM patients showed a reduced N2 and P2 amplitude over fronto-central and parietal electrodes.

The amplitude of the ULEPs was also reduced in the FMN patients, in a region restricted to the vertex and in the parietal and frontal regions of the AFM group (Figure 2).

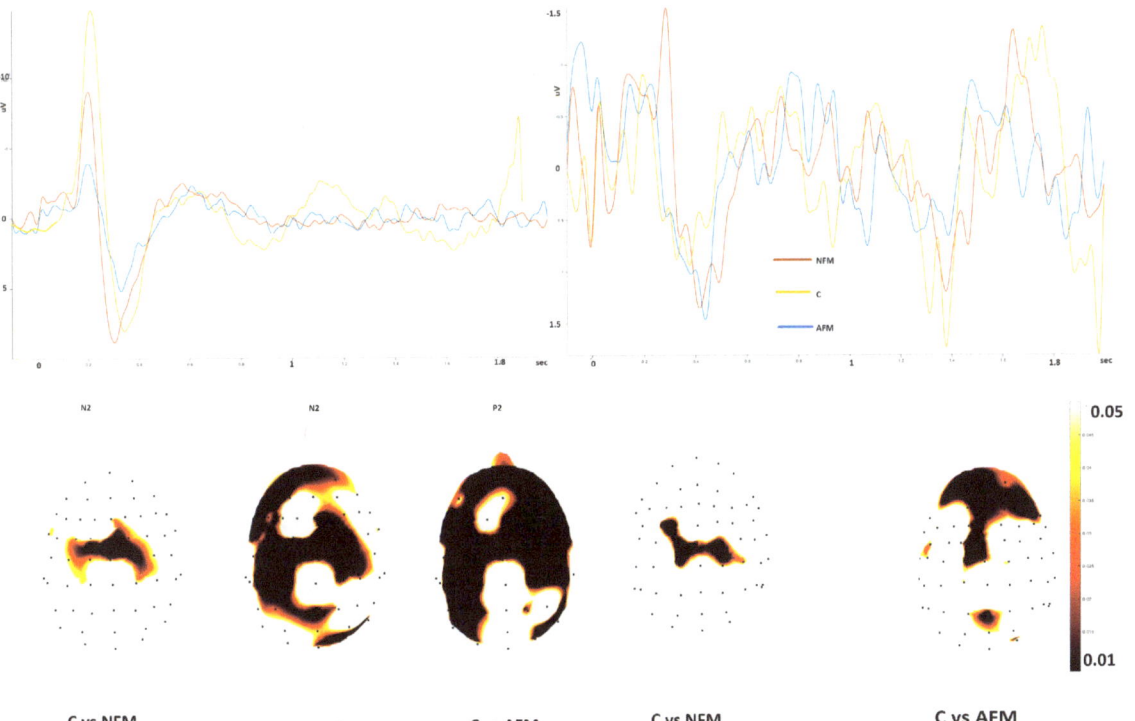

Figure 2. Left side: grand average of the N2–P2 complex from the hand in fibromyalgia with normal skin biopsy (NFM), abnormal skin biopsy (AFM) and controls (C). The lower part of the figure shows the statistical probability maps expressing the t-test. Right side: grand average of the ultralate responses obtained by hand in the three groups. The statistical probability maps express the results of the t-test applied to the ultralate positivity (t-test with cluster-based permutation was applied at a threshold of 0.05 and 2000 permutations).

The knee stimulation in the Aδ modality elicited an N2 wave with a reduced amplitude in the centro-parietal regions in FMN patients and a diffuse reduction in N2 and P2 waves in AFM patients compared to controls (Figure 3).

ULEPs appeared reduced in the AMF group compared to controls over the centro-frontal leads (Figure 3), whereas there was no significant difference in amplitude in the FMN group.

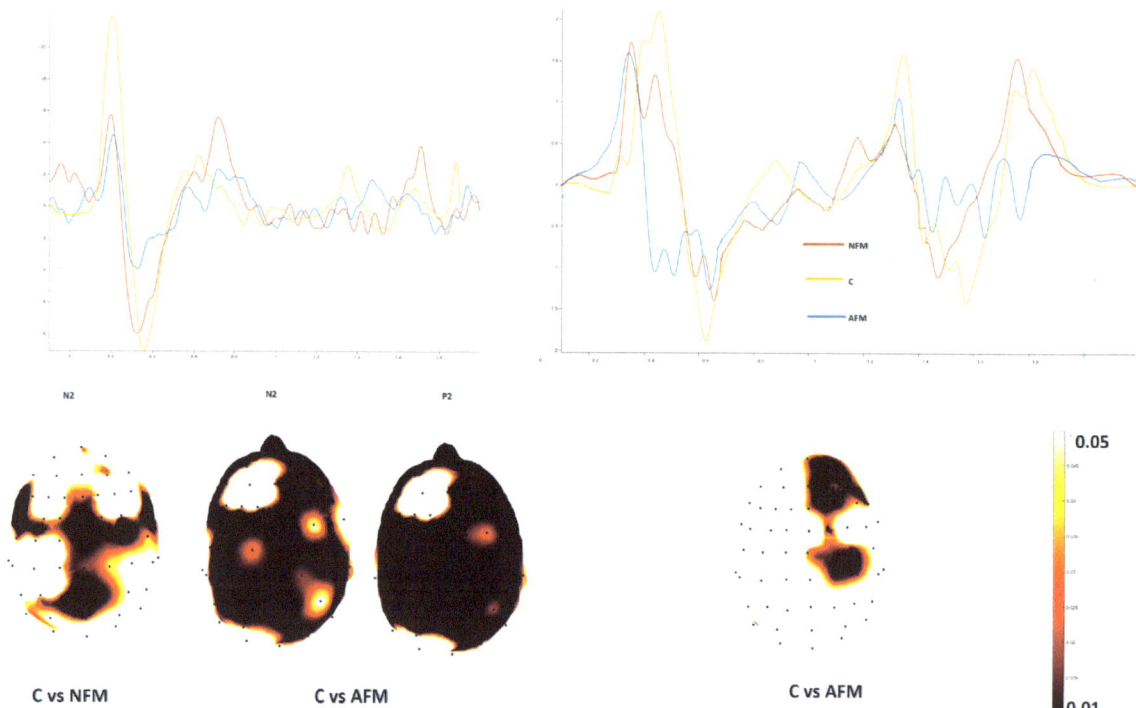

Figure 3. Left side: grand average of the N2–P2 complex from the thigh in fibromyalgia with normal skin biopsy (NFM), abnormal skin biopsy (AFM) and controls (C). Statistical probability maps expressing the *t*-test for the N2 and P2 components are shown in the lower part of the figure. Right side: grand average of the ultralate responses obtained by hand in the three groups. The statistical probability maps express the results of the *t*-test applied to the ultralate positivity (*t*-test with cluster-based permutation was applied at a threshold of 0.05 and 2000 permutations).

The foot stimulation in the Aδ modality resulted in a reduced P2 amplitude in the bilateral central leads in the AFM patients (Figure 4).

The ULEPs were absent in the AFM group and reduced in a limited zone within the central and parietal regions in the FMN group (Figure 4).

The latencies of LEPs and ULEPs, if present, were similar in the groups (Supplementary Table S3).

3.2. Correlation with Clinical Characteristics

The MANOVA analysis comparing the main clinical characteristics between the FM groups approached statistical significance (F 2.95 *p* 0.056). Notably, disease history was longer in the AFM group (patients with reduced IENFD had higher WPI scores (AFM 14 + 3.2; NFM 8.2 + 2.3 years F 4.79 *p* 0.01)) (Supplementary Table S3).

We found a positive correlation between the amplitude of knee-evoked ULEPs and the MAF score for fatigue (Pearson—0.71 *p* 0.05; linear regression test R^2 2.14 t 2.81 *p* 0.018). There was no relevant correlation between the IENFD values and the latencies and amplitudes of the LEPs and ULEPs.

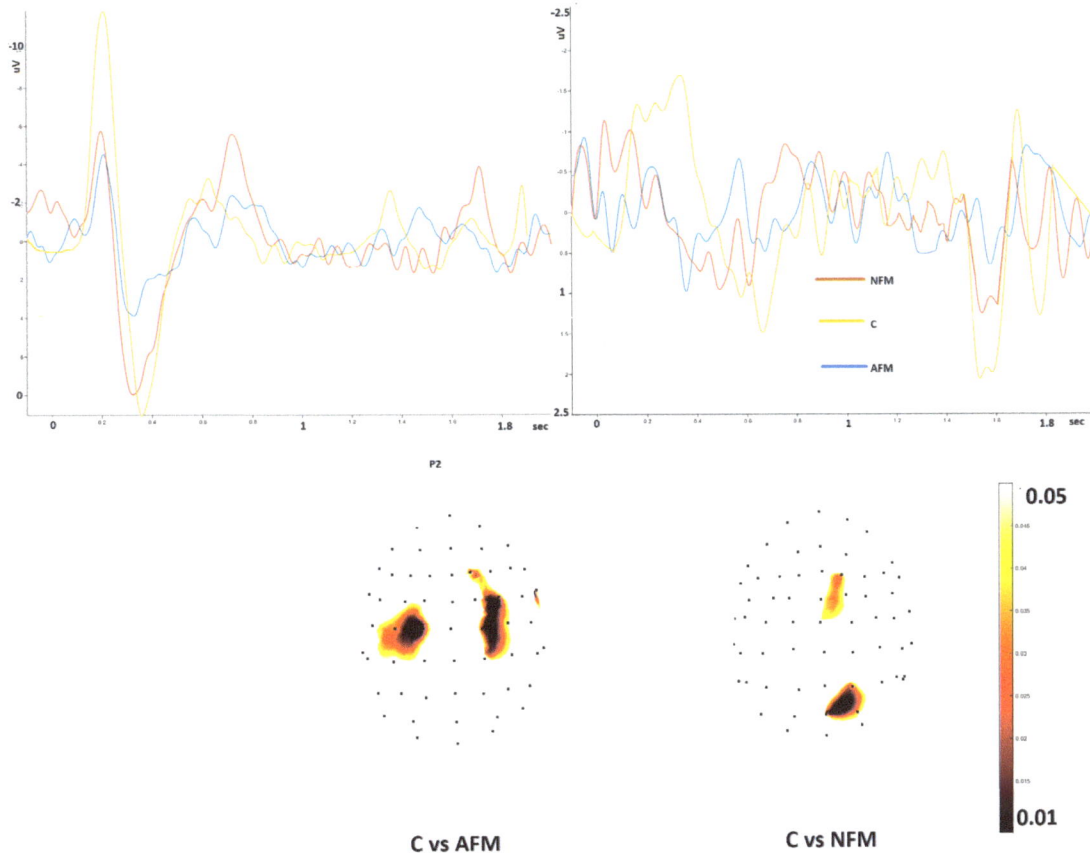

Figure 4. Left side: grand average of the N2–P2 complex from the foot in fibromyalgia with normal skin biopsy (NFM), abnormal skin biopsy (AFM) and controls (C). Statistical probability maps expressing the *t*-test for the P2 component are shown in the lower part of the figure. Right side: grand average of the ultralate responses obtained by hand in the three groups. The statistical probability maps express the results of the *t*-test applied to the ultralate positivity (*t*-test with cluster-based permutation was applied at a threshold of 0.05 and 2000 permutations).

4. Discussion

The present study followed on from a recent observation by our group on ultralate potentials elicited with the YAP laser at low intensity and an enlarged spot in normal controls [4]. In this study, we observed late responses in the trigeminal, upper and lower extremities in a congruent number of healthy subjects. Although they were preceded by an early positive–negative complex, indicating the probable coactivation of a-delta fibers during single sets of stimulation, their latency was consistent with the activation of C-fibers. Now, we wanted to test the same stimulation paradigm in patients with small fiber involvement confirmed through a recent skin biopsy. To this end, we studied patients with a clinical diagnosis of fibromyalgia who were divided into two subgroups, one with a normal and the other with a reduced IENFD in at least one site of the lower extremities, and an age-matched control group. We found that ULEPs were less common in FM patients than in control subjects, and that this was particularly evident in patients with abnormal IENFD values. At the sites where they were detectable, ULEPs were reduced in amplitude in both FM groups, but this tendency predominated in patients with abnormal skin biopsies. The reduction in the amplitude of ULEPs detected when the thigh was stimulated corresponded to a higher degree of fatigue in the entire FM sample. The following sections explained the results in detail.

4.1. Pain and Heat Threshold

Pain threshold was similar in both FM groups compared to controls, but pain perception was increased in both groups compared to controls on the thigh corresponding to the knee trigger point. This finding reproduced what has been described in previous studies [11,18], namely, a normal Aδ-fiber pinprick threshold in FM patients, with an enhancement in pain perception at critical points.

The heat threshold appeared to be slightly increased in FM patients with small fiber involvement, particularly at the hand and knee. However, this did not reach statistical significance, as the number of subjects was small and the subjective sensation of FM patients rarely corresponded to a neuropathic profile, a phenomenon that has been described in previous studies [18].

4.2. Presence of LEPs and ULEPs in FM Patients

While most FM patients, regardless of IENFD, had measurable LEPs on the hand and lower limbs, ULEPs were undetectable in a consistent group of FM patients with an abnormal skin biopsy, and even patients with a normal IENFD had a lower number of sites where ULEPs could be reliably detected compared to controls. According to previous studies on skin biopsies in FM patients [11,19,20], the predominant site of denervation was the proximal part of the leg. However, no patient with an abnormal skin biopsy showed ULEPs from the foot stimulation, probably because the generation of detectable ULEPs from the distal part of the leg might have required a constant number of activated C-fibers to bypass signal scattering along the afferent pathway. In this sense, a subtle C-fiber dysfunction in FM patients could also exist at the distal site of stimulation. ULEPs from the proximal leg stimulation site were present in a small number of patients with proximal small fiber denervation, albeit with a reduced amplitude, as we commented below. The complete absence of ULEPs at the somatic stimulation sites of the upper and lower limbs could be a sign of denervation of the small fibers in patients with FM, a statement that should be further confirmed in larger patient series.

4.3. LEP and ULEP Latencies and Amplitudes

In agreement with previous studies, we found no latency abnormalities of the cortical complex associated with the vertex Aδ and C in FM patients [11,19,20], as demyelination along the spino-thalamic tract is not typical of FM. In contrast to our recent study, we found a decrease in Aδ N2. In agreement with previous studies, we found no latency abnormalities of the cortical complex associated with vertex Aδ and C in FM patients [11,19,20], as demyelination along the spino-thalamic tract is not typical of FM. In contrast to our recent study, we found a decrease in the Aδ N2 amplitude upon the stimulation of the thigh and hand in FM patients with a normal skin biopsy [21], while the P2 amplitude was within normal values. In the present study, we used a statistical analysis with multiple channels, which could highlight the amplitude differences compared to a single-channel analysis. A visual inspection of the overall average revealed a reduced N2–P2 complex in NFM patients, but as discussed in previous studies [4,11], there is a large variability in FM patients for the phenomenon of reduced habituation with repeated stimulation. In this study, we did not calculate habituation across individual trials because we included ULEPs, which are rarely recognized as single responses [4]. In patients with an IENFD reduction, the amplitude of ULEPs was reduced at all stimulation sites compared to controls, indicating a dysfunction of Aδ fibers. The amplitude of ULEPs, when present, was reduced in patients with small fiber involvement, but also in patients with a normal IENFD, indicating a likely subtle and initial dysfunction of small fibers that could develop over time. Indeed, disease duration was shorter in patients with a normal skin biopsy than in patients with small fiber involvement.

4.4. Correlation with Clinical Features

In agreement with previous studies [11,18], involvement of the small fibers did not correspond to a more severe FM phenotype. FM is a complex syndrome which does not resemble a model of neuropathic pain but is rather an example of nociplastic pain in which phenomena of central sensitization may predominate over the purely neuropathic aspects of the disease. The correlation we found between the decrease in ULEP amplitude and fatigue confirmed previous findings of a possible influence of small fiber dysfunction on motor performance [22,23], even considering the limitation due to the small number of patients (see comments below).

4.5. Limitation of the Study

This was a pilot study to investigate the reliability of C-related ULEPs in patients with proven small fiber impairment. The number of patients was very small, as was the number of age-matched controls. Some comparisons approaching statistical significance could find confirmation in larger case series. We did not include the early N1 component as we wanted to focus on the main vertex components in the analysis. In agreement with previous findings [4], we observed an early vertex complex in patients and controls consistent with the coactivation of Aδ fibers also in the C modality of the stimulation, which was not included in the analysis due to its unclear origin. However, the presence of this early complex could reduce the reliability of somatic C-related ULEPs.

5. Conclusions

The present preliminary results may confirm the reliability of LEPs in detecting small fiber impairment, as the Aδ-related vertex complex amplitude reduction characterizes patients with small fiber impairment and likely predicts small fiber involvement during FM development. Although the signal-to-noise ratio of ULEPs elicited from somatic sites was low, they were detectable at a consistent number of stimulation sites in control subjects, and their complete absence in the upper and lower limbs, including distal sites, may underpin the findings of LEPs in patients with small fiber impairment.

Further prospective studies in larger case series could confirm the present findings on the sensitivity of LEP amplitude and ULEP imaging in detecting small fiber impairment and the development of IENFD in FM patients.

Supplementary Materials: The following supporting information can be downloaded at: https://www.mdpi.com/article/10.3390/jcm13113078/s1, Supplementary Methods, Table S1: Pain thresholds for a-delta fibers modality of stimulation in FM patients (J: joules, H: hand, K: knee and F: foot); Table S2: Stimulation parameters of C-LEPs (J: joules, H: hand, K: knee and F: foot); Table S3: Neurophysiological and clinical features in AFM and NFM patients. BPI Brain Pain Inventory. MAF; Multidimensional Assessment of Fatigue; NRS: Numerical Rating Scale; WPI Wide Pain Index IENFD Intraepidermal Nerve Fober Density.

Author Contributions: Conceptualization, M.d.T. and G.L.; methodology, G.T., E.A., S.G.Q. and R.L.; validation, E.L., A.S., E.L., S.G.Q. and E.A.; investigation, G.T., R.L., A.S., E.L., S.G.Q., E.A., M.d.T. and G.L.; writing, E.A., S.G.Q., M.d.T. and A.S.; visualization, A.S. and E.L.; supervision, M.d.T.; project administration, M.d.T.; funding acquisition, M.d.T. All authors have read and agreed to the published version of the manuscript.

Funding: This research was funded by #NEXTGENERATIONEU (NGEU) and funded by the Ministry of University and Research (MUR), National Recovery and Resilience Plan (NRRP), project MNESYS (PE0000006)—a multiscale integrated approach to the study of the nervous system in health and disease (DN. 1553 11.10.2022).

Institutional Review Board Statement: The study was approved by the ethical committee of the Policlinico General Hospital (Bari). The local ethics committee approved the study of LEP and skin biopsy for the first time in 2009 (n° 123/12 March 2009), then yearly authorized the prosecution of data collecting and updated the informed consent.

Informed Consent Statement: Written informed consent was obtained from all subjects involved in the study.

Data Availability Statement: Neurophysiological, skin biopsy and clinical data are available on request to corresponding author.

Conflicts of Interest: The authors declare no conflicts of interest. The funders had no role in the design of the study; in the collection, analyses or interpretation of data; in the writing of the manuscript or in the decision to publish the results.

Appendix A. Skin Biopsy

The skin biopsy involved the removal of a 3 mm skin flap from the thigh 20 cm below the anterior iliac spine and in the distal third of the leg (10 cm above the lateral malleolus in the area of the sural nerve). The procedure was performed under local anesthesia with an intradermal injection of lidocaine and required no sutures. The biopsy samples were processed to obtain a quantification of the small nerve fibers. The laboratory procedure described in the work of Devigili et al. [2] included a sample preparation phase: fixation with 2% paraformaldehyde lysine periodate at 4 °C overnight, cryoprotection, sectioning and finally immunostaining with the 9.5 anti-polyclonal protein product. The counting of small nerve fibers was performed with a semi-automatic counter on three non-consecutive central sections under a bright-field optical microscope [2]. The data obtained on the number of small nerve fibers were compared with normative values determined in adult subjects on the basis of gender and age groups [10].

Appendix B. Laser Stimulation

For this study, we used the STIMUL 1340 system from Electronic Engineering® (El.En. S.p.A., Florence, Italy). It was equipped with two laser sources: a neodymium:yttriumaluminum perovskite laser (Nd:YAP), which emits an infrared beam, and a coaxial diode laser source, which emits a visible red beam. The system works with a fiber optic conductor. We performed the recordings with a high-resolution EEG headset equipped with 62 recording electrodes (Micromed Brain Quick device, Micromed S.p.A., Treviso, Italy). The laser stimuli were administered at three sites on the right side of the body: on the dorsum of the hand, on the dorsum of the foot and on the proximal anterolateral segment of the lower limb near the knee. The stimulation procedure was similar to a previous study conducted in our laboratory [4]. In this case, only the right side was stimulated to increase compliance for this type of procedure, which is known for its relatively long duration (approximately 100 min in total) and discomfort, especially in individuals with altered pain perception, such as those with fibromyalgia.

The parameters were set to activate the small myelinated afferents (Aδ) or the unmyelinated afferents (C).

In brief, for each stimulated area and for each of the two modalities under study (Aδ and C), at least 25 consecutive stimulations were delivered with an interstimulus interval (ISI) of at least 10 s. To avoid the phenomenon of habituation and to minimize the skin damage caused by the laser beam, the laser beam was skillfully guided to nearby and never identical skin areas.

The Nd:YAP stimulator could elicit the stimulation of both types of small nerve fibers by modulating certain stimulation parameters: a higher stimulation intensity (10.19–26.74 J/cm^2), shorter duration (5 ms) and a small irradiated area (diameter 5 mm) to elicit the pinprick sensation; a lower intensity (7.46–13.37 J/cm^2), longer duration (10 ms) and a larger skin area (diameter 10 mm) to elicit only the heat sensation. The diameter of the illuminated area was measured with an infrared-sensitive paper and was 5 mm for Aδ-LEPs and 10 mm for C-LEPs. The threshold for delivered energy was individually adjusted and increased by 0.25 J per step until the subject clearly felt a pure warm sensation for C-fibers, whereas for the Aδ stimulation, after the initial sensation of a general feeling of pain, we delivered energy until the subjects clearly felt the corresponding stinging sensation on the pain rating scale with values between three and six.

Each subject was asked to pay attention to the two different types of sensations elicited by the stimulator: pinprick pain for the Aδ modality and pure heat sensations for the C modality. During the stimulation of the C fibers, the patient was instructed to alert the neurophysiology technician if they perceived any sensation other than warmth that may occur during the involuntary co-stimulation of the Aδ fibers, such as a stabbing or burning pain. Although we only had the skin biopsy results from the lower limb, we decided to test the upper limb with the YAP laser as well as the extremity, as the IENFD reduction could also affect this area [8]. The stimulation paradigm provided for randomization between sites and the modality of stimulation.

References

1. Devigili, G.; Di Stefano, G.; Donadio, V.; Frattale, I.; Mantovani, E.; Nolano, M.; Occhipinti, G.; Provitera, V.; Quitadamo, S.; Tamburin, S.; et al. Clinical criteria and diagnostic assessment of fibromyalgia: Position statement of the Italian Society of Neurology-Neuropathic Pain Study Group. *Neurol. Sci.* **2023**, *44*, 2561–2574. [CrossRef] [PubMed]
2. Devigili, G.; Tugnoli, V.; Penza, P.; Camozzi, F.; Lombardi, R.; Melli, G.; Broglio, L.; Granieri, E.; Lauria, G. The diagnostic criteria for small fibre neuropathy: From symptoms to neuropathology. *Brain* **2008**, *131*, 1912–1925. [CrossRef] [PubMed]
3. Truini, A.; Cruccu, G. Laser evoked potentials in patients with trigeminal disease: The absence of Aδ potentials does not unmask C-fibre potentials. *Clin. Neurophysiol.* **2008**, *119*, 1905–1908. [CrossRef]
4. Ammendola, E.; Tancredi, G.; Ricci, K.; Falcicchio, G.; Valeriani, M.; de Tommaso, M. Assessment of C Fibers Evoked Potentials in Healthy Subjects by Nd: YAP Laser. *Pain Res. Manag.* **2022**, *2022*, 7737251. [CrossRef] [PubMed]
5. Verdugo, R.J.; Matamala, J.M.; Inui, K.; Kakigi, R.; Valls-Solé, J.; Hansson, P.; Nilsen, K.B.; Lombardi, R.; Lauria, G.; Petropoulos, I.N.; et al. Review of techniques useful for the assessment of sensory small fiber neuropathies: Report from an IFCN expert group. *Clin. Neurophysiol.* **2022**, *136*, 13–38. [CrossRef] [PubMed]
6. de Tommaso, M.; Vecchio, E.; Nolano, M. The puzzle of fibromyalgia between central sensitization syndrome and small fiber neuropathy: A narrative review on neurophysiological and morphological evidence. *Neurol. Sci.* **2022**, *43*, 1667–1684. [CrossRef] [PubMed]
7. Evdokimov, D.; Frank, J.; Klitsch, A.; Unterecker, S.; Warrings, B.; Serra, J.; Papagianni, A.; Saffer, N.; zu Altenschildesche, C.M.; Kampik, D.; et al. Reduction of skin innervation is associated with a severe fibromyalgia phenotype. *Ann. Neurol.* **2019**, *86*, 504–516. [CrossRef] [PubMed]
8. Serra, J.; Collado, A.; Solà, R.; Antonelli, F.; Torres, X.; Salgueiro, M.; Quiles, C.; Bostock, H. Hyperexcitable C nociceptors in fibromyalgia. *Ann. Neurol.* **2014**, *75*, 196–208. [CrossRef] [PubMed]
9. Wolfe, F.; Clauw, D.J.; Fitzcharles, M.A.; Goldenberg, D.L.; Häuser, W.; Katz, R.L.; Mease, P.J.; Russell, A.S.; Russell, I.J.; Walitt, B. Revisions to the 2010/2011 fibromyalgia diagnostic criteria. *Semin. Arthritis Rheum.* **2016**, *46*, 319–329. [CrossRef]
10. Lauria, G.; Bakkers, M.; Schmitz, C.; Lombardi, R.; Penza, P.; Devigili, G.; Smith, A.G.; Hsieh, S.T.; Mellgren, S.I.; Umapathi, T.; et al. Intraepidermal nerve fiber density at the distal leg: A worldwide normative reference study. *J. Peripher. Nerv. Syst.* **2010**, *15*, 202–207. [CrossRef]
11. de Tommaso, M.; Nolano, M.; Iannone, F.; Vecchio, E.; Ricci, K.; Lorenzo, M.; Delussi, M.; Girolamo, F.; Lavolpe, V.; Provitera, V.; et al. Update on laser-evoked potential findings in fibromyalgia patients in light of clinical and skin biopsy features. *J. Neurol.* **2014**, *261*, 461–472. [CrossRef] [PubMed]
12. Johnson, E.W. Visual Analog Scale (VAS). *Am. J. Phys. Med. Rehabilitation* **2001**, *80*, 717. [CrossRef]
13. Zung, W.W. A self-rating depression scale. *Arch. Gen. Psychiatry* **1965**, *12*, 63–70. [CrossRef] [PubMed]
14. Zung, W.W. A Rating Instrument For Anxiety Disorders. *Psychosomatics* **1971**, *12*, 371–379. [CrossRef] [PubMed]
15. Bidari, A.; Hassanzadeh, M.; Mohabat, M.F.; Talachian, E.; Khoei, E.M. Validation of a Persian version of the Fibromyalgia Impact Questionnaire (FIQ-P). *Rheumatol. Int.* **2014**, *34*, 181–189. [CrossRef] [PubMed]
16. Belza, B.; Miyawaki, C.E.; Liu, M.; Aree-Ue, S.; Fessel, M.; Minott, K.R.; Zhang, X. A Systematic Review of Studies Using the Multidimensional Assessment of Fatigue Scale. *J. Nurs. Meas.* **2018**, *26*, 36–75. [CrossRef] [PubMed]
17. Caraceni, A.; Mendoza, T.R.; Mencaglia, E.; Baratella, C.; Edwards, K.; Forjaz, M.J.; Martini, C.; Serlin, R.C.; de Conno, F.; Cleeland, C.S. A validation study of an Italian version of the brief pain inventory (Breve questionario per la valutazione del dolore). *Pain* **1996**, *65*, 87–92. [CrossRef] [PubMed]
18. Fasolino, A.; Di Stefano, G.; Leone, C.; Galosi, E.; Gioia, C.; Lucchino, B.; Terracciano, A.; Di Franco, M.; Cruccu, G.; Truini, A. Small-fibre pathology has no impact on somatosensory system function in patients with fibromyalgia. *Pain* **2020**, *161*, 2385–2393. [CrossRef] [PubMed]
19. Vecchio, E.; Lombardi, R.; Paolini, M.; Libro, G.; Delussi, M.; Ricci, K.; Quitadamo, S.G.; Gentile, E.; Girolamo, F.; Iannone, F.; et al. Peripheral and central nervous system correlates in fibromyalgia. *Eur. J. Pain* **2020**, *24*, 1537–1547. [CrossRef]

20. Truini, A.; Aleksovska, K.; Anderson, C.C.; Attal, N.; Baron, R.; Bennett, D.L.; Bouhassira, D.; Cruccu, G.; Eisenberg, E.; Enax-Krumova, E.; et al. Joint European Academy of Neurology-European Pain Federation-Neuropathic Pain Special Interest Group of the International Association for the Study of Pain guidelines on neuropathic pain assessment. *Eur. J. Neurol.* **2023**, *30*, 2177–2196. [CrossRef]
21. Vecchio, E.; Quitadamo, S.G.; Ricci, K.; Libro, G.; Delussi, M.; Lombardi, R.; Lauria, G.; de Tommaso, M. Laser evoked potentials in fibromyalgia with peripheral small fiber involvement. *Clin. Neurophysiol.* **2022**, *135*, 96–106. [CrossRef] [PubMed]
22. Quitadamo, S.G.; Vecchio, E.; Delussi, M.; Libro, G.; Clemente, L.; Lombardi, R.; Modena, D.; Giannotta, M.; Iannone, F.; de Tommaso, M. Outcome of small fibers pathology in fibromyalgia: A real life longitudinal observational study. *Clin. Exp. Rheumatol.* **2023**, *41*, 1216–1224. [CrossRef] [PubMed]
23. Gentile, E.; Quitadamo, S.G.; Clemente, L.; Bonavolontà, V.; Lombardi, R.; Lauria, G.; Greco, G.; Fischetti, F.; De Tommaso, M. A multicomponent physical activity home-based intervention for fibromyalgia patients: Effects on clinical and skin biopsy features. *Clin. Exp. RHeumatol.* **2023**. [CrossRef] [PubMed]

Disclaimer/Publisher's Note: The statements, opinions and data contained in all publications are solely those of the individual author(s) and contributor(s) and not of MDPI and/or the editor(s). MDPI and/or the editor(s) disclaim responsibility for any injury to people or property resulting from any ideas, methods, instructions or products referred to in the content.

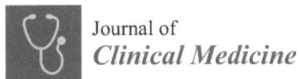
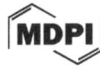

Article

Perspectives on Creating a Chronic Pain Support Line in Portugal: Results of a Focus Group Study among Patients and Healthcare Professionals

Mariana Cruz [1,2,*], Maria Inês Durães [3], Patrícia Azevedo [3], Célia Carvalhal [3], Simão Pinho [1,4] and Rute Sampaio [1,5]

1. Department of Biomedicine, Faculty of Medicine of University of Porto, Portugal Alameda Prof. Hernâni Monteiro, 4200-319 Porto, Portugal
2. Centro Hospitalar Universitário de Coimbra, Praceta Prof. Mota Pinto, 3004-561 Coimbra, Portugal
3. Administração Regional de Saúde do Norte, R. de Santa Catarina 1288, 4000-477 Porto, Portugal
4. Centro Hospitalar Tondela Viseu, Av. Rei Dom Duarte, 3504-509 Viseu, Portugal
5. CINTESIS@RISE, Rua Dr. Plácido da Costa, 4200-450 Porto, Portugal
* Correspondence: m.belo.cruz@gmail.com; Tel.: +351-936-576-346

Abstract: Background: Chronic pain (CP) patients frequently feel misunderstood and experience a lack of support. This led to the creation of support telephone lines in some countries. However, there is no scientific data grounding their development or evaluating their performance. Almost 37% of the Portuguese adult population suffers from CP, with great costs for patients and the healthcare system. **Methods**: To determine the viability of a support line for CP in Portugal, a qualitative study was designed, and online focus group meetings, with patients and healthcare professionals, were conducted. Their perspectives, beliefs, and expectations were evaluated and described. **Results**: This study revealed that a CP support line is a feasible project from the participants' perspective if its interventions are limited to active listening, emotional support, and tailored suggestions. **Conclusions**: It has the potential to generate a positive impact on healthcare services, while also contributing to greater equity of access to support.

Keywords: chronic pain; helpline; focus group; qualitative research

Citation: Cruz, M.; Durães, M.I.; Azevedo, P.; Carvalhal, C.; Pinho, S.; Sampaio, R. Perspectives on Creating a Chronic Pain Support Line in Portugal: Results of a Focus Group Study among Patients and Healthcare Professionals. *J. Clin. Med.* 2024, 13, 5207. https://doi.org/10.3390/jcm13175207

Academic Editor: Mariateresa Giglio

Received: 1 August 2024
Revised: 26 August 2024
Accepted: 27 August 2024
Published: 2 September 2024

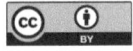

Copyright: © 2024 by the authors. Licensee MDPI, Basel, Switzerland. This article is an open access article distributed under the terms and conditions of the Creative Commons Attribution (CC BY) license (https://creativecommons.org/licenses/by/4.0/).

1. Introduction

The International Association for the Study of Pain (IASP) defines pain as "an unpleasant sensory and emotional experience associated with, or resembling that associated with, actual or potential tissue damage", identifying it as a leading cause of suffering and disability in the world [1–3]. Chronic pain (CP) was recognized by the European Federation of Pain (EFIC) as a pathology in 2001, whether isolated or accompanied by other disorders [4]. It is defined as pain that persists or recurs for longer than 3 months, associated with significant emotional distress or functional disability [2]. CP can be classified as primary CP (without an obvious cause) or secondary CP (as a symptom of an underlying pathology, including neuropathy, cancer, post-surgical, post-traumatic, orofacial, visceral, and musculoskeletal pain) [2].

The prevalence of CP is as high as 20% in the European adult population, while similar percentages can be found in the USA [5,6]. A Portuguese population-based study revealed that almost 37% of adults suffer from CP, making it a major public health issue [7]. The consequences of CP are vast, as they are both personal, economical, and societal, influencing absenteeism, social benefits, and early retirement costs. The annual cost of CP in Portugal amounts to EUR 5635.26 million; however, only 1% of Portuguese pain patients have access to specialized healthcare [8]. It has also been shown that, while patient access to care is somewhat restricted, when someone uses health services due to their pain, there is a propensity for overuse with no clinical gain [8]. Such findings make it pertinent to propose new intervention programs by bringing patients and healthcare professionals closer, empowering those who suffer, and maximizing the effective use of the available resources [7,8].

The creation of a CP support line (CPSL) can be one such program, making it possible to avoid some of the unjustified use of healthcare services (by providing patients with pain-preventing tools and self-management) and tackling major issues related to CP management, such as medication adherence (i.e., intaking the correct dosage of the right medicine in a timely manner and for the prescribed duration). Some pain support lines are functioning already, in countries such as Ireland, Canada, England, and Australia. Most were created by private organizations and operated by volunteers [9–13]. Even though this type of program seems to have a positive impact on patients with CP, with testimonies reinforcing the importance of human presence for those suffering, there is a lack of objective data on their effectiveness [9,14–16].

Using focus group methodology to gather an in-depth understanding of the perceptions and beliefs of patients with CP and healthcare professionals working in the field, we believe it to be possible to provide a truly objective ground for creating such a service. The focus group is characterized by a close interaction between the moderator and the group members and interactions between the participants themselves [17–20]. This methodology makes it possible to better understand the participants' perceptions on the topic under discussion and is particularly useful in the context of healthcare research, as most health-related conditions depend on the social environment and context [18,19]. Focus groups have been widely used to gather knowledge regarding patients' experiences with health services and healthcare providers' attitudes and needs [19,21].

This study aimed to describe the perspectives of both patients with CP and healthcare professionals regarding the creation of a CPSL in Portugal. To our knowledge, this is the first time the feasibility of a CP support line has been studied and structured within a scientific approach. Focus groups followed a previously published protocol [22], allowing for the development of a support line based on the reality of those living with the disease. Gathered data will also provide insight into the potential impact of a CPSL.

2. Materials and Methods

The present study is part of a larger project titled "Creating a pain support line in Portugal: feasibility, development and impact" and reports the results of focus groups carried out with patients with CP and healthcare professionals working in the field. The main objective was to evaluate the feasibility of creating such a support line, according to the participants' perspectives, beliefs, and expectations.

2.1. Study Design and Setting

To assess patients with CP and healthcare professionals' needs and expectations, an exploratory and phenomenological qualitative design based on focus group interviews was used, following the COREQ (Consolidated Criteria for Reporting Qualitative Research) guidelines [23,24]. An approach based on focus groups was considered to be the best option, as it allows researchers to obtain a varied array of perspectives, as close to everyday reality as possible, while providing participants with a safe and familiar environment to express their opinions and describe their experiences [19,21]. Due to COVID-19 pandemic restraints and post-pandemic time constraints, focus groups were arranged in an online setting, using the Zoom© videoconferencing platform. According to some authors, it is recommended that online focus groups do not exceed five to six participants because a fluid discussion is difficult to achieve [25,26]. The focus group dynamic and videoconference characteristics and requirements were presented before the meetings to both patients and healthcare professionals who volunteered to participate. All participants were informed that meetings were being video recorded for later transcription and analysis, under the Portuguese data protection laws.

Qualitative data were obtained and analyzed with the NVivo© software, version 12, and evidence was collected regarding the feasibility of developmental aspects of a support line.

2.2. Recruitment and Sampling

Patients registered in the *Força3P* pain association were invited to participate by e-mail, with the help of the association's representative. Following the same rationale, healthcare professionals working in public health units in Portugal were also invited by e-mail. The focus groups took place at a time conveniently arranged for most of the participants, who had previously communicated available timeframes for scheduling. All participants received a presentation explaining the study context and objectives and gave informed written consent after the presentation and prior to the interviews. Participants were selected through convenience sampling.

2.3. Participants

The inclusion criteria of participants consisted of them being 18 years old or older, having the ability to understand and communicate in Portuguese, being able to use technologies and to log into a Zoom© call, and being a patient with CP (diagnosed at least two years ago) or a healthcare professional working in Portuguese public healthcare units who attend to patients with CP.

2.3.1. Healthcare Professionals

In total, twenty-one medical doctors and nurses were contacted. Twelve volunteered to participate, one refused, and the others did not respond. They were e-mailed a short presentation of the project and a date suitable for the majority was arranged. Written consent was obtained prior to the meeting. Two of the volunteers were unexpectedly called to emergency cases; therefore, meetings occurred with the participation of a total of nine doctors and one nurse, within two meetings ($n = 4$ and $n = 6$). Within the specifications of qualitative research, we consider theme saturation to have been reached in these groups.

2.3.2. Patients with CP

Regarding patients with CP, seven volunteered to participate, but only six ($n = 6$) were effectively present. No further patients were recruited as theme saturation was reached.

2.4. Data Collection Procedures

The focus group meetings were held on the Zoom© platform (online videoconference) and led by two researchers. An entirely online approach was chosen to ensure safety and flexibility in the pandemic and post-pandemic era. The two researchers were present 30 min before the starting time to solve any technical issues. The facilitator was responsible for hosting and moderating the discussion, by asking questions from the discussion guide and ensuring adequate individual participation. The second moderator was responsible for recording major quotes, non-verbal interactions, and expressions, to add context to the recordings and aid the discussion of the transcripts later.

Questions related to the search topic were based on the literature regarding patients with CP and healthcare professionals' experiences, as well as related to technological potential and applications in medicine and CP [16,27–31]. The question guide used in each focus group was discussed in previous work [22] and did not limit the scope of the discussion; it was merely used to stimulate dialogue further.

The interview duration was one hour and forty minutes in the focus group of patients with CP and an average of one hour and thirty minutes for healthcare professionals' groups. All participants opted to display their real names, and all interviews were audio and video recorded. Everything was anonymized afterward. A total of three focus groups were carried out: one with patients and two with healthcare professionals. Data saturation was attained.

2.5. Analysis

The recordings were transcribed verbatim, anonymized, and codified; they were not returned to participants. Analysis was made according to the framework method [32,33]. Findings emerged directly from raw data, based on both inductive and deductive coding; each technique was applied independently for the patients' and healthcare professionals' focus groups in a systematic, sequential, and continuous way [34]. Data analysis with QRS NVivo© versions 12 and 14 software enabled identifying and organizing codes, categories, and themes. Coding of the segments of the transcriptions was made quotation by quotation [35]. The segments of coded text were synthesized into categories, which were further grouped into major themes [36,37]. Thematic analysis was performed through an iterative and reflexive process, carried out by three of the researchers, independently of each other. Afterward, comparative analysis between focus groups was carried out to better understand how the perspectives of patients with CP and healthcare practitioners converged or diverged in specific topics. All data were discussed and interpreted by at least two researchers; any disagreements were discussed with a third researcher until a consensus was reached. Participants were not asked for feedback on the findings. All quotes presented were transcribed from Portuguese to English and double-checked.

2.6. Data Sharing

Data retrieved from focus groups were recorded, transcribed, and completely anonymized. It includes the complete verbatim transcriptions, which will be made available upon request. The study protocol has been published [22]. There are no frequencies of categorical variables to report, as our approach primarily dealt with establishing concepts rather than specific wordings; this is because participants used different wording to convey the same concept, feeling, and/or opinion, and hence the importance of not limiting the analysis to a frequency determination. As stated previously, two coding methods were used (inductive and deductive), by manual codification with NVivo© software. There was no statistical analysis, the final data were analyzed through a comparative in-depth discussion by at least three researchers.

3. Results

In total, three focus group interviews were conducted. The majority of patients with CP were females (83%) and the same percentage were married. Fifty percent (50%) were unemployed and 33.3% had a university degree. Regarding the 10 healthcare professionals ($n = 10$): there was a nurse, an anesthesiologist, a stomatologist, a physical and rehabilitation medicine physician, and six family medicine physicians. The experience working with patients with CP ranged from 5 to 20 years.

After transcription, the data were coded, first inductively and then using the deductive method to confront the results and minimize bias. Four major themes emerged in both approaches and the three focus groups: (1) support available for patients, (2) perceived patients' difficulties, (3) perceived patients' necessities, and (4) creation of a chronic pain support line. The major theme "Perceived patients' difficulties" was discussed to a lesser extent in the healthcare professionals' groups. Descriptions can be found in Table 1.

Table 1. Main themes' descriptions.

Chronic Pain Patients	
Theme	Description
Support available for patients	Includes the existing support systems, their accessibility, and ideas on how to ameliorate them.
Perceived patients' difficulties	Refers to the many difficulties patients with CP face, from the diagnostic to living with the disease for years.
Perceived patients' necessities	Includes the main perceived needs to be addressed, identified by patients with CP.

Table 1. *Cont.*

Chronic Pain Patients	
Creation of a chronic pain support line	Includes opinions, characteristics that must be present, what must be avoided, and foreseeable difficulties from a patient perspective
Healthcare professionals	
Theme	Description
Support available for patients	Includes the existing support systems, their accessibility, and ideas on how to ameliorate them.
Perceived patients' necessities	Includes the main perceived needs to be addressed, identified by healthcare professionals during their activity.
Creation of a chronic pain support line	Includes opinions, characteristics that must be present, what must be avoided, and foreseeable difficulties from a healthcare profession perspective.

As for the minor themes, some appeared only with deductive coding, reinforcing their less significant role. These themes are related mainly to two topics: the daily living of patients and the importance of treatment adherence on pain control. This last theme was only discussed in the healthcare groups but its relevance for pain management and its dependency on the doctor–patient relationship and proper communication was vehemently reinforced.

3.1. Theme 1: Support Available for Patients

Under Theme 1, four types of support were identified: Hospital pain units; Family physician (FP), which was much more valued by healthcare professionals than by patients; Emergency Services, which were solely mentioned by patients (even though with a negative outlook on their efficacy) but never mentioned by professionals; and Information available about CP, which was considered to be insufficient by patients while healthcare professionals regard it as adequate. All in all, perspectives slightly diverged between the two groups, and examples of the two can be found in Table 2.

Table 2. Perspectives of patients and healthcare professionals: excerpts.

Theme 1: Support Available for Patients
1.1 Hospital pain units
"I go to my pain doctor. It's in the hospital, we have to call or if we show up we talk to the nurse. We always end up being attended to."—Patient 1
"We also have a phone line for our patients (...) that turns out to be much more of a kind of psychological and emotional support."—Professional 2
1.2 Family physician
"That's what's important, is that at the Pain Unit they talk to us. The FP is very different; there is not much time for talking, as the doctor is overworked (...) giving the impression that he doesn't even look at us."—Patient 5
"(...) there is a minimal percentage of patients who are followed up in Pain Units. We dare say everyone else is followed by their FP."—Professional 1
1.3 Emergency services
"Going to the emergency services is a mistake because the professional who is there does not know how to assess our pain. If we have any other disease, he does not even waste time trying to understand what kind of pain the person has."—Patient 1
1.4 Information available about CP
"(...) because nobody talks to you about pain dedicated appointments, not in hospitals nor in primary health care centers."—Patient 5
"I tell them to research this topic, consult this website (...). In our unit we have some leaflets that explain a little about pain and how to adapt to the pain situation, how the Pain Unit works, etc."—Professional 2

Table 2. *Cont.*

Theme 2: Perceived patients' difficulties
2.1 Feeling misunderstood "I used to go to the doctor, I complained of pain, but as I could not explain what I was feeling or verbalize the intensity and cause of the pain, it ended making me feel blocked (...)."—Patient 3 "I think people feel misunderstood. And since it's not a visible thing, it is a problem that exists even within the family, is it not? The husband does not understand, the parents do not understand, nobody understands."—Professional 2
2.2 Difficulty in asking for help "Experiencing what I was experiencing and what I was feeling was very complicated... asking for help? No way (...) what I have also seen is that people in this situation, especially in the early stages, are somewhat reluctant to seek healthcare."—Patient 3 "I think people have difficulty...they think like "it's pain, just bear it" and do not seek help (...)."—Patient 1
2.3 Misjudgment of complaints and delay of diagnosis "From the moment the person starts to feel it and looking for health professionals because she feels constant pain, until having a diagnosis, many years pass. First, they will investigate and discard all possibilities, until they decide we have CP because of an X or Y pathology. With all this, around 6 years go by."—Patient 3
2.4 Difficulty accepting the diagnosis "I will give my example: before I was diagnosed and before I accepted CP I was angry, so for me a CP diagnosis was not seen with good eyes, despite actually having pain."—Patient 3
2.5 Gender bias "If we are treated by male doctors, they have the idea that women are melodramatic, and very emotional, and the first thing they think of is always depressive syndrome. Sorry but this is true."—Patient 2
Theme 3: Perceived patients' necessities
3.1 Emotional and psychological support "In times of crisis and pain, we would just like to have someone we could talk to, to calm us down (...)."—Patient 2 "We also have a line for our patients (...) with strong psychological and emotional support, a lot of listening, giving expression to, allowing the expression of feelings"—Professional 2
3.2 Effective communication skills "Of course, listening is essential. The person on the other end must have an exceptional ability to listen, to respect the silences, have communication techniques, some psychotherapy tools."—Patient 7
3.3 Scientifically reliable information "Dialogue is really important (...), and scientific information. Hence the importance of scales and pain assessment. (...) people must have scientific knowledge, I have no doubt about that."—Patient 2
3.4 Advice and coping mechanisms "Sometimes we are so desperate and confused that the fact that a professional is asking basic and logical questions makes us open our minds and realize "I still haven't done everything I could". (...) I would like for the person to be an advisor and say: "Look, try this, try that, do this, apply hot water, apply cold water...", a person who would guide us."—Patient 1 "Just listening is not enough, if we do not implement strategies with our patient and try to get him to establish other focuses of attention, make him find other anchors in life besides his pain (...)."—Professional 1
3.5 Limitless support "I would have to know that there will be someone who knows how to listen and help during the entire process, without time limitations. (...) I want to feel that the person on the other end is holding my hand and will not let go until I am ok."—Patient 7
3.6 Opportunity for sharing common experiences "I think that a group session/appointment would be a good option to consider. Chronic pain patients frequently state the need they have to feel understood, sharing experiences and stories would be a great option."—Professional 4
Theme 4: Creation of a CPSL
4.1 Support line functionality "It is fundamental to have someone who deals with pain closely, because dealing with something is very different from learning about it and that makes all the difference (...). It would be good for those on the other end of the line to have knowledge."—Patient 3 "We have to have very well-prepared people on the other end of the line, who understands what this concept of CP is, so as not to be immediately alarmed if the patient says he has 7 or 8 pain intensity."—Professional 1 "Whoever is on the other end of the line has to have a very good understanding of analgesic schemes (...)."—Professional 2" The issue with algorithms, for me, is that they will only lead to very clinical, very medical things, and we want listening, empathy, all not so mechanical (...). This [the scope of action of the line] must be extremely well-defined (...) we need to define it, so that there are no doubts on the part of the patient who calls (...). There must be clinical safety for both patients and professionals."—Professional 5

Table 2. Cont.

4.2 Support line requirements
"The support line should act throughout the entire process. (...) Whoever is on the line must know how to direct and adapt the advice given to the patient and his pathology."—Patient 3
"It would be essential to be able to provide good quality information [to the patients]."—Patient 2
"(...) being able to ask for help anonymously and always respecting me as a person in pain."—Patient 7 *"Men may also want to be attended to by men... we have issues of daily life and sexuality."*—Patient 6 (Male)
4.3 What to avoid in a support line
"The line could never give an authorization to do something, it should only give the correct information to the patient."—Patient 7
"It makes sense if there is mostly active listening, coping mechanisms, not much more than that."—Professional 2
4.4 Foreseeable difficulties
"There needs to be someone, 24/7, available to answer calls. This part of the operationalization may be difficult to plan, it is necessary to mobilize a lot of people (...) and sponsorship to pay for the line. Oh, money, money!"—Patient 2
"Yes, it is important to have permanent possibility of contact, but in terms of resources it will be quite complicated."—Patient 7
"But we have to beware, because superimposed on a well diagnosed CP can be an exacerbation of another disease, and that is a completely different story!"—Professional 1
4.5 Support line feasibility
"Yes, I would use the line and try for the person [answering my call], in addition to the psychological support, to be my mentor (...)."—Patient 1
"For me the line makes sense like this [empathic listening and coping mechanisms] (...). I think that this line is not to solve problems, that is not the goal here."—Professional 2
"I often hear the nurses complaining that we have patients who call there constantly, I do not say daily, but they do call two or three times a week."—Professional 2

3.2. Theme 2: Perceived Patients' Difficulties

Five categories emerged under the perceived patients' difficulties: Feeling misunderstood, which was identified as a major drawback by both patients and professionals; Difficulty in asking for help, admitted by almost all patients but unnoticed by healthcare professionals; the majority of patients mentioned Misjudgment of complaints and delay of diagnosis, which was also recognized by health professionals, who described patients with CP as frequently having undergone multiple medical assessments and treatments achieving no effective response nor adequate follow-up, which contributes to the feeling of discredit; Difficulty accepting the diagnosis, which is seen as a source of suffering for patients, but somewhat overlooked by professionals; and Gender bias, a common complaint among female patients, failed to be mentioned by healthcare professionals. Examples of these opinions are described in Table 2.

3.3. Theme 3: Perceived Patients' Necessities

Patients and healthcare professionals discussed six major necessities: Emotional and psychological support was identified as a crucial need, mainly during pain exacerbations; Effective communication skills, such as active listening, empathy, and avoidance of a patronizing attitude were mentioned as essential qualities of healthcare professionals; Scientifically reliable information was also identified as an important need, with all three groups stating it should be provided by professionals and easily available for patients. Regarding this topic, healthcare professionals highlighted the need for adequate training and on-the-job opportunities to keep updating their knowledge; Advice and coping mechanisms on how to deal with pain and its exacerbations, as well as how to prevent them, were mentioned in all groups; and Limitless support, as all participants agreed that there is a need to have permanent access to support because pain exacerbations are impossible to anticipate. Both patients and professionals emphasized the Opportunity for sharing common experiences, as it seems to be a source of relief and understanding for patients. Excerpts of these topics are listed in Table 2.

3.4. Theme 4: Creation of a CPSL

With respect to the creation of a CPSL, five topics emerged: Support line functionality was a recurrent topic in which participants reinforced the importance of adequate skill training for those operating the line, such as having pharmacological knowledge and high-level communication skills. Professionals considered the possibility of creating an algorithm-based CPSL not to be feasible, as it would narrow the scope of the support line, which must also be very well defined. All three groups identified various Support line requirements: the permanent availability of support and the possibility of receiving video calls, and the option for patients to remain anonymous. Moreover, callers should have the opportunity to choose the sex of the operator and the advice given should not only be evidence-based but also tailored to the individual. Participants also said that a CPSL ought to be able to connect them to a CP Patient Association or provide them with tools to contact fellow CP patients (which reinforces the importance of sharing common experiences). Healthcare professionals also mentioned that professionals must have adequate training and that the line should act as a bidirectional way of exchanging information (e.g., sharing information with the patient's family physician). As for What to avoid in a support line, patients and professionals clearly stated that a CPSL must never act as a replacement for an appointment with a doctor: diagnosing illnesses is unacceptable and the prescription of medications must never occur. Another reiterated idea was that patients' complaints must never be dismissed. Foreseeable difficulties included the sizeable need of staff, which must be adequately trained and possess the necessary knowledge, the guarantee of availability without imposing limitations in call duration, and funding. Professionals also mentioned the fact that the only source of information during a call would be the patient, which would necessarily add subjectivity to the interaction and potentially impair one's ability to provide adequate advice. Regarding Support line feasibility, patients stated that creating a support line is not only feasible but also desirable, to create equity among all patients. Healthcare professionals maintained the idea that a CPSL would be useful and could potentially contribute to lessening their burden. Examples can be found in Table 2.

Besides the main themes described so far, two other minor themes emerged. Among professionals, Healthcare professionals' current difficulties were discussed: the participants mentioned having too many patients on their lists, too much administrative workload, and the fact that they often feel overburdened, particularly from an emotional perspective; when trying to help their patients, family doctors feel that they frequently give too much of themselves.

> "Because it is often the doctor acting as a therapeutic tool (...),I present myself full of energy, full of positivism, full of optimism, full of ideas, that I will be able to change the patient's life (...). At the end of the day, I am a wreck!"—Professional 2

> "I often feel empty... Completely consumed."—Professional 1

Healthcare professionals also mentioned difficulties in accessing patients' information regarding their chronic pain, suggesting that an integrated data platform should be created and shared by all potential health services so that it would be possible to know the patient history of assessments and treatments. On the same rationale, healthcare professionals pointed out the absence of protocols or guidelines to support clinical practice regarding CP, as well as a lack of opportunities to keep on learning and improve their skillset in relation to the field.

> "(...) It is true, the lack of health education, not only among patients but also among us, professionals, makes it all the more difficult."—Professional 3

Among patients, the *Use of information technologies to support patients with CP* was discussed, relating to the idea of increasing healthcare access equality. Patients considered the use of information technologies to be an inexpensive widespread means to deliver support to more remote areas of the country.

"(. . .) this line could be a way of having more equality, as it can be accessible anywhere in the country."—Patient 5

4. Discussion

This study describes the perspectives, needs, and difficulties that both patients with chronic pain and healthcare professionals experience on a daily basis. It also shows that creating a chronic pain support line for patients is considered valuable, as long as such a line operates under well-defined guidelines.

When coding focus group data, four major themes emerged. There was no difference in major themes when comparing patients' and healthcare professionals' focus groups. The fact that coding was made both inductively and deductively and that inductive coding was applied first strengthens the validity of collected data and increases the reliability of the findings, as bias was significantly reduced.

By analyzing the first main theme, Support available for patients, one can find interesting distinctions between patients' and professionals' perspectives of CP support. Firstly, both groups agreed that Hospital Pain Units are the best available support system for patients with CP. This is somewhat expected, as these units have teams specialized in dealing with CP; nevertheless, healthcare professionals highlighted that these units have very long waiting lists. The second most mentioned support system was family physicians. Here, opinions start to differ: healthcare professionals assume that, besides being responsible for most Portuguese patients with CP, FPs are mostly successful in managing their pain. This notion is corroborated by a previous study, which stated that 85% of Portuguese patients with CP are managed by FPs [38]. However, patients with CP have less trust in FPs' ability to manage their pain, stating that they do not have the necessary knowledge about CP. Patients' perspective is more in line with what has been demonstrated in previous studies [39,40]. Their lack of trust in their FPs leads them to resort to emergency services when experiencing pain exacerbations, even though they complain that these too are unsatisfactory support services. This is unsurprising since emergency services are designed to manage acute and at times life-threatening situations and CP patients' needs are very different, so much so that healthcare professionals did not even consider emergency services to be a type of support for CP management. These findings show that patients often have misconceptions regarding the role of emergency services, which leads to their overuse, as the previous literature has described [16,38]. Another relevant inconsistency between patients' and professionals' perspectives concerns available information about CP and its management tools: patients refer to it as insufficient and difficult to access, whereas healthcare professionals believe the resources provided are enough. This may indicate an important gap in communication.

The second main theme discussed, Perceived patients' difficulties, understandably had a greater emotional significance in the patient group. This is aligned with the Self-Regulation Model of Leventhal: when confronted with illness, people tend to process the information emotionally and cognitively to give it meaning and then cope with it [41]. As everyone has a unique illness representation, it is not surprising that a lack of understanding is perceived as a major issue, with patients revealing that they deal with other specific struggles in their everyday life that professionals failed to mention. A frequently discussed problem was the inhibition patients show in asking for help. This is a complex issue that may be partially explained by cultural beliefs regarding pain [9,39,40]. Misjudgment and dismissal of complaints, with consequent diagnosis delays, was another obstacle identified. This seems to be more frequent among women, who highlighted that male doctors are more prone to interpret their symptoms as secondary to psychiatric pathology [39,40]. This finding seems to suggest that there is a gender bias in CP management. Although this bias is not new, further studies are needed to clarify the motives behind these perceptions [40]. For different reasons, men also mentioned that it would be important to them to be able to choose the gender of the person they interact with. In their case, the main reason for this is that they feel there are sensitive themes they are not comfortable discussing with someone of the opposite sex, such as sexual dysfunction secondary to chronic pain. Finally, patients are also assumed to experience some reluctance in accepting their diagnosis once it is made. This may seem like a somewhat peculiar and even paradoxical notion at first, given the fact that the same patients complained about the excessive time to diagnosis; however, when one takes into account the fact that CP is a serious, often permanent, and difficult to manage diagnosis, it is easier to understand their reluctance.

Regarding the third major theme, Perceived patients' necessities, there was greater unanimity. Both patients and healthcare professionals identified emotional and psychological support as the main necessity for those who suffer from CP. This seems to be linked to the misunderstanding of patients' feelings, as well as to the burden of the disease itself [39,40,42]. Similarly, both groups mentioned the need for reliable and scientific information, which highlights the importance of adequate counseling and coping mechanisms: these can greatly help patients self-manage, besides aiding them in preventing their pain from becoming worse [16,39,43]. Patients also mentioned the importance of having support with no time limitations and good communication skills, ideas that have been widely discussed in previous studies [43,44]. Patients and healthcare professionals also noted the importance of being able to be in contact with people who have experienced similar situations and hardship.

Lastly, regarding the fourth main theme, Creation of a CPSL, there was also a significant alignment of ideas. Both groups agreed that those operating a CPSL must have proper training and experience in CP in particular [3]. Likewise, pharmacological knowledge is essential to help avoid mistakes and answer frequent questions. The possibility of creating contact points between patients and their peers or CP patients' associations was also mentioned as an interesting service for a CPSL to provide; the importance of this approach has been discussed in previous studies [9,42,43]. Choosing the gender of the operator and making video calls were also mentioned as very significant positives from patients' perspectives. The importance of video calls has become particularly relevant in recent years [45]. As for what to avoid, it was clear that the line must not make therapeutic interventions and must never act as a substitute for the doctor or nurse. Healthcare professionals added that algorithms are not reasonable in a support line that aims to support the experience of the disease and not the disease itself, as they would render the approach mechanical and almost exclusively directed at medical decisions, something that should be avoided, given the aim of such a project. Its purpose should be to complement already available support systems, with the potential to relieve the burden of the Pain Units and promote equality in CP support access. Both patients and professionals agreed on the feasibility of a CPSL. Professionals considered it a good system to relieve their work overload by making emotional and psychological support easily accessible to all patients. This idea has emerged in a previous study [16].

Despite the volume of data collected, participants rarely discussed medication adherence. It was only addressed by professionals after the facilitator mentioned it. Although this is an important factor in CP mismanagement, patients do not regard treatment adherence as relevant; as for healthcare professionals, they considered the assessment of medication adherence to be of major significance and openly assumed its dependency on the quality of the communication established with the patient, as described in previous studies [8].

This study has some limitations. The most obvious and major limitation was the sampling method; participants' characteristics may be very similar regardless of their number, and thus the sample may not comprehensively represent the population being studied [34,46]. In this study, there were some societal groups that were underrepresented in the patients' group: people from rural areas, males, and people with less than a secondary education. Nonetheless, the group included elements ranging from very talkative to very quiet, as well as people with diverging opinions on several topics, which enhances sample representativity. Regarding the study's methodology, some aspects should be noted. Ideally, focus group meetings would have been conducted in person. This would allow us to better identify alternative sources of information such as participants' body language and posture.

However, it was necessary to opt for an entirely online approach to guarantee participants' safety during the COVID-19 pandemic and more flexibility to enhance participation during post-pandemic restrictions.

The dropout rate was 14.3% for patients with CP, which is a relatively low number, compared to previous studies [47]. The higher participation rate might be explained by the logistical characteristics of online focus groups: they are easier to attend to and scheduling conflicts are less of a restriction [47]. Healthcare professionals' numbers are compliant with the numbers reported in previous focus group studies, which accounted for a 52% dropout rate [47]. These findings confirm that a complete online approach to focus group methodology is valid and has the potential to enable research projects that would otherwise be impossible to undertake.

Despite these limitations, our findings provide insight into how receptive stakeholders are to the creation of a CPSL and how comprehensively it may respond to their needs.

To the authors' knowledge, this is the first study supporting the development of a CPSL from a scientific standpoint; the project has the potential to have a positive impact on access equality and enhancement of quality of life for all patients with CP, while also contributing to more efficient use of healthcare services and healthcare professionals' wellbeing.

5. Conclusions

Overall, the present study identified similar perceived needs between patients and professionals. However, two themes marked a distinct perception among the groups: gender bias regarding CP diagnosis and management (unidentified by healthcare professionals and not anticipated by researchers) and the need for more comprehensive health education among the Portuguese population, in order to prevent the overuse of emergency services associated with CP. Furthermore, bettering communication standards between patients and healthcare professionals also emerged as being of paramount importance. It also revealed that the creation of a CPSL is welcomed by both patients and healthcare professionals, as long as its development is accomplished in accordance with the identified needs and in close collaboration with all implied stakeholders. Both groups were also able to anticipate major difficulties in attaining a 24h support line, such us staff requirements and training needs, as well as the significance of the costs implicated in operating this type of support system.

Author Contributions: Conceptualization, M.C. and R.S.; methodology, M.C., S.P. and R.S. formal analysis, M.C., S.P. and M.I.D.; investigation, M.C., S.P., M.I.D., P.A., C.C. and R.S.; data curation, M.C., S.P. and C.C.; writing—original draft preparation, M.C., M.I.D. and P.A.; writing—review and editing, M.C., S.P. and R.S.; supervision, R.S.; project administration, R.S.; funding acquisition, R.S. All authors have read and agreed to the published version of the manuscript.

Funding: This research was supported by Cátedra de Medicina da Dor at the Faculty of Medicine of University of Porto.

Institutional Review Board Statement: The study and its protocol were conducted in accordance with the Declaration of Helsinki and approved by the Ethics Committee of Centro Hospitalar Universitário de São João (protocol code 109-21, 19 March 2021).

Informed Consent Statement: Informed consent was obtained from all subjects involved in the study.

Data Availability Statement: The data that support the findings of this study are available from the corresponding author, MC, upon reasonable request.

Acknowledgments: The authors of this study are most grateful to the "Força 3P" (Chronic Pain Patient Association) for their support, time, and patience. We are also deeply grateful to all healthcare professionals who agreed to contribute with their knowledge and experience working with patients with CP.

Conflicts of Interest: The authors declare no conflicts of interest.

References

1. Treede, R.D. The International Association for the Study of Pain definition of pain: As valid in 2018 as in 1979, but in need of regularly updated footnotes. *Pain Rep.* **2018**, *3*, e643. [CrossRef]
2. Treede, R.D.; Rief, W.; Barke, A.; Aziz, Q.; Bennett, M.I.; Benoliel, R.; Cohen, M.; Evers, S.; Finnerup, N.B.; First, M.B.; et al. Chronic pain as a symptom or a disease: The IASP Classification of Chronic Pain for the International Classification of Diseases (ICD-11). *Pain* **2019**, *160*, 19–27. [CrossRef] [PubMed]
3. Cohen, S.P.; Vase, L.; Hooten, W.M. Chronic pain: An update on burden, best practices, and new advances. *Lancet* **2021**, *397*, 2082–2097. [CrossRef]
4. Raffaeli, W.; Arnaudo, E. Pain as a disease: An overview. *J. Pain. Res.* **2017**, *10*, 2003–2008. [CrossRef] [PubMed]
5. van Hecke, O.; Torrance, N.; Smith, B.H. Chronic pain epidemiology and its clinical relevance. *Br. J. Anaesth.* **2013**, *111*, 13–18. [CrossRef]
6. Yong, R.J.; Mullins, P.M.; Bhattacharyya, N. Prevalence of chronic pain among adults in the United States. *Pain* **2022**, *163*, e328–e332. [CrossRef] [PubMed]
7. Azevedo, L.F.; Costa-Pereira, A.; Mendonça, L.; Dias, C.C.; Castro-Lopes, J.M. Epidemiology of chronic pain: A population-based nationwide study on its prevalence, characteristics and associated disability in Portugal. *J. Pain* **2012**, *13*, 773–783. [CrossRef]
8. Azevedo, L.F.; Costa-Pereira, A.; Mendonça, L.; Dias, C.C.; Castro-Lopes, J.M. The economic impact of chronic pain: A nationwide population-based cost-of-illness study in Portugal. *Eur. J. Health Econ.* **2016**, *17*, 87–98. [CrossRef]
9. Finlay, K.A.; Elander, J. Reflecting the transition from pain management services to chronic pain support group attendance: An interpretative phenomenological analysis. *Br. J. Health Psychol.* **2016**, *21*, 660–676. [CrossRef]
10. Canada Pain Support Line. Available online: https://painbc.ca/find-help/pain-support-line (accessed on 23 November 2023).
11. Ireland Chronic Pain Support Line. Available online: https://www.chronicpain.ie/ (accessed on 12 November 2022).
12. UK Pain Support Line. Available online: https://painconcern.org.uk/helpline/ (accessed on 5 February 2023).
13. Australia Pain Support Services. Available online: https://www.painaustralia.org.au/find-support/care-in-community-1/painaustralia-support-groups-help-lines (accessed on 5 February 2022).
14. Matthias, M.S.; Evans, E.; Porter, B.; McCalley, S.; Kroenke, K. Patients' Experiences with Telecare for Chronic Pain and Mood Symptoms: A Qualitative Study. *Pain Med.* **2020**, *21*, 2137–2145. [CrossRef]
15. Bushey, M.A.; Kroenke, K.; Weiner, J.; Porter, B.; Evans, E.; Baye, F.; Lourens, S.; Weitlauf, S. Telecare management of pain and mood symptoms: Adherence, utility, and patient satisfaction. *J. Telemed. Telecare* **2019**, *26*, 619–626. [CrossRef] [PubMed]
16. Varsi, C.; Solem, I.K.L.; Eide, H.; Børøsund, E.; Kristjansdottir, O.B.; Heldal, K.; Waxenberg, L.B.; Weiss, K.E.; Schreurs, K.M.G.; Morrison, E.J.; et al. Health care providers' experiences of pain management and attitudes towards digitally supported self-management interventions for chronic pain: A qualitative study. *BMC Health Serv. Res.* **2021**, *21*, 275. [CrossRef] [PubMed]
17. Kinalski, D.D.; Paula, C.C.; Padoin, S.M.; Neves, E.T.; Kleinubing, R.E.; Cortes, L.F. Focus group on qualitative research: Experience report. *Rev. Bras. Enferm.* **2017**, *70*, 424–429. [CrossRef]
18. Traynor, M. Focus group research. *Nurs. Stand.* **2015**, *29*, 44–48. [CrossRef]
19. Ping, W.L. Focus group discussion: A tool for health and medical research. *Singap. Med. J.* **2008**, *49*, 256.
20. Tausch, A.P.; Menold, N. Methodological Aspects of Focus Groups in Health Research: Results of Qualitative Interviews with Focus Group Moderators. *Glob. Qual. Nurs. Res.* **2016**, *3*, 2333393616630466. [CrossRef]
21. Stalmeijer, R.E.; McNaughton, N.; Van Mook, W.N. Using focus groups in medical education research: AMEE Guide No. 91. *Med. Teach.* **2014**, *36*, 923–939. [CrossRef]
22. Cruz, M.; Pinho, S.; Castro-Lopes, J.; Sampaio, R. Patients and healthcare professionals perspectives on creating a chronic pain support line in Portugal: A qualitative study protocol. *PLoS ONE* **2022**, *17*, e0273213. [CrossRef]
23. Cleland, J.A. The qualitative orientation in medical education research. *Korean J. Med. Educ.* **2017**, *29*, 61–71. [CrossRef]
24. Tong, A.; Sainsbury, P.; Craig, J. Consolidated criteria for reporting qualitative research (COREQ): A 32-item checklist for interviews and focus groups. *Int. J. Qual. Health Care* **2007**, *19*, 349–357. [CrossRef]
25. Wettergren, L.; Eriksson, L.E.; Nilsson, J.; Jervaeus, A.; Lampic, C. Online Focus Group Discussion is a Valid and Feasible Mode When Investigating Sensitive Topics Among Young Persons with a Cancer Experience. *JMIR Res. Protoc.* **2016**, *5*, e86. [CrossRef] [PubMed]
26. Zwaanswijk, M.; van Dulmen, S. Advantages of asynchronous online focus groups and face-to-face focus groups as perceived by child, adolescent and adult participants: A survey study. *BMC Res. Notes* **2014**, *7*, 756. [CrossRef] [PubMed]
27. Solem, I.K.L.; Varsi, C.; Eide, H.; Kristjansdottir, O.B.; Mirkovic, J.; Børøsund, E.; Haaland-Øverby, M.; Heldal, K.; Schreurs, K.M.; Waxenberg, L.B.; et al. Patients' Needs and Requirements for eHealth Pain Management Interventions: Qualitative Study. *J. Med. Internet Res.* **2019**, *21*, e13205. [CrossRef]
28. Nøst, T.H.; Steinsbekk, A.; Riseth, L.; Bratås, O.; Grønning, K. Expectations towards participation in easily accessible pain management interventions: A qualitative study. *BMC Health Serv. Res.* **2017**, *17*, 712. [CrossRef] [PubMed]
29. Kong, T.; Scott, M.M.; Li, Y.; Wichelman, C. Physician attitudes towards-and adoption of-mobile health. *Digit. Health* **2020**, *6*, 2055207620907187. [CrossRef] [PubMed]
30. Currie, M.; Philip, L.J.; Roberts, A. Attitudes towards the use and acceptance of eHealth technologies: A case study of older adults living with chronic pain and implications for rural healthcare. *BMC Health Serv. Res.* **2015**, *15*, 162. [CrossRef]

31. Dueñas, M.; Ojeda, B.; Salazar, A.; Mico, J.A.; Failde, I. A review of chronic pain impact on patients, their social environment and the health care system. *J. Pain Res.* **2016**, *9*, 457–467. [CrossRef]
32. Gale, N.K.; Heath, G.; Cameron, E.; Rashid, S.; Redwood, S. Using the framework method for the analysis of qualitative data in multi-disciplinary health research. *BMC Med. Res. Methodol.* **2013**, *13*, 117. [CrossRef]
33. Srivastava, P.; Hopwood, N. A Practical Iterative Framework for Qualitative Data Analysis. *Int. J. Qual. Methods* **2009**, *8*, 76–84. [CrossRef]
34. Doody, O.; Slevin, E.; Taggart, L. Focus group interviews part 3: Analysis. *Br. J. Nurs.* **2013**, *22*, 266–269. [CrossRef]
35. Stemler, S.; Colors, P. An overview of content analysis, Practical Assessment. *Res. Eval.* **2001**, *7*, 1–6.
36. Ulin, P.R.; Robinson, E.T.; Tolley, E.E. *Qualitative Methods in Public Health: A Field Guide for Applied Research*, 1st ed.; Jossey-Bass: San Francisco, CA, USA, 2005.
37. Mays, N.; Pope, C.; Popay, J. Systematically reviewing qualitative and quantitative evidence to inform management and policy-making in the health field. *J. Health Serv. Res. Policy* **2005**, *10* (Suppl. S1), 6–20. [CrossRef] [PubMed]
38. Azevedo, L.F.; Costa-Pereira, A.; Mendonça, L.; Dias, C.C.; Castro-Lopes, J.M. Chronic pain and health services utilization: Is there overuse of diagnostic tests and inequalities in nonpharmacologic treatment methods utilization? *Med. Care* **2013**, *51*, 859–869. [CrossRef]
39. Upshur, C.C.; Bacigalupe, G.; Luckmann, R. "They don't want anything to do with you": Patient views of primary care management of chronic pain. *Pain Med.* **2010**, *11*, 1791–1798. [CrossRef] [PubMed]
40. Driscoll, M.A.; Knobf, M.T.; Higgins, D.M.; Heapy, A.; Lee, A.; Haskell, S. Patient Experiences Navigating Chronic Pain Management in an Integrated Health Care System: A Qualitative Investigation of Women and Men. *Pain Med.* **2018**, *19*, S19–S29. [CrossRef]
41. Cameron, L.; Leventhal, H. *The Self-Regulation of Health and Illness Behaviour*; Routledge: New York, NY, USA, 2003.
42. Matthias, M.S.; Kukla, M.; McGuire, A.B.; Bair, M.J. How Do Patients with Chronic Pain Benefit from a Peer-Supported Pain Self-Management Intervention? A Qualitative Investigation. *Pain Med.* **2016**, *17*, 2247–2255. [CrossRef]
43. Farr, M.; Brant, H.; Patel, R.; Linton, M.J.; Ambler, N.; Vyas, S.; Wedge, H.; Watkins, S.; Horwood, J. Experiences of Patient-Led Chronic Pain Peer Support Groups After Pain Management Programs: A Qualitative Study. *Pain Med.* **2021**, *22*, 2884–2895. [CrossRef]
44. Vermeir, P.; Vandijck, D.; Degroote, S.; Peleman, R.; Verhaeghe, R.; Mortier, E.; Hallaert, G.; Van Daele, S.; Buylaert, W.; Vogelaers, D. Communication in healthcare: A narrative review of the literature and practical recommendations. *Int. J. Clin. Pract.* **2015**, *69*, 1257–1267. [CrossRef]
45. Brown, J.; Doherty, D.; Claus, A.P.; Gilbert, K.; Nielsen, M. In a Pandemic That Limits Contact, Can Videoconferencing Enable Interdisciplinary Persistent Pain Services and What Are the Patient's Perspectives? *Arch. Phys. Med. Rehabil.* **2021**, *103*, 418–423. [CrossRef]
46. Andrade, C. The inconvenient truth about convenience and purposive samples. *Indian J. Psychol. Med.* **2021**, *43*, 86–88. [CrossRef]
47. Halliday, M.; Mill, D.; Johnson, J.; Lee, K. Let's talk virtual! Online focus group facilitation for the modern researcher. *Res. Social. Adm. Pharm.* **2021**, *17*, 2145–2150. [CrossRef] [PubMed]

Disclaimer/Publisher's Note: The statements, opinions and data contained in all publications are solely those of the individual author(s) and contributor(s) and not of MDPI and/or the editor(s). MDPI and/or the editor(s) disclaim responsibility for any injury to people or property resulting from any ideas, methods, instructions or products referred to in the content.

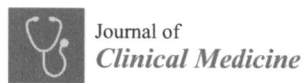 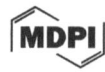

Article

To Be in Pain: Pain Multidimensional Questionnaire as Reliable Tool to Evaluate Multifaceted Aspects of Pain

Giuseppe Forte [1], Francesca Favieri [1,*], Vilfredo De Pascalis [2] and Maria Casagrande [1]

[1] Department of Dynamic and Clinical Psychology and Heath Studies, "Sapienza" University of Rome, 00185 Rome, Italy; g.forte@uniroma1.it (G.F.); maria.casagrande@uniroma1.it (M.C.)
[2] Department of Psychology, "Sapienza" University of Rome, 00185 Rome, Italy; vilfredo.depascalis@uniroma1.it
* Correspondence: francesca.favieri@uniroma1.it

Abstract: Background/Objectives: Pain is a multidimensional experience influenced by sensory, emotional, and cognitive factors. Traditional pain assessments often fail to capture this complexity. This study aimed to develop and validate the Pain Multidimensional Questionnaire (Pa-M-QU), a new self-report tool designed to assess pain catastrophizing, sensitivity, and coping strategies. **Methods:** Two independent samples of Italian-speaking participants, aged 18 and above, were recruited online. The first sample (n = 392; mean age = 29.36) was used for exploratory factor analysis (EFA), and the second sample (n = 123; mean age = 28.0) for confirmatory factor analysis (CFA). Pearson's correlations and convergent validity analyses were conducted. **Results:** From an initial pool of 59 items identified through focus group discussions, 35 items were removed based on reliability analysis. The final 24-item Pa-M-QU features a three-factor structure: catastrophizing, pain sensitivity, and coping with pain. **Conclusions:** The Pa-M-QU offers a rapid, non-invasive assessment that captures the multidimensional nature of pain. It is a starting point to develop tools for both clinical and research settings, aiding in evaluating pain in healthy individuals and predicting acute and chronic pain disorders. Future research should focus on refining the Pa-M-QU for broader clinical applications and exploring its potential to complement or replace traditional pain assessments, thereby advancing pain management and research.

Keywords: pain; questionnaire; validation; pain sensitiveness; factorial structure

Citation: Forte, G.; Favieri, F.; De Pascalis, V.; Casagrande, M. To Be in Pain: Pain Multidimensional Questionnaire as Reliable Tool to Evaluate Multifaceted Aspects of Pain. *J. Clin. Med.* **2024**, *13*, 5886. https://doi.org/10.3390/jcm13195886

Academic Editors: Felice Eugenio Agro and Mariateresa Giglio

Received: 11 August 2024
Revised: 23 September 2024
Accepted: 1 October 2024
Published: 2 October 2024

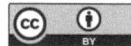

Copyright: © 2024 by the authors. Licensee MDPI, Basel, Switzerland. This article is an open access article distributed under the terms and conditions of the Creative Commons Attribution (CC BY) license (https://creativecommons.org/licenses/by/4.0/).

1. Introduction

"I focus on the pain. The only thing that's real". Johnny Cash

Since its foundation, the International Association for the Study of Pain (IASP) has been faced with the challenge of establishing definitions of pain that needed simultaneously to align with the significant advances in the scientific basis of nociception and to be pragmatic for individuals experiencing a spectrum of pain conditions, from acute to chronic [1]. A first definition considered pain as "an unpleasant sensory and emotional experience associated with actual or potential tissue damage or described in terms of such damage" [1]. However, understanding and explaining the experience of pain is a challenging endeavor, especially when considering its verbal communication [2]. As suggested by Cohen and colleagues, individuals experiencing pain have no direct language in which to express that experience to themselves and others [3]. Consequently, they tend to rely on metaphorical and comparative language. This linguistic issue also arises in clinical practice where, for oversimplification, pain is commonly defined as a correlation between organic damage and pain reported by the patients. This definition excludes cases where there is pain without evident tissue damage. Pain is a more complex phenomenon than the relationship with damage. Pain can be considered, in its nature and intensity, a critical component of conscious experience, affecting thoughts, emotions, and overall mental state. Accordingly, a recent theorization considers pain as a personal distressing experience characterized by multiple sensory, emotional, and cognitive components, which are associated with actual or potential damage [4,5]. In this sense, the subjective experience of pain is relevant because it highlights the existence of interindividual variability in pain perception, even in the case of similar injuries. Furthermore, it marks the influence of biological, psychological, and social factors on pain experience [6].

In this context, the concept of pain sensitivity became central. The substantial interindividual variability in pain sensitivity [7] has received increasing attention in recent years [8]. For example, higher sensitivity was observed in experimental models of induced pain in individuals with chronic pain disorders (e.g., chronic tension-type headache, fibromyalgia, temporomandibular dysfunction, and chronic low back pain), which raises the question of whether the response to an acute nociceptive stimulation may indicate a predisposition to develop a chronic pain disorder or if the reported pain sensitivity in an experimental setting increases during the course of the disease [9]. The assessment of pain sensitivity and its components is of crucial importance in the context of clinical pain conditions. Several tools have been developed for the evaluation of these aspects in conditions beyond the experimental setting. This aspect is relevant because a manipulated setting, such as that of an experimental model, allows for the indirect evaluation of pain perception and sensitivity, which may not fully reflect the ecological and real-life components [10]. Moreover, sensitivity is only one aspect that should be considered. For example, negative cognition related to the experienced pain (i.e., pain catastrophizing) as well as the ability to manage pain would provide a more comprehensive framework for understanding pain experience, given their close relationship to both the perception of the experience and the therapeutic outcomes. These aspects, which have been reported in previous studies in association with pain sensitivity, involve both cognitive and emotional variables that are interrelated. Despite its pervasive impact on quality of life and the significant burden that it places on healthcare systems, a standardized and reliable method for assessing pain sensitivity that encompasses all these aspects is still lacking. This is especially true when considering the trait dimension of pain experience rather than the state dimension that is associated with the current and real state of pain. This gap poses a significant challenge for researchers and clinicians, as it hampers the accurate diagnosis of pain-related conditions, the management of chronic pain, and the evaluation of therapeutic interventions. Notable limitations [11] were reported for current methods of pain assessment, including self-report scales like the Visual Analog Scale (VAS) and the Numeric Rating Scale (NRS), as well as observational tools such as the Behavioral Pain Scale (BPS). The self-reported experience of pain is susceptible to variability and potential bias in pain measurement due to individual differences in perception and expression, as well as the physical condition of the subject during the assessment [12]. Furthermore, these tools often fail to capture the multidimensional nature of pain, which encompasses sensory, emotional, and cognitive components [13]. New tools should be developed and tested to provide a consistent metric that could help in measuring the features that may affect our response and management of pain, both acute and chronic. This would facilitate more rigorous research into pain mechanisms and treatments [14]. This approach would not only improve patient outcomes but also facilitate advancement in our understanding of the underlying mechanisms of pain. The development of a reliable and valid measure of pain sensitivity requires an interdisciplinary approach [15]. The present study aims to develop a brief self-report instrument for the preliminary assessment of multifaceted aspects of pain, as well as for the assessment of pain experience reported in non-current pain. Accordingly, we have devised a self-rating instrument, the Pain Multidimensional Questionnaire (Pa-M-QU), which is based on several dimensions of pain. Following an examination of previous studies on pain and pain sensitivity assessment, we identified three main and recurrent dimensions that comprise pain experience [2,3,5], i.e., (i) catastrophizing pain, which is characterized by an exaggeration and dramatization of pain and pain consequences and management, (ii) pain sensitivity, which is define as a trait rather than state of pain, and (iii) pain interferes and coping, which is defined as the aspects that may justify coping with pain and that are useful for describing the individual's pain experience independently by the state of pain. We selected these aspects because a conceptual model could account for the diverse correlates and the consequences of pain might also be useful in a complex explanatory model in the area of mental health related to pain perception. The instrument was assessed for its reliability and validity. The Pa-M-QU was designed with the specific intention of facilitating a more comprehensive assessment of the multifaceted nature of pain experiences.

2. Materials and Methods

2.1. Participants

Two independent samples were recruited to conduct exploratory factor analysis (EFA) and confirmatory factor analysis (CFA). A first version of the questionnaire for EFA was spread via a KoboToolbox, v. 2.023, survey to collect data from the Italian-speaking population. Only completed surveys were included in the analyses. Participants could withdraw from the study at any time without providing any justification. The sole criterion for inclusion was that the participants be over the age of 18 years. A sample of 362 respondents was included in the analyses (mean age = 29.36; SD = 12.88; female = 72%). CFA was carried out on a sample of 123 respondents (mean age = 28.0; SD = 13.2; female = 74%) who completed a second survey.

2.2. Measures

Demographic Questionnaire. A demographic questionnaire collected information about age, gender, and level of education. Moreover, a survey for CFA, which included preliminary information on the diagnosis of chronic illness and or chronic pain, pharmacological treatment, frequency of nociceptive pain experience, common pain type, and physical extensivity of pain expedite, was collected (see Table 1).

Table 1. Results of EFA and Factor Loading for each item of the scales. Each item is presented in English, with the original Italian version provided in parentheses.

Catastrophizing of Pain		Pain Sensitivity		Pain Interferes and Coping	
KMO = 0.80 Bartlett X^2 = 322; $p < 0.0001$ Cronbach's alpha = 0.70		KMO = 0.83 Bartlett X^2 = 408; $p < 0.0001$ Cronbach's alpha = 0.72		KMO = 0.83 Bartlett X^2 = 532; $p < 0.0001$ Cronbach's alpha = 0.77	
	Factor Loading		Factor Loading		Factor Loading
1. I can tolerate physical pain with relative ease. (Il dolore fisico per me è facilmente sopportabile)	0.48	1. People close to me often tell me that I am too sensitive to pain. (Le persone a me vicine spesso mi dicono che sono troppo sensibile al dolore)	0.34	1. When I experience even minimal pain, it prevents me from performing normal activities of daily living (e.g., doing household chores, going to work, studying, etc.). (Quando provo dolore, anche minimo, questo mi impedisce di svolgere le normali attività di vita quotidiana (ad es. svolgere le attività casalinghe, andare al lavoro, studiare, ecc.)	0.37
2. Immediately upon experiencing even the slightest pain, I contact the physician to request a prescription for pain medication. (Appena inizio ad avvertire anche un minimo dolore, contatto subito il medico affinché possa prescrivermi dei farmaci antidolorifici.)	0.47	2. I think I would be able to have a minor medical procedure (such as a few stitches) without worry. (Penso che riuscirei a sottopormi a una piccola operazione (per es. pochi punti di sutura) senza nessuna preoccupazione.	0.57	2. When I feel physical pain, I am forced to stay in bed all day. (Quando inizio a percepire un dolore fisico, sono costretto a stare a letto per tutta la giornata.)	0.59

Table 1. Cont.

Catastrophizing of Pain		Pain Sensitivity		Pain Interferes and Coping	
KMO = 0.80		KMO = 0.83		KMO = 0.83	
Bartlett X^2 = 322; p < 0.0001		Bartlett X^2 = 408; p < 0.0001		Bartlett X^2 = 532; p < 0.0001	
Cronbach's alpha = 0.70		Cronbach's alpha = 0.72		Cronbach's alpha = 0.77	
	Factor Loading		Factor Loading		Factor Loading
3. When I feel pain, I am forced to think about it all the time. (Quando provo dolore non riesco a fare a meno di pensarci)	0.40	3. It is very easy for me to feel pain. (È molto facile per me sentire dolore).	0.33	3. When I have pain, my focus is on the pain. (Quando provo dolore non riesco a fare a meno di concentrarmi su ciò che mi fa male)	0.55
4. When I feel pain, I feel that this will never end (Quando provo dolore sento che questo non finirà più)	0.43	4. If I happen to bump a part of my body against the edge of a hard surface (like a table), the pain is hardly sustainable for me. (Quando mi capita di urtare una parte del mio corpo contro il bordo di una superficie dura (ad esempio un tavolino) il dolore è per me difficilmente sostenibile)	0.51	4. When I feel pain, I think I can handle it. (Quando provo dolore, penso di poterlo gestire)	0.67
5. When I feel pain, I am always afraid that this will increase (Quando provo dolore ho sempre paura che questo possa aumentare)	0.53	5. I can't eat food that's too hot because it causes me pain. (Non riesco a mangiare cibi troppo caldi perché questo mi crea dolore)	0.57	5. I often think about how pain causes me suffering. (Penso spesso a quanto il dolore mi provochi sofferenza)	0.36
6. When I feel pain, I feel that everything is useless, and the pain is about to overwhelm me (Quando provo dolore sento che tutto sia inutile e che il dolore stia per sopraffarmi)	0.50	6. I experience a lot of pain if I happen to irritate my eyes with soap while taking a bath or shower. (Provo molto dolore se mi capita di irritarmi gli occhi con del sapone mentre mi faccio il bagno o la doccia)	0.47	6. When I feel pain, I cannot concentrate on other activities (Quando provo dolore non riesco a concentrarmi su altre attività)	0.41
7. When I feel pain, it is hard for me to think of anything besides pain. (Quando provo dolore, è difficile per me pensare a qualcosa oltre al dolore)	0.51	7. I feel a lot of pain when I have a muscle cramp. (Provo molto dolore quando ho un crampo muscolare)	0.60	7. When I feel pain, I can't sleep (Quando provo dolore non riesco a dormire)	0.82
8. When I feel pain, I can't think of anything else to overcome it (Quando provo dolore non riesco a pensare ad altro che superarlo)	0.57	8. I experience a lot of pain when I undergo a blood draw (Provo molto dolore quando mi sottopongo a un prelievo ematico)	0.65	8. When I experience pain, I am unable to engage in distracting activities. (Quando provo dolore non riesco a distrarmi)	0.61

Rating scale of the questionnaire was developed on a 5-point scale from 0 (absolutely false) to 4 (absolutely true). KMO: Kaiser–Meyer–Olkin test.

Pain Multidimensional Questionnaire (Pa-M-QU). A focus group comprising clinical psychologists, cognitive psychologists, and neuropsychologist screened 138 items. All items encompass multiple aspects of pain (for a review, see Main, 2016 [16]), with a particular focus on the characteristics of pain sensitivity, pain catastrophizing, and coping with pain. From these items, a pool of 59 items was then selected. Subsequently, according to the hypotheses of this study, the items were divided into three different independent scales, which were subjected to three independent exploratory factor analyses and sensitivity analyses (see Results Section). The participants were instructed to reflect on their own painful experiences and indicate the degree to which they had experienced each of the thoughts or feelings represented by the items when experiencing pain on a 5-point scale from 0 (absolutely false) to 4 (absolutely true). The final version of the questionnaire provided respondents with the following instruction: "The following definitions refer to the condition of physical pain and to experiences or states that may be experienced or felt in life contexts related to pain. Please indicate on a scale from 0 (absolutely false) to 4 (absolutely true) the extent to which each definition represents your individual experience with pain". For further details on the final version of the questionnaire, refer to the Results Section.

Pain catastrophizing. The term "pain catastrophizing" is used to describe a cognitive and emotional process whereby individuals experience a heightened sense of distress and anxiety in response to pain. The Italian validation of the Pain Catastrophizing Scale (PCS) [17] was used to evaluate the extent of catastrophic thinking about pain and to assess the convergent validity of the new questionnaire. The PCS is composed of 13 items on a five-point Likert scale (ranging from 0 = "not at all" to 4 = "all the time"), developed for use with both clinical and non-clinical populations. The Italian version of the scale, which assesses the helplessness, rumination, and magnification dimensions of catastrophizing, has satisfactory psychometric properties, consistent with those observed in the original version (Cronbach's α range for 0.56 to 0.89). The total score ranges from 0 to 52, with higher scores indicating higher levels of pain catastrophizing (Cronbach's α = 0.92).

2.3. Procedure

A two-step data collection process was employed. In the first phase of the study, data were collected to perform an exploratory analysis (EFA) via an online survey (using KoboToolbox), which was disseminated on the main social media platforms to all potential respondents aged 18 and above. A second independent sample of volunteers completed a second survey, employing similar strategies, to confirm the psychometric aspects via confirmatory factor analysis (CFA). To ensure anonymity, no personal information that could allow the identification of participants was collected. The procedure was approved by the ethical committee of the Department of Dynamic and Clinical Psychology and Health Studies ("Sapienza" University of Rome; protocol number: 0001168, 21 August 2019) and conformed to the Helsinki Declaration.

2.4. Data Analysis

A three-step analysis was conducted to test the reliability and validity of the instrument. The focus group identified specific items for each scale of the questionnaire and included them in the appropriate scales. Then, different strategies were adopted to select the most reliable items for each scale [18]: (a) removing items that allow improving Cronbach's alpha, (b) removing any item with an item–total correlation lower than 0.20, and (c) ranking the remaining items with the removal of one of the similar items if they correlate highly (>0.75). This strategy enabled us to maximize homogeneity. Following the removal of items through item analysis, psychometric properties were tested. The factorial structure of the scales was examined using both exploratory (EFA) and confirmatory factor analyses (CFA) for each scale proposed by the focus group (i.e., catastrophizing of pain, pain sensitivity, coping with pain). These analyses were conducted on two independent samples. Oblimin rotation was used in EFAs because there was no reason to assume that the extracted factors were orthogonal. A scree plot was used to determine the number of extracted factors. However, each factor with an eigenvalue equal to or higher than 1 was considered. The number of factors suggested by the EFAs was then cross-validated in the CFA. Maximum likelihood (ML) estimation was employed in the CFA. Goodness-of-fit was assessed using chi-square, the Comparative Fit Index (CFI), the Tucker–Lewis Index (TLI) and the Standardized Root Mean Square Residual (SRMR) and Root Mean Square Error of Approximation (RMSEA) indices. The cut-off criteria for determining the fit indices were based on Kline's suggestions [19].

Pearson's r correlations were calculated to describe the relationship between some of the sample's characteristics (age, years of education) and the Pa-M-QU global score. Moreover, the convergent validity of the construct was evaluated through the correlations with the PCS. Jamovi and open-source software R (R-Core, 2018 [20]) were used to perform statistical analyses in the current study.

3. Results

3.1. Items Analysis

From the pool of 59 items identified by the focus group, 14 were included in the Catastrophizing scale, 21 in the Pain Sensitivity scale, and 17 in the Pain Interferes and

Coping scale. Then, the analysis of reliability indicated that 35 items should be removed. The final scale consists of 24 items.

3.2. Reliability and Exploratory Factor Analysis

Cronbach's alpha coefficients for all scales suggested good reliability (see Table 1). An examination of the scree plots and the percentages of variance accounted for revealed the presence of a single factor for each scale. The KMO and Bartlett's test statistics for each scale indicated that the data were suitable for factor analytic procedures [21] (Table 1).

3.3. Reliability and Confirmatory Factor Analysis

The CFA confirmed the three monofactorial structures with optimal fit indices (see Table 2).

Table 2. Results of CFA.

Catastrophizing of Pain	Pain Sensitivity	Pain Interferes and Coping
CFI = 0.93;	CFI = 0.98;	CFI = 0.98;
TLI = 0.90;	TLI = 0.97;	TLI = 0.97;
SRMR = 0.04;	SRMR = 0.03;	SRMR = 0.03
RMSA = 0.05 (CI 90% = 0.03–0.07)	RMSA = 0.04 (CI 90% = 0.001–0.06)	RMSA = 0.04; (CI 90% = 0.005–0.06)

CFI: Comparative Fit Index; TLI: Tucker–Lewis Index; SRMR: Standardized Root Mean Square Residual; RMSEA: Root Mean Square Error of Approximation.

3.4. Convergent Validity and Inter-Correlations

Person's linear correlations were carried out between the scores of each scale of the Pa-M-QU and the total score of the PCS and the three monofactorial structures positively correlated with each other and with the PCS (see Table 3).

Table 3. Correlations between the Pa-M-QU scales and the PCS.

	Catastrophizing of Pain	Pain Sensitivity	Pain Interferes and Coping
Pain Sensitivity	0.61 **	-	
Coping with Pain	0.77 **	0.67 **	-
PCS	0.63 **	0.62 **	0.78 **

** $p < 0.001$. PCS: Pain Catastrophizing Scale.

3.5. Characteristics of the Sample and Consideration of the Scale

Table 4 shows the main characteristics of the sample considering pain-related information and experience. Table 5 shows quantitative results for each scale and distribution of the scores across the participants.

Table 4. Characteristics of pain in the sample for CFA.

	n (%)
Chronic Pathologies	
Yes	15 (12.2)
No	108 (87.8)
Chronic Pain Diseases	
Yes	1 (0.8)
No	122 (99.2)
Pharmacological Treatment for Pain	
Yes	12 (9.8)
No	111 (90.2)
Frequency of Experiencing Pain	
Almost Never	2 (1.6)
Sometimes	37 (30.1)
Frequently	75 (61.0)
Mostly	9 (7.3)

Table 5. Mean and standard deviation of the scales of the Pa-M-QU, according to the items reported by the CFA.

	Catastrophizing of Pain	Pain Sensitivity	Pain Interferes and Coping	PCS
Mean and Std.Dev.	9.30 (4.37)	7.84 (5.04)	8.52 (5.90)	15.04 (9.58)
Scores over 2 Std.Dev	18.04	17.92	20.32	34.2
% of participant overcoming 2 Std.Dev.	4 (5/123)	4 (5/123)	5 (6/123)	

Here, 2/123 (2% of respondents) overcome the average of the sample of 2 Std.Dev. for all the three scales of the Pa-M-QU.

4. Discussion

Our study was conducted within a framework that emphasized the multifaceted nature of pain. The development of the Pa-M-QU was centered on the attempt to assess this complexity by screening some of the multiple components that may influence the self-reported experience of pain, i.e., catastrophizing of pain, pain sensitivity, and pain interferes and coping. The tool demonstrated good reliability in a three-monofactorial structure. Moreover, the fit indices of the CFA yielded highly satisfactory results, indicating a notable degree of stability of the questionnaire in the analysis of the questionnaire pain components in the general Italian population.

4.1. Pain Sensitivity

Regarding sensitivity, our scale is not intended to quantify localized pain perception, which previous works have assessed in overt states of pain or experimental conditions through self-rating measures of pain (for a review, see [11]). Instead, in accordance with other authors, our scale aims to improve understanding of general pain sensitivity. Two existing questionnaires, the Central Sensitization Inventory (CSI) [22] and the Pain Sensitivity Questionnaire (PSQ) [10], have been previously developed to assist in the identification of pain sensitivity. The authors considered these questionnaires to be relevant for both clinical purposes in chronic pain conditions and for the assessment of pain intensity in healthy subjects experiencing pain-induced conditions. The PSQ addresses different body sites and pain modalities, requesting respondents to imagine pain. The CSI is a self-report measure designed to identify patients with symptoms that may be related to Central Sensitization (e.g., fibromyalgia and temporomandibular disorders). Given that pain sensitivity is not unidimensional [23], we included a scale of pain sensitivity in a questionnaire that globally considers different facets of pain experience. Further, this scale encompasses both bodily (e.g., Item 4: "When I happen to hit a part of my body against the edge of a hard surface (such as a table) the pain is hardly tolerable for me"; Item 5: "I can't eat foods that are too hot because this results in pain") and central dimensions of pain sensitivity (e.g., Item 1: "People who are close to me often tell me that I am too sensitive to pain"; Item 3:"It is very easy for me to feel pain"). The present study thus would suggest the utility of the Pa-M-QU for a rapid assessment of general pain sensitivity. Potential future applications include experimental pain sensitivity assessments in healthy subjects and the prediction of acute pain (e.g., post-operative pain) or chronic pain disorders. It is also relevant to consider pain sensitivity from a cognitive perspective. Indeed, recent findings suggest an increasing association between cognitive aspects and pain sensitivity, pain threshold, and tolerance [24–26]. Cognitive factors, such as attention, expectation, and emotional regulation, can significantly influence pain perception and modulation. A comprehensive assessment of pain sensitivity requires understanding the interplay between cognitive, social, and physiological factors. This understanding can inform the development of more effective pain management interventions. Further studies can adopt this screening tool to detect cognitive and affective components of pain further.

4.2. Catastrophizing Pain

The term "catastrophizing" is used to describe a maladaptive cognitive style involving the occurrence of exaggerated negative thoughts and emotions during actual or anticipated instances of pain. In previous studies, different foci were directed toward the exaggeration or dramatization of threat or pain [27] or pain-related worry and fear, with an inability to divert attention from pain [28]. From these definitions of pain catastrophizing, research focused on developing reliable self-report instruments for the assessment of this phenomenon. For example, the Coping Strategies Questionnaire (CSQ) by Rosentiel and Keefe included a subscale for helplessness and pessimism in pain contexts [29], which was expanded by Sullivan et al. [30] with the Pain Catastrophizing Scale (PCS), assessing helplessness, rumination, and magnification associated with pain experience. Also, our purpose was to improve the measurement of pain catastrophizing, including it in a screening scale for evaluating this construct in the general population incorporating multiple aspects of pain catastrophizing (e.g., Item 3: "When I feel pain, I can't help but think about it."; Item 5: "When I feel pain, I am always afraid that this will increase"; and Item 6: "When I feel pain, I feel that everything is useless and that the pain is about to overwhelm me."). This is crucial because accurately evaluating catastrophizing can inform treatment strategies and improve patient outcomes. By understanding how and to what degree individuals magnify pain threats and experience helplessness, clinicians can adapt their interventions to mitigate these maladaptive thoughts and behaviors, which may ultimately reduce the overall burden of chronic pain. Furthermore, the Pa-M-QU correlates with measures of catastrophizing (i.e., PCS score), thus providing a viable and brief alternative.

4.3. Pain Interferes and Coping

Effective pain management is of crucial importance for improving patient outcomes and quality of life. An understanding of the ways in which individuals manage pain and cope with it is essential and requires a focus on cognitive, emotional, and behavioral strategies. Several well-established questionnaires are used for the evaluation of pain management techniques, each with its particular strengths and limitations. For example, the Coping Strategies Questionnaire (CSQ; [29]) includes subscales for evaluating cognitive and behavioral coping strategies, such as diverting attention, reinterpreting pain sensations, and using positive self-statements. Also, the Pain Self-Efficacy Questionnaire (PSEQ; [31]) measures the confidence of individuals in performing activities despite their pain.

In this regard, the PSEQ shows the impact of self-efficacy on pain management. Nevertheless, despite the usefulness of these questionnaires, several critical aspects highlight the need for developing additional tools. One significant limitation is the inadequate consideration of the social and contextual factors that influence pain management. Pain management is a multifaceted process affected by social support, cultural background, and environmental context. Comprehensive assessment tools that capture these dimensions are essential for holistic pain management [32]. Another critical aspect is the dynamic nature of pain management strategies. Individuals may change their coping strategies over time in response to treatment, psychological state, and social interactions. The development of tools capable of tracking changes in pain management strategies longitudinally and providing real-time data would be helpful in pain studies [33]. The experience of pain may fluctuate depending on the activities in question. For example, an individual with chronic back pain may experience an exacerbation of symptoms following a day spent seated at a desk and a subsequent improvement following a yoga class. A significant limitation of many pain assessments is that they only reflect the intensity of pain experienced or reacted to during the test session without providing any insight into the subject's overall pain experience at the time of the test. In this sense, a functional perspective can be the analysis of individual response to different representations of pain experience from early and less severe forms of pain to generalized response to pain (e.g., Item 1: "When I experience even minimal pain, this prevents me from carrying out normal activities of daily living (e.g., doing household chores, going to work, studying, etc.)."; Item 3: "When I experience pain, I can't help but focus on what hurts."; and Item 6: "When I feel pain, I cannot sleep").

4.4. General Considerations and Limitations

The three-monofactorial structure of this questionnaire, including three independent but correlated scales assessing different features of pain with a limited number of items, represents a key objective achieved by this study. The aim of this study was to develop a brief but reliable screening tool for pain experience, including more than just a single domain, such as pain sensitivity or pain catastrophizing. As previous studies have indicated, a multidimensional analysis of how individuals feel and react to pain is relevant. This analysis should be conducted independently of the current presence of pain, as it is particularly relevant in clinical practice. Although this tool needs further studies to verify its reliability in clinical practice as a possible screening questionnaire for pain sensitivity, and to evaluate a possible cut-off, which is relevant to cover a limitation that emerged in this work, we found promising evidence on pain's multifactorial nature.

The Pa-M-QU, especially as suggested by the CFA, is a valid tool for this purpose but some limitations should be reported. Firstly, the monofactorial structure of the scales included in the questionnaire precludes the possibility of identifying a global score of pain experience on which the scales may converge. However, this is not possible because pain is a multifaceted phenomenon with many definitions and expressions, which makes it challenging to measure its experience as a global and univocal dimension. Another limitation of this study is represented by the absence of a sample of individuals experiencing clinical pain, specifically those with chronic pain conditions. In fact, despite 61 percent of respondents reporting frequent experience of nociceptive pain, only one respondent indicated a diagnosis of a chronic pain condition. The inclusion of such a sample would have provided valuable insights when compared with a group of individuals without chronic pain. This is because the components investigated by the scales may interact bidirectionally with the chronic pain diagnosis. This could result in the exacerbation and perpetuation of the catastrophizing of pain, alteration in its sensitivity, and an influence on its management [34,35]. Further studies should provide the inter-rater and test–retest reliability of the Pa-M-QU in multiple clinical populations. Finally, pain may be a causal factor in the development of negative emotional reactions, such as transient or chronic anger, depression, loneliness, and anxiety [36–38], also in the absence of a chronic clinical condition. This is evidenced by studies that have demonstrated that such emotional states can modify the subjective experience of pain, amplifying the processing of pain signals. Therefore, further studies could also consider these variables in relation to Pa-M-QU scores.

5. Conclusions

The Pa-M-QU has demonstrated a significant and adequate fit index for evaluating some aspects of pain in healthy subjects. If its reliability is confirmed in further study, the Pa-M-QU would provide a rapid, straightforward, and non-invasive approach to assessment with good psychometric propriety. The evidence reported in this work may be extended in the analysis of acute pain and in the investigation of pain sensitivity as a potential risk factor for the development of chronic pain disorders. In line with the cognitive–behavioral model of pain treatment, aspects such as pain experience, coping mechanisms, and other psychological components may highly affect outcomes. Future research should focus on evaluating to extend the research on the Pa-M-QU as an alternative or supplementary method to traditional experimental pain assessments in these contexts. Finally, the goal is to develop a reliable instrument for measuring the efficacy of pain interventions in clinical settings.

Author Contributions: Conceptualization, G.F., V.D.P. and M.C.; methodology, G.F. and F.F.; validation, G.F., F.F. and M.C.; formal analysis, G.F. and F.F.; investigation, G.F. and F.F.; resources, M.C.; data curation, G.F., F.F., V.D.P. and M.C.; writing—original draft preparation, G.F., F.F., V.D.P. and

M.C.; writing—review and editing, G.F., F.F., V.D.P. and M.C.; supervision, M.C.; funding acquisition, M.C. All authors have read and agreed to the published version of the manuscript.

Funding: This research was funded by "Sapienza" University of Rome, "Progetti di Ricerca Grandi"; protocol number: RG1221816C3B6C27.

Institutional Review Board Statement: This study was conducted in accordance with the Declaration of Helsinki and approved by the Ethics Committee of the Department of Dynamic and Clinical Psychology and Health Studies, "Sapienza" University of Rome (protocol code: 0001168, 21 August 2019).

Informed Consent Statement: Written informed consent was obtained from all subjects involved in this study.

Data Availability Statement: Data are available by contacting corresponding author.

Conflicts of Interest: The authors declare no conflicts of interest.

References

1. Ladder, W.A. International Association for the Study of Pain®. 2022. Available online: https://www.iasp-pain.org/ (accessed on 10 August 2024).
2. Raja, S.N.; Carr, D.B.; Cohen, M.; Finnerup, N.B.; Flor, H.; Gibson, S.; Keefe, F.J.; Mogil, J.S.; Ringkamp, M.; Sluka, K.A.; et al. The revised International Association for the Study of Pain definition of pain: Concepts, challenges, and compromises. *Pain* **2020**, *161*, 1976–1982. [CrossRef]
3. Cohen, M.; Weisman, A.; Quintner, J. Pain is not a "thing": How that error affects language and logic in pain medicine. *J. Pain* **2022**, *23*, 1283–1293. [CrossRef]
4. Craig, K.D.; MacKenzie, N.E. What is pain: Are cognitive and social features core components? *Paediatr Neonatal Pain* **2021**, *3*, 106–118. [CrossRef] [PubMed]
5. Williams, A.C.D.C.; Craig, K.D. Updating the definition of pain. *Pain* **2016**, *157*, 2420–2423. [CrossRef]
6. Trachsel, L.A.; Munakomi, S.; Cascella, M. *Pain Theory*; StatPearls Publishing: Treasure Island, FL, USA, 2019.
7. Dionne, R.A.; Bartoshuk, L.; Mogil, J.; Witter, J. Individual responder analyses for pain: Does one pain scale fit all? *Trends Pharm. Sci.* **2005**, *26*, 125–130. [CrossRef]
8. Edwards, R.R.; Sarlani, E.; Wesselmann, U.; Fillingim, R.B. Quantitative assessment of experimental pain perception: Multiple domains of clinical relevance. *Pain* **2005**, *114*, 315–319. [CrossRef]
9. Edwards, R.R. Individual differences in endogenous pain modulation as a risk factor for chronic pain. *Neurology* **2005**, *65*, 437–443. [CrossRef] [PubMed]
10. Ruscheweyh, R.; Marziniak, M.; Stumpenhorst, F.; Reinholz, J.; Knecht, S. Pain sensitivity can be assessed by self-rating: Development and validation of the Pain Sensitivity Questionnaire. *Pain* **2009**, *146*, 65–74. [CrossRef] [PubMed]
11. Breivik, H.; Borchgrevink, P.C.; Allen, S.M.; Rosseland, L.A.; Romundstad, L.; Breivik Hals, E.K.; Stubhaug, A. Assessment of pain. *Br. J. Anaesth.* **2008**, *101*, 17–24. [CrossRef]
12. Jensen, M.P.; Karoly, P. Self-report scales and procedures for assessing pain in adults. In *Handbook of Pain Assessment*; Turk, D.C., Melzack, R., Eds.; The Guilford Press: New York, NY, USA, 2011; Volume 3, pp. 19–44.
13. Melzack, R.; Katz, J. *Wall & Melzack's Textbook of Pain*; Saunders: London, UK, 2013.
14. Colloca, L.; Ludman, T.; Bouhassira, D.; Baron, R.; Dickenson, A.H.; Yarnitsky, D.; Raja, S.N. Neuropathic pain. *Nat. Rev. Dis. Primers* **2017**, *3*, 17002. [CrossRef]
15. Tracey, I.; Mantyh, P.W. The cerebral signature for pain perception and its modulation. *Neuron* **2007**, *55*, 377–391. [CrossRef] [PubMed]
16. Main, C.J. Pain assessment in context: A state of the science review of the McGill pain questionnaire 40 years on. *Pain* **2016**, *157*, 1387–1399. [CrossRef] [PubMed]
17. Monticone, M.; Baiardi, P.; Ferrari, S.; Foti, C.; Mugnai, R.; Pillastrini, P.; Vanti, C. Development of the Italian version of the Pain Catastrophising Scale (PCS-I): Cross-cultural adaptation, factor analysis, reliability, validity and sensitivity to change. *Qual. Life Res.* **2012**, *21*, 1045–1050. [CrossRef] [PubMed]
18. Moshki, M.; Khajavi, A.; Sadeghi-Bazargani, H.; Vahedi, S.; Pour-Doulati, S. Developing Pedestrians' Red-light Violation Behavior Questionnaire (PRVBQ); Assessment of Content Validity and Reliability. *Bull. Emer. Trauma* **2020**, *8*, 98.
19. Kline, R. Exploratory and confirmatory factor analysis. In *Applied Quantitative Analysis in Education and the Social Sciences*; Routledge: London, UK, 2013; pp. 171–207.
20. RStudio Team. *RStudio: Integrated Development for R*; RStudio: Boston, MA, USA, 2020; Available online: http://www.rstudio.com/ (accessed on 10 August 2024).
21. Tinsley, H.E.M.; Tinsley, D.J. Uses of factor analysis in counseling psychology research. *J. Couns. Psych.* **1987**, *34*, 414. [CrossRef]
22. Mayer, T.G.; Neblett, R.; Cohen, H.; Howard, K.J.; Choi, Y.H.; Williams, M.J.; Gatchel, R.J. The development and psychometric validation of the central sensitization inventory. *Pain Pract.* **2012**, *12*, 276–285. [CrossRef]

23. Baamer, R.M.; Iqbal, A.; Lobo, D.N.; Knaggs, R.D.; Levy, N.A.; Toh, L.S. Utility of unidimensional and functional pain assessment tools in adult postoperative patients: A systematic review. *Br. J. Anaesth.* **2022**, *128*, 874–888. [CrossRef]
24. Forte, G.; Giuffrida, V.; Scuderi, A.; Pazzaglia, M. Future treatment of neuropathic pain in spinal cord injury: The challenges of nanomedicine, supplements or opportunities? *Biomedicines* **2022**, *10*, 1373. [CrossRef]
25. Forte, G.; Troisi, G.; Favieri, F.; De Pascalis, V.; Langher, V.; Casagrande, M. Inhibition and heart rate variability in experimentally Induced Pain. *J. Pain Res.* **2023**, *16*, 3239–3249. [CrossRef]
26. Forte, G.; Troisi, G.; Pazzaglia, M.; Pascalis, V.D.; Casagrande, M. Heart rate variability and pain: A systematic review. *Brain Sci.* **2022**, *12*, 153. [CrossRef]
27. Chaves, J.F.; Brown, J.M. Spontaneous cognitive strategies for the control of clinical pain and stress. *J. Behav. Med.* **1987**, *10*, 263–276. [CrossRef]
28. Spanos, N.P.; Radtke-Bodorik, H.L.; Ferguson, J.D.; Jones, B. The effects of hypnotic susceptibility, suggestions for analgesia, and the utilization of cognitive strategies on the reduction of pain. *J. Abn. Psych.* **1978**, *88*, 282. [CrossRef] [PubMed]
29. Rosenstiel, A.K.; Keefe, F.J. The use of coping strategies in chronic low back pain patients: Relationship to patient characteristics and current adjustment. *Pain* **1983**, *17*, 33–44. [CrossRef] [PubMed]
30. Sullivan, M.J.; Bishop, S.R.; Pivik, J. The pain catastrophizing scale: Development and validation. *Psych. Assess.* **1995**, *7*, 524. [CrossRef]
31. Nicholas, M.K. The pain self-efficacy questionnaire: Taking pain into account. *Eur. J. Pain* **2007**, *11*, 153–163. [CrossRef]
32. Cascella, M.; Schiavo, D.; Cuomo, A.; Ottaiano, A.; Perri, F.; Patrone, R.; Migliarelli, S.; Bignami, E.G.; Vittori, A.; Cutugno, F. Artificial Intelligence for Automatic Pain Assessment: Research Methods and Perspectives. *Pain Res. Manag.* **2023**, *28*, 6018736. [CrossRef] [PubMed]
33. Majid, M.; Yahya, M.; Ansah Owusu, F.; Bano, S.; Tariq, T.; Habib, I.; Kumar, B.; Kashif, M.; Varrassi, G.; Khatri, M.; et al. Challenges and Opportunities in Developing Tailored Pain Management Strategies for Liver Patients. *Cureus* **2023**, *15*, e50633. [CrossRef]
34. Janssen, J.; Abou-Assaly, E.; Rasic, N.; Noel, M.; Miller, J.V. Trauma and pain sensitization in youth with chronic pain. *Pain Rep.* **2022**, *7*, e992. [CrossRef]
35. Speed, T.J.; Jung Mun, C.; Smith, M.T.; Khanuja, H.S.; Sterling, R.S.; Letzen, J.E.; Campbell, C.M. Temporal association of pain catastrophizing and pain severity across the perioperative period: A cross-lagged panel analysis after total knee arthroplasty. *Pain Med.* **2021**, *22*, 1727–1734. [CrossRef]
36. IsHak, W.W.; Wen, R.Y.; Naghdechi, L.; Vanle, B.; Dang, J.; Knosp, M.; Louy, C. Pain and depression: A systematic review. *Harv. Rev. Psychiatry* **2018**, *26*, 352–363. [CrossRef]
37. Zhuo, M. Neural mechanisms underlying anxiety–chronic pain interactions. *Trend Neurosci.* **2016**, *39*, 136–145. [CrossRef] [PubMed]
38. McHugh, R.K.; Kneeland, E.T.; Edwards, R.R.; Jamison, R.; Weiss, R.D. Pain catastrophizing and distress intolerance: Prediction of pain and emotional stress reactivity. *J. Behav. Med.* **2020**, *43*, 623–629. [CrossRef] [PubMed]

Disclaimer/Publisher's Note: The statements, opinions and data contained in all publications are solely those of the individual author(s) and contributor(s) and not of MDPI and/or the editor(s). MDPI and/or the editor(s) disclaim responsibility for any injury to people or property resulting from any ideas, methods, instructions or products referred to in the content.

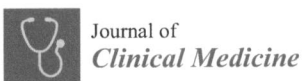

Review

Treating Anxiety-Based Cognitive Distortions Pertaining to Somatic Perception for Better Chronic Pain Outcomes: A Recommendation for Better Practice in the Present Day and the Cyber Age of Medicine

Marcelina Jasmine Silva [1,2,3]

[1] The Focus on Opioid Transitions (FOOT Steps) Program, Walnut Creek, CA 94598, USA; msilva7@touro.edu
[2] The Focus on Opioid Transitions (FOOT Steps) Program, Capitola, CA 95010, USA
[3] Touro University College of Osteopathic Medicine, Vallejo, CA 94592, USA

Abstract: Anxiety-based cognitive distortions pertaining to somatic perception (ABCD-SPs)—primarily catastrophizing, fear avoidance, and kinesiophobia—have been repeatedly linked to worsening chronic, non-cancer pain (CNCP) outcomes of increased disability, amplified pain, ineffective opioid use, and opioid misuse. Several studies have suggested that treating ABCD-SPs can improve pain outcomes, yet identification and targeting of ABCD-SPs are not part of the standard medical pain assessment and treatment plan. Utilizing a narrative review of proposed mechanisms, published patient perspectives, and study correlations connecting these cognitive distortions with CNCP outcomes, an approach for better practice in the delivery of standard medical CNCP care can be deduced and formulated into a Belief and Behavior Action Plan (BBAP) for medical clinicians treating CNCP to implement into initial and maintenance care planning. These recommendations require relatively few resources to implement and have the potential to disseminate more effective CNCP treatment on a large scale now and in the future with the new frontier of cognitive computing in medicine.

Keywords: chronic pain; catastrophizing; fear avoidance; kinesiophobia; opioids; anxiety; depression; artificial intelligence

1. Introduction

Chronic, non-cancer pain (CNCP) is estimated to affect more than 100 million adults in the United States [1,2]. The prevalence of this condition is so high that the Centers for Disease Control have declared that efforts to improve the lives of people with CNCP are a public health imperative [1]. Although an array of medical and interdisciplinary pain specialists exist and are trained to offer their respective complementary, interdisciplinary, pharmaceutical, interventional, and surgical pain treatments, CNCP diagnosis and treatment is most often delivered in the primary care setting [3]. Further, there is a disproportionate amount of high-impact pain (defined as pain severity high enough to interfere with activities of daily living) [4] reported in under-resourced and underserved communities that rely upon primary care for all of their medical needs [5].

Limited specialist involvement is only one of the problems within the current CNCP management climate in the Unites States. Recent CNCP treatment standards have resulted in secondary problems for the individual patient, and in the greater public health and managed care arenas. Such problems include ostracizing patient stigma [6,7], morbidity and mortality from adverse medication effects [8], the rise and reign of the opioid epidemic [9], and skyrocketed costs of managed care [7]. The financial burden of morbidity related to CNCP alone is more than that of the afflictions of heart disease and cancer combined, and has been tallied to be over USD 600 billion per year in the US [2].

Identifying more effective and efficient care approaches for those who suffer with CNCP continues to be a priority need in US healthcare, especially approaches that will

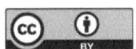

have enduring relevancy as medicine advances into the cyber age. Artificial intelligence (AI) and machine learning (ML) are rapidly being integrated into everyday healthcare experiences in an effort to reduce healthcare costs [10]. Early estimates of the cost-saving impact of AI use in medicine project a spending reduction between 5% and 10%, saving roughly USD 200 billion to USD 360 billion a year [11]. Improved approaches that can be widely disseminated and implemented in low-resourced areas by the first line of medical clinicians assessing and treating CNCP are urgently needed now. The present time also offers a uniquely primed opportunity in medical history to articulate and integrate these improved approaches into conscious computing medical interfaces. Current efforts to this end have the potential to broaden CNCP treatment accessibility, and to have a resounding effect as the basis for the future of CNCP care.

Pain catastrophizing is the most common cognitive distortion seen in patients with chronic pain, and severe catastrophizing is prevalent for nearly 40% of people experiencing CNCP [12,13]. This belief paradigm has been linked to maladaptive behavior and resulting negative CNCP sequelae [14] exemplified by increased disability [15–21], pain intensity [22,23], emotional distress [15], absenteeism [19], and ineffective opioid use [22,24]. Cognitive distortions are defined as faulty or inaccurate thinking, perceptions, or beliefs [14]. Catastrophizing is characterized by the belief that the worst possible outcome will occur when in a setting that may be serious and upsetting but is not necessarily disastrous [9]. Pain catastrophizing is associated with feelings of helplessness to succumb to a catastrophic outcome, as well as hypervigilance to behave in a way that avoids stimuli that may insight discomfort in painful areas [25]. The pervasiveness of this symptomatology within the chronic pain experience—in both frequency and influence—identifies it as a target of high relevance when looking to improve the quality of CNCP treatment.

Opioid misuse and ineffective use (referred to in this manuscript as opioid use that does not facilitate adequate analgesic and functional results, or that does not achieve desired medical results that outweigh the burden of adverse medication effects) are contributors to poor patient outcomes and to larger public health concerns regarding the opioid epidemic [7,8,22–24,26]. The adverse effects of full mu agonist long-term opioid therapy (LTOT) are numerous and well documented, and are amplified if patients fail to experience reasonable functional and analgesic satisfaction from such therapy. Adverse effects that may occur range from immediate [27] (constipation, dry mouth, cognitive impairment, and abuse liability, potentially fatal respiratory depression, and—in the case of methadone—cardiac arrhythmias [28]) to long term and insidious (hypogonadism [29], immune compromise [30–32], and hyperalgesia [33,34]). The chronicity incurred from LTOT use can be burdensome not only to the individual but to society as a whole in the form of increased managed care charges [7], longer lengths of disability [9], and a nationally decreased life expectancy due to fatal opioid-related overdoses [9,35–37].

Due to abundant evidence of the negative synergy between pain-related catastrophizing and the morbidity of CNCP, care planning to assess and address this cognitive distortion should be a foundational part of CNCP treatment now and in future digital and cyber iterations of care delivery. Utilizing a narrative review of proposed mechanisms, published patient perspectives, and study correlations connecting this cognitive distortion with disability, pain levels, and/or ineffective opioid use or misuse, an approach for better practice among pain clinicians can be deduced—one rooted in holistic clinical assessment, abundant patient education, supportive fear quiescence, and therapeutic confrontation of concerns. This new approach requires few resources to implement and has the potential to lead to a more effective CNCP treatment on a large scale now and in the future.

2. Anxiety-Based Cognitive Distortions Pertaining to Somatic Perception (ABCD-SPs)

More than one assessment scale has been validated in an attempt to quantify the clinical significance of the contribution of pain-related catastrophizing to the morbidity of CNCP. Most of the literature examines the relationship between CNCP sequelae as related to this cognitive distortion via one of the following: the Fear-Avoidance Beliefs Questionnaire (FAB), the Pain Catastrophizing Scale (PCS), and the Tampa Scale of Kinesiophobia (TSK) (Table 1). Due to the plurality of these validated tools, this paper has adopted an encompassing term to discuss the significance of their contributions to the morbidity of CNCP: anxiety-based cognitive distortions pertaining to somatic perception (ABCD-SPs).

Table 1. Table of Assessments for anxiety-based cognitive distortions pertaining to somatic perception (ABCD-SPs).

Fear-Avoidance Beliefs Questionnaire—Work and Physical Activity (FAB-W and -PA) [16,22,38]	Two subscales (FAB-W: 0–42; FAB-PA 0–24) in which higher scores indicate more severe pain and disability due to fear-avoidance beliefs about work and physical activity, respectively. Various score thresholds have been documented as associated with clinical relevancy and specific negative chronicity of CNCP. Higher scores have been associated with poor physical and manual therapy results and low return-to-work rates after an injury.
Tampa Scale of Kinesiophobia (TKS) [39,40]	A measure of fear of movement and reinjury. Scores range from 17 to 68, with higher scores being of higher severity. Higher TKS scores have been correlated with higher disability and pain scores.
Pain Catastrophizing Scale (PCS) [24,41,42]	Assesses levels of catastrophizing. In initial validation, a score of 30 or more correlated with high unemployment, self-declared "total" disability, and clinical depression. However, various lower score thresholds have been documented as associated with clinical relevancy for specific negative chronicity of CNCP.

2.1. An Overview of the Role of ABCD-SPs in the Negative Sequelae of CNCP

ABCD-SPs in the setting of CNCP have been repeatedly linked to worsening pain outcomes. Such beliefs, and resulting maladaptive behaviors, have been associated with increased disability [15–21], pain intensity [22,23], emotional distress [15], and absenteeism [19]. Studies have shown that fear of movement and reinjury is a better predictor of self-reported disability and treatment failure than biomedical findings, or pain intensity levels [43–45]. ABCD-SPs have also been documented to affect opioid use in terms of prolonging postoperative use, increasing opioid craving, and contributing to general misuse [22,46–49].

Objectively, improvements in ABCD-SPs can be visualized on functional MRI, and improvements correlate with a decreased pain state [50,51]. Catastrophizing has been shown to recruit regions of the brain that evoke a more intense suffering response to mild pain and an inability to decouple and suppress more intense pain when compared to controls [50]. A successful decrease in catastrophizing via cognitive behavioral therapy (CBT) has been shown on functional MRI to increase the mass of a subject's gray matter—an anatomical substance known to generally be reduced in volume and density in patients who suffer with chronic pain [51].

Perhaps most persuasive regarding the import of ABCD-SPs to CNCP-related morbidity are the studies that suggest treating ABCD-SPs can reverse some of the negative sequelae associated with CNCP. It has been documented that treatment campaigns targeting ABCD-SPs can have a positive effect on the clinical outcomes of somatic symptom prevalence and the length of pain episodes when effectively reduced [38,52–54]. Some studies have shown efficacy in harnessing ABCD-SP education to affect positive change in disability length related to CNCP [52,55].

2.2. ABCD-SP Validated Assessment Tools

2.2.1. The Fear-Avoidance Beliefs Questionnaire (FAB)

The Fear-Avoidance Beliefs Questionnaire (FAB) was designed to measure fear-avoidance beliefs about physical activity and work, and it has strongly correlated these beliefs with work loss and pain [16]. The FAB consists of two subscales: Work (FAB-W) and Physical Activity (FAB-PA). Several studies have investigated the reliability of the FAB for the assessment of fear avoidance among patients with various etiologies of CNCP [38,43,56–58]. A higher FAB score has consistently been shown to correlate with an increased probability of current and future work loss and disability [16,19,20], as well as social withdrawal [21]. While the relationship between an elevated FAB score and increased disability and pain remain correlated, the optimal cut off for determining a significant FAB score in relation to negative chronicity in CNCP has varied with the pain context [16,38,52,56,58–60]. Higher FAB scores have also been shown to significantly predict treatment failure [56,57]. FAB analysis has also been used to determine which clinical interventions have a better likelihood of a successful outcome to decrease patient-reported disability and pain [56–58,61]. An elevated FAB-PA has been shown to be a strong correlate with the inability to cease ineffective LTOT use, more so than morphine equivalent levels and elevated Current Opioid Misuse Measure scores [22].

Several studies have examined the relationship between improved disability and treatment of CNCP via graded exposures that confront fear-avoidant beliefs and behaviors to improve patient self-efficacy and overall disability [62–68]. FAB-targeted educational campaigns have had positive effects on beliefs and clinical outcomes [38,52–54]. Specifically, one study found that successfully lowering fear-avoidance scores in patients with chronic back pain through an educational campaign resulted in subsequently decreased patient reports of disability [52].

2.2.2. The Pain Catastrophizing Scale (PCS)

The PCS determines a patient's level of pain catastrophizing, which is tested by assessing the elements of rumination, magnification, and helplessness [42]. It was created to better assess the relationship between greater pain intensity, negative pain-related thoughts, and greater emotional distress. Higher scores have been shown to significantly correlate with a prediction of pain intensity and emotional distress [42,46,48,55,57,69], and have also been implicated as a risk factor for increased disability length [48,54,58], pain interference [69], and delayed return to work [41]. Preoperative catastrophizing can even predict higher postoperative pain levels and poorer patient-reported postoperative satisfaction following minimally invasive implantations [70] and surgery [71–74]. It has been postulated that this correlation may contribute to increased use of healthcare services, and higher costs to the healthcare system [75].

Targeted therapy to improve catastrophizing has been shown to significantly improve pain outcomes. Pain intensity and disability have been shown to improve with improved PCS scores when maladaptive beliefs were challenged via education and cognitive restructuring, even when such interventions occurred on a purely theoretical and cognitive level [62]. Combined physical therapy (PT) with treatment to minimize psychological catastrophizing barriers improves return-to-work rates [55,66]. One study reported this treatment combination had a 25% higher return-to-work rate than physical therapy alone [55]. PCS score improvements have also been correlated with successful cessation of ineffective LTOT in a population for whom cessation had not been previously achievable through usual care methods [23].

2.2.3. The Tampa Scale of Kinesiophobia (TSK)

The TSK is a measure of fear of movement, injury, or reinjury [39] and has been validated for use in assessing comorbidities of chronic pain from multiple etiologies including backpain, neck pain, lower-limb complaints [76,77], and fibromyalgia [17,39,78]. Increased TSK scores are implicated in decreased physical performance and increased pain intensity, depressive symptoms, pain-related anxiety, and disability [17,79]. Like the PCS and FAB, the TSK has also been associated with ineffective opioid use and misuse [22–24]. Several studies have shown that high kinesiophobia is an independent risk factor for less satisfactory treatment outcomes [76,77,80]. Also, similar to the other ABCD-SP assessments, studies show that targeted cognitive exercises for decreasing kinesiophobia can improve disability [80] and pain [81] when combined with PT better than PT alone [82–84], and can improve pain intensity and physical function [85–87].

3. Pathology of Anxiety-Based Cognitive Distortions Pertaining to Somatic Perception—Proposed Mechanisms

The Fear-Avoidance Belief and Behavior Model (Figure 1) [16,22,56,57] can be visually represented to illustrate the different trajectories for patients with a low fear reaction versus patients with a catastrophizing reaction to their pain experience. The basic tenet of the model is that the way in which pain is interpreted leads to two potential pathways. When pain is perceived as non-threatening, or low threat, patients are likely to behave in a way that confronts real, or perceived, factors that limit their pursuit of meaningful endeavors. This step of confrontation is imperative to eventually overcome those limitations and move toward recovery. In the case of opioid use, the low-fear pathway leads to the use of only a short course of opioids before decreasing use, or ceasing use altogether, thus minimizing or eliminating adverse medication effects [22].

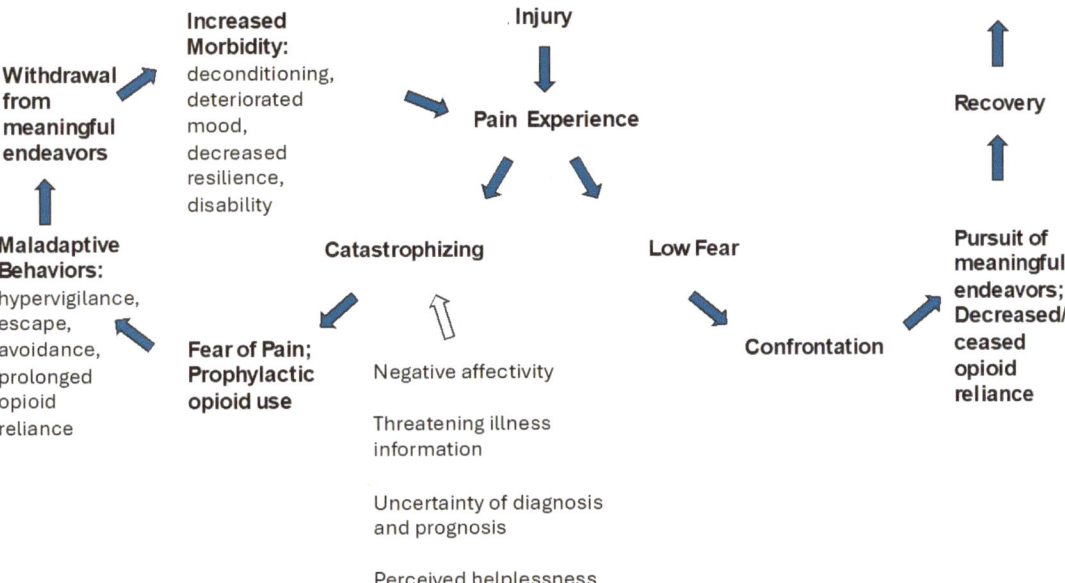

Figure 1. The Fear-Avoidance Belief and Behavior Model [16,22,56,57].

In contrast, a maladaptive cycle may be initiated when pain is perceived through a catastrophizing lens. Catastrophizing entails, among other things, a sense of feeling overwhelmed and powerless to succumb to external, negative forces and experiences [14,62]. This gives rise to pain-related fear, activity avoidance, experience escape (including prolonged opioid use, or misuse), and a negativity-biased hypervigilance. These propensities lead to a progressive withdrawal from meaningful activities and an eventual decline in the physical and emotional capability to access resiliency-building experiences and tools, as previously identified activities of meaning become less attainable. While avoiding the stimuli suspected, or proven, to provoke pain can be adaptive in the acute pain stage, it paradoxically entrenches disability and reliance upon opioids in the subacute and chronic stages of pain. Eventually, the long-term consequences of deconditioning due to disuse [88] and mood deterioration [26,46,89–91] result in increased morbidity [9,36] and decreased ability to recruit and access alternative, resilience-building chronic pain coping mechanisms [22].

Several things can accelerate and amplify the maladaptive cycle. Receiving threatening information about a diagnosis can understandably send a patient's focus to worst-case scenario possibilities. However, uncertainty about a diagnosis can be just as disturbing as threatening information [16,92]. Lack of understanding about the significance of pain is one of the main reasons patients with CNCP go to the Emergency Department (ED) [93]. Negative affectivity and mood disorders, especially anxiety and depression [94,95], coexisting in the patient promote and propel the catastrophizing cycle via a distortion of negativity bias [92]. Also, a history of trauma—even if it precedes the inciting pain event—can propel this maladaptive cycle. A large body of evidence shows that numerous morbidities are accelerated, if not generated, by exposures to adverse childhood experiences (ACEs) [96]. ACE exposure fosters general hypervigilance and negativity bias in daily experiences, resulting in increased catastrophizing and pain-related suffering, among multiple other poor health outcomes [97].

Fear avoidance of movement due to pain, from the stance of learning theory, is a self-perpetuating dynamic in which a small sensory insult—or even the threat of such an insult—can propel anticipation of hyperbolized potential consequences. This anticipation can create—and reinforce—global, habitual, and maladaptive behavior [98], and hinder trials of adaptive activity. If the expectation of catastrophic pain is not confronted, it cannot be disproved. This leads to further maladaptive beliefs and behaviors, deconditioning, and disability [16,22,99,100]. As Vlaeyen et al. state in their paper describing the Fear-Avoidance Model, "Avoidance can be used as a source of information to derive danger, for example: "I am avoiding, therefore there must be danger". The relief that the expected threat did not occur may reinforce avoidance behavior, and hence maintain it [92].

This uninterrupted cyclic dynamic is also applicable in the context of problematic LTOT usage, as many patients associate the action of taking a scheduled opioid with that of prophylactically avoiding or escaping pain. In this pattern, the unadulterated experience of physical nociception is rarely confronted, and patients can spiral deeper into habitual opioid administration, and the possible adverse effects of LTOT use. This dynamic is compounded in opioid use, as it is triply reinforced by dopaminergic incentivization and abrupt abstinence syndrome disincentivization [22].

4. The Call for a Belief and Behavior Action Plan—Theoretical Considerations

Using a reverse-engineering approach to the Fear-Avoidance Belief and Behavior Model, entry points for promoting a more healthful ABCD-SP dynamic in the pursuit of better CNCP outcomes emerge for the pain clinician (Figure 2). The maladaptive cycle is amplified and accelerated when the patient perceives threatening illness information, uncertainty of diagnosis and prognosis, and the perception of powerlessness to succumb to an overwhelming amount of negative sequelae. Thus, initial and ongoing quality communication between a medical clinician and patient about pain etiology, treatment, and prognosis is substantive to the patient's pain experience and treatment outcome potential. Much as the technique of motivational interviewing has been a highly effective and relatively easy treatment technique to disseminate to improve significant measures in multiple chronic physical and psychological diseases [101], there is an opening for a simple—yet sophisticated—change in clinicians' approach to communication with patients experiencing CNCP. Specifically needed is a patient-centered, individualized approach to treatment planning that develops empowered agency and supports therapeutic ABCD-SP identification and confrontation within the scope of patient-identified endeavors of meaning. This treatment approach should address patient-disclosed fears, concerns, and misconceptions in a supportive, open-ended, and ongoing manner. The goal should be to culminate the clinical visit with a patient-specific Belief and Behavior Action Plan (BBAP) for CNCP treatment.

To begin to formulate what a BBAP for CNCP would entail, we must first look beyond data and diagrams to the patient perspective. Numerous reports have documented patients' dislike of—and frank objection to—medical discussions involving "catastrophizing" and like terms. Many patients have called the concept of categorizing their pain experience in this way—as a maladaptive psychological response and behavior—as condescending, and even disenfranchising [102]. Some feel that validated terms currently used within the medical community to assess and address ABCD-SPs carry connotations of "pain shame" [103]. Patients have reported that the label of "catastrophizer" is perceived as unempathetic, stigmatizing, blaming, judgmental, dismissive, minimizing, and weaponizable as a tool to selectively restrict treatment [102]. Some have even contended that the term "catastrophizing" can harbor systemic racism and microaggression, especially when a care plan has failed to distinguish between an ABCD-SP and a generalized stress response to the overall institution of medicine, which for some is a construct fraught with inaccessibility [104], injustice, inequality, and discrimination [105,106]. Some scholars have set about renaming the phenomena of catastrophizing altogether [107]. Despite the mounting volume of these valid and important voices, many feel resigned that stigma will eventually undermine any nomenclature revision attempt to create a patient-centered term used to describe the ABCD-SPs that are a prominent feature in the CNCP experience, and that the stigma lies with the way that people categorize the phenomena [108].

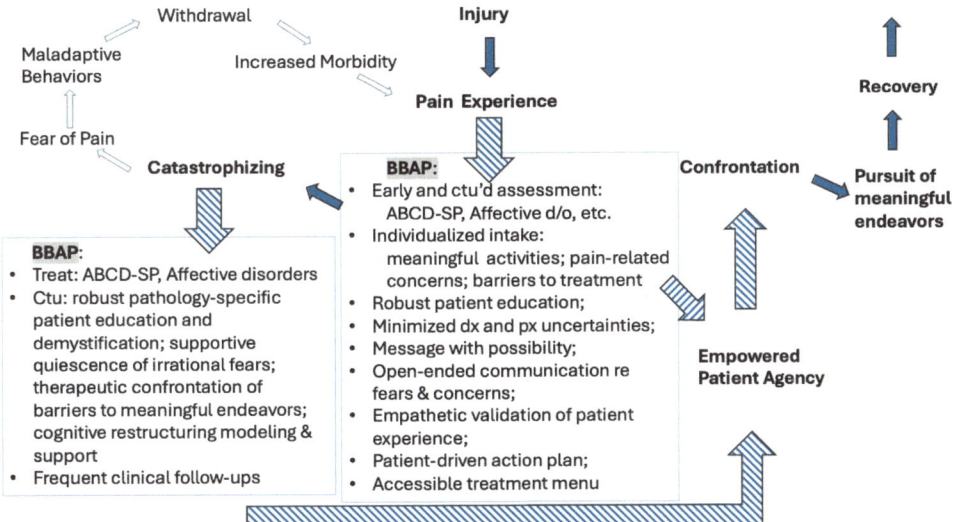

Figure 2. Belief and Behavior Action Plan (BBAP) for CNCP: The better-practice treatment approach is recommended to be inserted by clinicians at specifically identified care plan intervals—indicated by striped arrows—in order to shunt treatment outcomes toward more adaptive outcomes. Abbreviations: ctu/ctu'd = continue/continued; d/o = disorders; dx = diagnostic; px = prognostic.

Semantically, the notion of categorizing ABCD-SPs experienced by so many with CNCP as an added pathology is arguably redundant, if not excessively persecutory—a point that has also been made by patients and advocacy groups [102,103]. Pain is defined as, "An unpleasant sensory and emotional experience associated with actual or potential tissue damage, or described in terms of such damage" [109]. Literally, the emotional experience associated with potential tissue damage is real pain, and consequently, treating the ABCD-SP should be conceived of as providing holistic pain care. Thus, ABCD-SPs should be evaluated for, and addressed, like other associated pain symptoms and features—such as radicular symptoms or paresthesia—in every case of CNCP. Each of these features should be associated with the appropriate treatment line item in a comprehensive care plan, just as a different medication class might be used for neuropathic versus axial pain.

The above discussion begins to illuminate the need for a paradigm shift in the conceptual construct of not only the patient but also the medical provider. First and foremost, patients need to be approached with empathy. While this may seem self-evident, empathy is not a universal patient experience for patients with CNCP, who have likely experienced diagnosis-associated discrimination and marginalization from the general and medical communities [110]. Aside from maintaining the integrity of the Hippocratic Oath, empathy and trust are imperative to bring about fertile ground for true cognitive, physical, and prognostic change for patients with CNCP [111]. While it is difficult for clinicians to focus on a patients' suffering because of the accompanying sense of clinical impotence, and frequent lack of objective solutions, simply witnessing the patient's subjective suffering experience may decrease suffering in itself [112]. Further, in a cohort study that included 1470 adults with chronic lower back pain, physician empathy was more strongly associated with favorable outcomes pertaining to pain, function, and quality of life than were nonpharmacological treatments, opioid therapy, and lumbar spine surgery [113]. This approach bears particular portent in the contemporary environment where many patients have become "opioid refugees" [114–116]. This dynamic is compounded for populations experiencing generalized discrimination due to racial, ethnic, gender, or sexual backgrounds or identities that differ from that of their clinician [117–120].

5. Creating a Belief and Behavior Action Plan—Clinical Considerations

Creating a comprehensive and empathetic BBAP for CNCP begins with thorough information gathering on the part of the clinician. An effective pain evaluation and assessment must go far beyond the "OPQRST" (Onset, Palliation/Provocation, Quality, Radiation, Severity, Timing) that is taught in training. It should include a comprehensive mood assessment as well as a healthcare literacy reconciliation between what the patient has been told and what the patient understands—and believes—about their diagnosis and prognosis. Also included should be a cataloging and recording of the patient's pain-related concerns; a recollection of the patient's similar past experiences; and adequate time to discuss expectations about potentially affected patient-identified meaningful activities. A thorough clinician will also be cognizant of a potential history of actual or perceived disenfranchisement, discrimination, or implicit bias on the part of the medical system toward the patient [119,120]. It has been postulated that inquiring about this last experience openly and early may help avoid repeat offenses on the part of unintending clinicians, and facilitate a more equitable and effective therapeutic relationship [105]. Any, and all, of the factors above—and potentially more—can result in anxiety that can ignite and fuel the fear-avoidance belief and behavior cycle [18,92,105], and each symptom—and associated belief and behavior—should be documented, triaged, and revisited every visit as part of the symptomatology requiring palliative and restorative CNCP care planning.

The goal of the BBAP for CNCP should be to end with a patient-empowering care plan strongly rooted in patient self-efficacy. The patient and clinician should work together to create a menu of patient treatment options, independent of the part of the care plan that relies upon a medical, rehabilitative, or behavioral health clinician, which should not be usurped by the efforts invested in the making of the BBAP. To assign the appropriate patient-administered actions to the BBAP, the patient's descriptions of symptoms should be cataloged in terms of levels of severity and physical and emotional distress, along with an associated detailing of the default patient behavioral reaction to these symptoms. These scenarios should then be examined individually and optimized when effective, and gently challenged and replaced when they have been ineffective in the past. The end result is that the patient should leave every clinical visit with an approachable and navigable treatment action plan documenting several ways in which they have control and agency to access pressure release valves for the full spectrum of pain flare severity that may occur. These BBAP interventions should include features that are accessible when in and out of the home, and which represent treatment modalities from a variety of dimensions, including behavioral, physical, social, medical, spiritual, and occupational.

6. Creating a Belief and Behavior Action Plan—Recommendations and Practical Considerations

The following is a synopsis of clinical and practical better-practice recommendations to create a BBAP for CNCP, derived from current evidence (Figure 2):

I. Utilize standardized assessments and short-answer questionnaires upon initial evaluation, and periodically in follow-up, to assess and monitor the potential for ABCD-SPs to interfere with rehabilitation:
   a. Standardized assessments:
      i. Assess for high ABCD-SP via one of the frequently used, validated assessments (FAB, PCS, or TSK) [16,22,24,42,57,92,102].
      ii. Assess for mood disorders that can be independent risk factors for ABCD-SP escalations, especially depression and anxiety [22,24,94,95].
      iii. Offer a validated instrument assessing perceived discrimination and/or trauma history [96,105,121].
   b. Short-answer questionnaires to catalog patients' perceptions regarding the following:
      i. Concerns and fears related to their pain or treatment [57,92].
      ii. Perceived barriers to accessing helpful pain treatment [104,122].
      iii. Activities of meaning, which can help accomplish the following goals:
         1. Lay the groundwork to create an individualized care plan.
         2. Strategize support and diminish negative impact on these activities.
         3. Better motivate patient participation [24].
         4. Apply to cognitive restructuring exercises [57,92].
         5. Aid in decreasing treatment plans rooted in implicit bias for populations heralding from a race, culture, gender, sexuality, or age group that differs from the provider [123].
      iv. Satisfaction with their current and previous pain treatment, e.g., which interventions, medications, therapies, etc., have been perceived as the most helpful, which were the most problematic and why [22,24].

II. Implement an intentional BBAP inquiry and communication strategy and style in the clinical visit:
   a. Invest heavily in the first visit by performing a deep exploration and inquiry into the patient's pain experience and their current pain-related beliefs and resulting behaviors (much of which can be initiated via the short-answer format suggested above) [101].
   b. Demonstrate empathy [113,124].
   c. Use validating active listening, which has been shown to increase patient adherence to care planning [125].
   d. Lean into, and address head-on, patient's accounts of suffering and fear in the clinical setting to achieve the following:
      i. Dispel the ability of these sentiments to hijack adaptive recovery processes when the patient ruminates alone [93].
      ii. Decrease the suffering of invisibility that patients with CNCP often face. While it is difficult for clinicians to focus on a patients' suffering because of the accompanying sense of clinical impotence, and frequent lack of objective solutions, it has been suggested that simply witnessing the patient's subjective suffering experience may decrease the severity of the same suffering [112].
   e. Be cognizant of both the implicit and explicit messaging inherent in communications imparted by the clinician to the patient about diagnosis and prognosis. Positive self-perceptions and health-related optimism correlate with improved pain suffering, pain-related disability [92,95,97,126–128], and even increased longevity [129]. When possible and appropriate, choose vocabulary and descriptors that de-escalate the patient's perceived threat of nociceptive input, and which highlight functional and meaningful possibility.

- f. Message with mindfulness of potential emotional trauma-affected hyperarousal and increased sensitivity to pain [130].
- g. Temper areas of diagnostic uncertainty and remaining investigation with clear descriptions of the investigative next steps, while explicitly outlining the activities that are safe to pursue in the interim [57,92].
- h. Increase healthcare literacy and promote pathology demystification:
    - i. Ask patients to paraphrase their understanding of their injury, pain, and pathology. Note terminology used and connect medical terminology to patient's perceptions and descriptions to promote demystification [57,92]. Correct misconceptions while maintaining patient-generated frame of reference and terminology, when appropriate.
    - ii. Consider inviting a call and paraphrased repeat opportunity between the clinician and the patient to improve comprehension of pathology and related care plan.
    - iii. Assuming the standard use of language interpreters to bridge translation barriers, also employ visual aids and physical models to engage multiple patient learning style preferences to explain not only pathology but also the mechanisms of pain symptomatology in an effort to demystify and decrease anxiety related to somatic perceptions.
- i. Orient to when fear of catastrophe is warranted.
    - i. Debrief previous urgent, or emergent, clinical visits to seek pain treatment. Discuss causational factors and a care plan for future episodes in the form of improved medication organization, strategized BBAP interventions, a change in medication regimen for more effective analgesia, a change in formulary or treatment type for improved access, etc.
    - ii. Orient to "red flag" signs and symptoms that medically warrant emergent attention and educate to differentiate from chronic, stable stimuli.

III. BBAP components should include the following:
- a. Cultivate an empowering, patient-driven action plan (to complement the encompassing medical and interdisciplinary treatment plan) containing the following elements:
    - i. Facilitation of a menu of active, self-care options to address various pain levels and flares. Include features accessible in and out of the home, and which represent treatment modalities from a variety of psychosocial domains: behavioral, physical, social, medical, spiritual, occupational, etc.
    - ii. Minimized barriers and avoidance of the "gate keeper" perception of clinical treatment options where possible—within the confines of evidence-based care—which inherently promote a role of helplessness, perceptions of scarcity, and an external locus of control. Instead, promote care planning options that are autonomously administered and are rooted in patient agency, including the following:
        1. Prescribe medications and self-administered devices that can be safely used as needed for specific indications [22,24].
        2. Orient to a home exercise program that de-amplifies pain suffering via an assortment of activities rooted in multiple psychosocial domains [62].
        3. Plan a care regimen creatively, and individually, around potential socioeconomic barriers to treatment access (transportation, mobility, coverage, cost, etc.) by choosing generic medications, refilling for longer durations, providing telemedicine, etc. [131].

b. Use a patient-controlled mechanism to maintain a continuous log of worries and fears associated with pain symptomatology in the CBT-based exercise of cognitive restructuring [132], which has been shown to be helpful for CNCP outcomes even when self-administered [133,134].

c. Carry out frequent routine clinical follow-ups to consistently support the ABCD-SP cognitive restructuring process in the model of treatment recommended for somatoform disorders [135,136], as catastrophizing and somatoform disorders share many clinical features and frequently co-exist [137].

7. Discussion

7.1. Anticipated Objections to BBAP Implementation—Financial Disincentivization

Clinical efficiency and the demands of billable time have been cited as a barriers to more encompassing CNCP care planning [138]. Cultivating a BBAP that fosters patient empowerment and autonomy, and adequately addresses patient-specific healthcare literacy and individualized concerns, requires time and resources that clinicians are often disincentivized to employ during their limited billable minutes. However, this nearly ubiquitous impediment of limited clinical facetime stems from an unbalanced and short-sighted cost–benefit equation. A minimally invasive surgery or procedure may take as much time—and reimburse exponentially better—than a thorough face-to-face conversation with a patient seeking palliation for a pain complaint. Similarly, a clinician can complete several billable prescription refill visits in the time it takes to thoroughly communicate with one patient. The ironic counterproductivity of this dynamic is illustrated by research that suggests that patients will be less satisfied with the outcomes of these same interventions [70], surgeries [71–74], and medications [22] if their ABCD-SPs are not adequately addressed first. Thus, a dynamic of high prescription and procedural implementation has been created and perpetuated, often accompanied by dissatisfaction with treatment outcomes. Ultimately, attempts to conserve clinician resources by delaying holistic pain care rooted in emotional resiliency building, stress reduction, and health education in a human-centered approach has resulted in higher overall managed care costs regarding patients with CNCP [7].

Further, much like incorporating motivational interviewing has been found to have a favorable cost–benefit ratio for treatment outcomes of various etiologies in multiple medical settings [139,140], implementing a potentially more efficacious treatment that simply involves a change in communication strategy, such as a BBAP, requires very little resource investment. Considering the current financial and opportunity costs inherent in the standard care approach to treating CNCP in the US, incorporating a BBAP would only require a relatively small investment in medical clinician training hours. Additionally, a BBAP is a care planning strategy that can equally serve populations that are abundantly resourced or under-resourced, alike, potentially bridging some of the inequities currently seen in populations who disproportionately suffer with high-impact CNCP.

7.2. Anticipated Objections to BBAP Implementation—Scope of Practice Creep

The significant role that psychologists and allied professionals contribute to the myriad facets of CNCP treatment via an interdisciplinary care plan is not meant to be replaced, or undermined, by the recommendation for the pain clinician to create a BBAP. In fact, most studies have shown greatest success when addressing ABCD-SPs via multimodal efforts, especially when including physical therapies, CBT, and/or acceptance and commitment therapy [141]. However, CNCP is frequently associated with—and compounded by—limited access to such resources [131]. Thus, the recommendation to implement a BBAP for CNCP is non-exclusive in regard to behavioral health specialist collaboration, and is designed to benefit from the more in-depth and expansive behavioral health treatment that a specialist in that field can provide, if accessible.

Further, a BBAP has the potential to champion interdisciplinary care offered by available behavioral health clinicians. Patient buy-in of behavioral health treatment is often improved when medical clinicians specifically endorse and provide education to help patients better understand the far-reaching implications of behavioral health efforts in their medical treatment and recovery [142]. Also, removing some of the figurative partition siloing the physical from the psychological symptoms and treatment of CNCP can help decrease the stigma of psychological suffering related to CNCP, which has the potential to improve outcomes, as described above.

7.3. BBAP Relevance and Potential: Medicine in the Cyber Age

Artificial intelligence (AI) and machine learning (ML) are rapidly being integrated into everyday healthcare experiences in an effort to reduce healthcare costs [10,11]. Harnessing the potential for improved treatment outcomes via a BBAP-informed AI algorithm could augment healthcare savings even further in the costly field of CNCP by enhancing outcome improvement and increasing spending returns, not just reducing healthcare costs. It is imperative that the medical community lays a foundation of effective and human-centered design into patient interfaces, as they may be programed into conscious computing perpetuity. This is a uniquely primed time in history to consider which strategies are working well to deliver preferred medical outcomes, and which need improvement, as we enter this new cyber frontier of medical practice.

The integration of cognitive computing in healthcare presents an interesting potential for advancement in crafting personalized medical and psychological treatment plans, and to improve patient and clinician satisfaction [10,11]. Artificial intelligence (AI) can employ algorithms to process standardized screening assessments and generate comprehensive treatment strategies that address both medical and psychological aspects of patient care. AI algorithms are already supporting clinical decision making in many medical disciplines [143] and have the potential to streamline the holistic assessment recommended in a BBAP to drive more efficient, effective, and individualized care planning. Natural language processing (NLP), machine learning (ML), and specified design principles have the potential to customize the patient interface while adhering to a consistent communication strategy, congruent with that of a BBAP. All of this has the potential to be available to adapt and respond with the real-time needs of the patient.

Once again, one can look to the example of motivational interviewing to envision the potential of BBAP propagation in the cyber age. AI is being successfully used to train physicians to better demonstrate the technique of motivational interviewing in their patient visits [144]. This suggests that AI may be a promising avenue of disseminating continuing medical education for BBAP implementation. Programmers and AI developers are also harnessing AI, NLP, and ML to perform digital and AI-assisted motivational interviewing [145–147]. It follows that these same cyber techniques could successfully generate and support the individualized, human-centered design of a BBAP.

8. Limitations

The aim of this article is to utilize a narrative review of currently available evidence and observations to recommend a better-practice approach to CNCP care, as chronic pain management is an area identified as being in great need of improvement in terms of related public health, individual medical outcomes, and national financial impact. A recommendation for better practice based on such observations has the inherent limitations of not being directly tested or proven as an intervention, as would be the gold standard. Also inherent in the limitations of validating the benefits of a BBAP is the fact that the nature of a BBAP is highly individualized so as to be nearly universal in its applicability. Standardizing a randomized controlled trial for such an approach would be challenging. Future research is encouraged in the form of initial case studies and pilot programing to better understand the impact possibilities of BBAP implementation.

9. Conclusions

Due to abundant evidence of the negative synergy between ABCD-SPs and worsening sequelae of CNCP, care planning to assess and address ABCD-SPs via a BBAP should be a foundational part of CNCP treatment. While a multidisciplinary approach is ideal, the role of the individual pain clinician is poised to have a profound effect on a patient's formation—and either maintenance or dissipation—of ABCD-SP, which is a determinant of CNCP severity and morbidity. CNCP is a multifaceted bio-psycho-social diagnosis, and treatment requires a complex, holistic approach. Maximizing every treatment avenue available is imperative to improve CNCP-related outcomes on the individual and public health fronts. Utilizing a better-practice BBAP is a low-risk, low-investment intervention that currently has the potential to yield high gains on individual and public health levels, and is a strategy that also may be of high relevance in the cyber age of medicine.

Funding: This research received no external funding.

Conflicts of Interest: The author declares no conflicts of interest.

References

1. Rikard, S.M. Chronic Pain Among Adults—United States, 2019–2021. *MMWR Morb. Mortal. Wkly. Rep.* **2023**, *72*, 379–385. [CrossRef] [PubMed]
2. Smith, T.J.; Hillner, B.E. The Cost of Pain. *JAMA Netw. Open* **2019**, *2*, e191532. [CrossRef] [PubMed]
3. Von Korff, M.; Scher, A.I.; Helmick, C.; Carter-Pokras, O.; Dodick, D.W.; Goulet, J.; Hamill-Ruth, R.; LeResche, L.; Porter, L.; Tait, R.; et al. United States National Pain Strategy for Population Research: Concepts, Definitions, and Pilot Data. *J. Pain.* **2016**, *17*, 1068–1080. [CrossRef] [PubMed]
4. Bifulco, L.; Anderson, D.R.; Blankson, M.L.; Channamsetty, V.; Blaz, J.W.; Nguyen-Louie, T.T.; Scholle, S.H. Evaluation of a Chronic Pain Screening Program Implemented in Primary Care. *JAMA Netw. Open* **2021**, *4*, e2118495. [CrossRef] [PubMed]
5. Dahlhamer, J.; Lucas, J.; Zelaya, C.; Nahin, R.; Mackey, S.; DeBar, L.; Kerns, R.; Von Korff, M.; Porter, L.; Helmick, C. Prevalence of Chronic Pain and High-Impact Chronic Pain Among Adults—United States, 2016. *MMWR Morb. Mortal. Wkly. Rep.* **2018**, *67*, 1001–1006. [CrossRef]
6. MPR. Opioid Refugees: Patients Adrift in Search of Pain Relief. Available online: https://www.empr.com/home/mpr-first-report/painweek-2013/opioid-refugees-patients-adrift-in-search-of-pain-relief/ (accessed on 6 May 2020).
7. Silva, M.J.; Kelly, Z. The Escalation of the Opioid Epidemic Due to COVID-19 and Resulting Lessons About Treatment Alternatives. *Am. J. Manag. Care* **2020**, *26*, e202–e204. [CrossRef]
8. Silva, M.J.; Coffee, Z.; Goza, J.; Rumril, K. Microinduction to Buprenorphine from Methadone for Chronic Pain: Outpatient Protocol with Case Examples. *J. Pain Palliat. Care Pharmacother.* **2022**, *36*, 40–48. [CrossRef]
9. Dowell, D.; Haegerich, T.M.; Chou, R. CDC Guideline for Prescribing Opioids for Chronic Pain—United States, 2016. *MMWR Recomm. Rep.* **2016**, *65*, 1624–1645. Available online: https://www.cdc.gov/mmwr/volumes/65/rr/rr6501e1.htm (accessed on 20 September 2024). [CrossRef]
10. Davenport, T.; Kalakota, R. The potential for artificial intelligence in healthcare. *Future Healthc. J.* **2019**, *6*, 94–98. [CrossRef]
11. Sahni, N.; Stein, G.; Zemmel, R.; Cutler, D.M. *The Potential Impact of Artificial Intelligence on Healthcare Spending 2023*; National Bureau of Economic Research: Cambridge, MA, USA, 2023; Available online: https://papers.ssrn.com/abstract=4334926 (accessed on 10 September 2024).
12. Alcon, C.; Bergman, E.; Humphrey, J.; Patel, R.M.; Wang-Price, S. The Relationship between Pain Catastrophizing and Cognitive Function in Chronic Musculoskeletal Pain: A Scoping Review. *Pain Res. Manag.* **2023**, *2023*, 5851450. [CrossRef]
13. Brouwer, B.; Waardenburg, S.; Jacobs, C.; Overdijk, M.; Leue, C.; Köke, A.; Kuijk, S.V.; Van Kleef, M.; Van Zundert, J.; De Meij, N. Biopsychosocial baseline values of 15,000 patients suffering from chronic pain: Dutch DataPain study. *Reg. Anesth. Pain Med.* **2020**, *45*, 774–782. [CrossRef] [PubMed]
14. APA Dictionary of Psychology. Available online: https://dictionary.apa.org/ (accessed on 19 July 2024).
15. PCSManual_English.pdf. Available online: http://sullivan-painresearch.mcgill.ca/pdf/pcs/PCSManual_English.pdf (accessed on 8 May 2020).
16. Waddell, G.; Newton, M.; Henderson, I.; Somerville, D.; Main, C.J. A Fear-Avoidance Beliefs Questionnaire (FABQ) and the role of fear-avoidance beliefs in chronic low back pain and disability. *Pain* **1993**, *52*, 157–168. [CrossRef] [PubMed]
17. Neblett, R.; Hartzell, M.M.; Mayer, T.G.; Bradford, E.M.; Gatchel, R.J. Establishing clinically meaningful severity levels for the Tampa Scale for Kinesiophobia (TSK-13). *Eur. J. Pain* **2016**, *20*, 701–710. [CrossRef] [PubMed]
18. Sullivan, M.J.L.; Martel, M.O.; Tripp, D.; Savard, A.; Crombez, G. The relation between catastrophizing and the communication of pain experience. *Pain* **2006**, *122*, 282–288. [CrossRef] [PubMed]
19. Linton, S.J.; Shaw, W.S. Impact of Psychological Factors in the Experience of Pain. *Phys. Ther.* **2011**, *91*, 700–711. [CrossRef]
20. Waddell, G.; Somerville, D.; Henderson, I.; Newton, M. Objective clinical evaluation of physical impairment in chronic low back pain. *Spine* **1992**, *17*, 617–628. [CrossRef]
21. Philips, H.; Jahanshahi, M. The components of pain behaviour report. *Behav. Res. Ther.* **1986**, *24*, 117–125. [CrossRef]

22. Silva, M.J.; Coffee, Z.; Ho Alex Yu, C.; Martel, M.O. Anxiety and Fear Avoidance Beliefs and Behavior May Be Significant Risk Factors for Chronic Opioid Analgesic Therapy Reliance for Patients with Chronic Pain—Results from a Preliminary Study. *Pain Med.* **2021**, *9*, 2106–2116. [CrossRef]
23. Silva, M.J.; Coffee, Z.; Yu, C.H.A.; Hu, J. Changes in Psychological Outcomes after Cessation of Full Mu Agonist Long-Term Opioid Therapy for Chronic Pain. *J. Clin. Med.* **2023**, *12*, 1354. [CrossRef]
24. Silva, M.J.; Coffee, Z.; Yu, C.H. Prolonged Cessation of Chronic Opioid Analgesic Therapy: A Multidisciplinary Intervention. *Am. J. Manag. Care* **2022**, *28*, 60–65. [CrossRef]
25. Borkum, J. Maladaptive Cognitions and Chronic Pain: Epidemiology, Neurobiology, and Treatment. *J. Ration.-Emotive Cogn.-Behav. Ther.* **2010**, *28*, 4–24. [CrossRef]
26. Silva, M.J.; Coffee, Z.; Yu, C.H. The Correlation of Psychological Questionnaire Response Changes after Cessation of Chronic Opioid Analgesic Therapy in Patients with Chronic Pain. 2020; *Manuscript Submitted for Publication*.
27. National Institute on Drug Abuse. Prescription Opioids DrugFacts. Available online: https://www.drugabuse.gov/publications/drugfacts/prescription-opioids (accessed on 19 October 2020).
28. Wedam, E.F.; Bigelow, G.E.; Johnson, R.E.; Nuzzo, P.A.; Haigney, M.C.P. QT-interval effects of methadone, levomethadyl, and buprenorphine in a randomized trial. *Arch. Intern. Med.* **2007**, *167*, 2469–2475. [CrossRef] [PubMed]
29. Antony, T.; Alzaharani, S.Y.; El-Ghaiesh, S.H. Opioid-induced hypogonadism: Pathophysiology, clinical and therapeutics review. *Clin. Exp. Pharmacol. Physiol.* **2020**, *47*, 741–750. [CrossRef] [PubMed]
30. Eisenstein, T.K.; Rogers, T.J. Drugs of Abuse. In *Neuroimmune Pharmacology*; Ikezu, T., Gendelman, H.E., Eds.; Springer International Publishing: Cham, Switzerland, 2017; pp. 661–678. [CrossRef]
31. Lei, L.; Gong, X.; Wen, C.; Zeng, S.; Lei, Q. Research progress on the effects of opioids on the immune system. *Trends Anaesth. Crit. Care* **2024**, *57*, 101372. [CrossRef]
32. NORCO® Hydrocodone Bitartrate and Acetaminophen Tablet. Available online: https://www.accessdata.fda.gov/drugsatfda_docs/label/2019/040099s023lbl.pdf (accessed on 20 September 2024).
33. Chu, L.F.; Angst, M.S.; Clark, D. Opioid-induced hyperalgesia in humans: Molecular mechanisms and clinical considerations. *Clin. J. Pain* **2008**, *24*, 479–496. [CrossRef]
34. Lee, M.; Silverman, S.M.; Hansen, H.; Patel, V.B.; Manchikanti, L. A comprehensive review of opioid-induced hyperalgesia. *Pain Physician* **2011**, *14*, 145–161. [CrossRef]
35. Rudd, R.A. Increases in Drug and Opioid-Involved Overdose Deaths—United States, 2010–2015. *MMWR Morb. Mortal. Wkly. Rep.* **2016**, *65*, 1445–1452. [CrossRef]
36. Xu, J. Mortality in the United States, 2018. *NCHS Data Briefs* **2020**, *8*, 355.
37. National Institute on Drug Abuse. Overdose Death Rates. Available online: https://www.drugabuse.gov/drug-topics/trends-statistics/overdose-death-rates (accessed on 9 June 2021).
38. George, S.Z.; Fritz, J.M.; Bialosky, J.E.; Donald, D.A. The effect of a fear-avoidance-based physical therapy intervention for patients with acute low back pain: Results of a randomized clinical trial. *Spine (Phila Pa 1976)* **2003**, *28*, 2551–2560. [CrossRef]
39. Miller, R.P.; Kori, S.H.; Todd, D.D. The Tampa Scale: A Measure of Kinisophobia. *Clin. J. Pain* **1991**, *7*, 51. [CrossRef]
40. Hudes, K. The Tampa Scale of Kinesiophobia and neck pain, disability and range of motion: A narrative review of the literature. *J. Can. Chiropr. Assoc.* **2011**, *55*, 222–232. [PubMed]
41. Adams, H.; Ellis, T.; Stanish, W.D.; Sullivan, M.J.L. Psychosocial factors related to return to work following rehabilitation of whiplash injuries. *J. Occup. Rehabil.* **2007**, *17*, 305–315. [CrossRef] [PubMed]
42. Sullivan, M.J.L.; Bishop, S.R.; Pivik, J. The Pain Catastrophizing Scale: Development and Validation. *Psychol. Assess.* **1995**, *7*, 524–532. [CrossRef]
43. Vlaeyen, J.W.; Kole-Snijders, A.M.; Rotteveel, A.M.; Ruesink, R.; Heuts, P.H. The role of fear of movement/(re)injury in pain disability. *J. Occup. Rehabil.* **1995**, *5*, 235–252. [CrossRef]
44. Crombez, G.; Vlaeyen, J.W.; Heuts, P.H.; Lysens, R. Pain-related fear is more disabling than pain itself: Evidence on the role of pain-related fear in chronic back pain disability. *Pain* **1999**, *80*, 329–339. [CrossRef] [PubMed]
45. Wertli, M.M.; Eugster, R.; Held, U.; Steurer, J.; Kofmehl, R.; Weiser, S. Catastrophizing—A prognostic factor for outcome in patients with low back pain: A systematic review. *Spine J.* **2014**, *14*, 2639–2657. [CrossRef]
46. Helmerhorst, G.T.T.; Vranceanu, A.-M.; Vrahas, M.; Smith, M.; Ring, D. Risk Factors for Continued Opioid Use One to Two Months after Surgery for Musculoskeletal Trauma. *JBJS* **2014**, *96*, 495–499. [CrossRef] [PubMed]
47. Arteta, J.; Cobos, B.; Hu, Y.; Jordan, K.; Howard, K. Evaluation of How Depression and Anxiety Mediate the Relationship between Pain Catastrophizing and Prescription Opioid Misuse in a Chronic Pain Population. *Pain Med.* **2016**, *17*, 295–303. [CrossRef] [PubMed]
48. Martel, M.O.; Jamison, R.N.; Wasan, A.D.; Edwards, R.R. The Association Between Catastrophizing and Craving in Patients with Chronic Pain Prescribed Opioid Therapy: A Preliminary Analysis. *Pain Med.* **2014**, *15*, 1757–1764. [CrossRef]
49. Martel, M.O.; Wasan, A.D.; Jamison, R.N.; Edwards, R.R. Catastrophic thinking and increased risk for prescription opioid misuse in patients with chronic pain. *Drug Alcohol. Depend.* **2013**, *132*, 335–341. [CrossRef]
50. Seminowicz, D.A.; Davis, K.D. Cortical responses to pain in healthy individuals depends on pain catastrophizing. *Pain* **2006**, *120*, 297–306. [CrossRef] [PubMed]

51. Seminowicz, D.A.; Shpaner, M.; Keaser, M.L.; Krauthamer, G.M.; Mantegna, J.; Dumas, J.A.; Newhouse, P.A.; Filippi, C.G.; Keefe, F.J.; Naylor, M.R. Cognitive-behavioral therapy increases prefrontal cortex gray matter in patients with chronic pain. *J. Pain* **2013**, *14*, 1573–1584. [CrossRef] [PubMed]
52. Burton, A.K.; Waddell, G.; Tillotson, K.M.; Summerton, N. Information and advice to patients with back pain can have a positive effect. A randomized controlled trial of a novel educational booklet in primary care. *Spine* **1999**, *24*, 2484–2491. [CrossRef]
53. Vlaeyen, J.W.S.; Morley, S. Cognitive-behavioral treatments for chronic pain: What works for whom? *Clin. J. Pain* **2005**, *21*, 1–8. [CrossRef]
54. Jellema, P.; van der Horst, H.E.; Vlaeyen, J.W.S.; Stalman, W.A.B.; Bouter, L.M.; van der Windt, D.A.W.M. Predictors of Outcome in Patients with (Sub)Acute Low Back Pain Differ across Treatment Groups. *Spine* **2006**, *31*, 1699–1705. [CrossRef] [PubMed]
55. Sullivan, M.J.L.; Adams, H.; Rhodenizer, T.; Stanish, W.D. A psychosocial risk factor–targeted intervention for the prevention of chronic pain and disability following whiplash injury. *Phys. Ther.* **2006**, *86*, 8–18. [CrossRef] [PubMed]
56. Vlaeyen, J.W.; Linton, S.J. Fear-avoidance and its consequences in chronic musculoskeletal pain: A state of the art. *Pain* **2000**, *85*, 317–332. [CrossRef]
57. Leeuw, M.; Goossens, M.E.J.B.; Linton, S.J.; Crombez, G.; Boersma, K.; Vlaeyen, J.W.S. The fear-avoidance model of musculoskeletal pain: Current state of scientific evidence. *J. Behav. Med.* **2007**, *30*, 77–94. [CrossRef]
58. Fritz, J.M.; George, S.Z. Identifying psychosocial variables in patients with acute work-related low back pain: The importance of fear-avoidance beliefs. *Phys. Ther.* **2002**, *82*, 973–983. [CrossRef]
59. George, S.Z.; Fritz, J.M.; Erhard, R.E. A comparison of fear-avoidance beliefs in patients with lumbar spine pain and cervical spine pain. *Spine* **2001**, *26*, 2139–2145. [CrossRef]
60. George, S.Z.; Fritz, J.M.; McNeil, D.W. Fear-avoidance beliefs as measured by the fear-avoidance beliefs questionnaire: Change in fear-avoidance beliefs questionnaire is predictive of change in self-report of disability and pain intensity for patients with acute low back pain. *Clin. J. Pain* **2006**, *22*, 197–203. [CrossRef]
61. Cleland, J.A.; Fritz, J.M.; Brennan, G.P. Predictive validity of initial fear avoidance beliefs in patients with low back pain receiving physical therapy: Is the FABQ a useful screening tool for identifying patients at risk for a poor recovery? *Eur. Spine J.* **2008**, *17*, 70–79. [CrossRef] [PubMed]
62. Ryum, T.; Stiles, T.C. Changes in pain catastrophizing, fear-avoidance beliefs, and pain self-efficacy mediate changes in pain intensity on disability in the treatment of chronic low back pain. *Pain Rep.* **2023**, *8*, e1092. [CrossRef] [PubMed]
63. Boersma, K.; Linton, S.; Overmeer, T.; Jansson, M.; Vlaeyen, J.; de Jong, J. Lowering fear-avoidance and enhancing function through exposure in vivo. A multiple baseline study across six patients with back pain. *Pain* **2004**, *108*, 8–16. [CrossRef] [PubMed]
64. Besen, E.; Gaines, B.; Linton, S.J.; Shaw, W.S. The role of pain catastrophizing as a mediator in the work disability process following acute low back pain. *J. Appl. Biobehav. Res.* **2017**, *22*, e12085. [CrossRef]
65. De Jong, J.R.; Vlaeyen, J.W.S.; Onghena, P.; Goossens, M.E.J.B.; Geilen, M.; Mulder, H. Fear of movement/(re)injury in chronic low back pain: Education or exposure in vivo as mediator to fear reduction? *Clin. J. Pain* **2005**, *21*, 9–17, discussion 69–72. [CrossRef]
66. Ryum, T.; Hartmann, H.; Borchgrevink, P.; De Ridder, K.; Stiles, T.C. The effect of in-session exposure in Fear-Avoidance treatment of chronic low back pain: A randomized controlled trial. *Eur. J. Pain* **2021**, *25*, 171–188. [CrossRef]
67. Vlaeyen, J.W.S.; de Jong, J.; Geilen, M.; Heuts, P.H.T.G.; van Breukelen, G. The treatment of fear of movement/(re)injury in chronic low back pain: Further evidence on the effectiveness of exposure in vivo. *Clin. J. Pain* **2002**, *18*, 251–261. [CrossRef]
68. Simons, L.E. Fear of pain in children and adolescents with neuropathic pain and complex regional pain syndrome. *Pain* **2016**, *157*, S90. [CrossRef]
69. Yuan, Y.; Schreiber, K.; Flowers, K.M.; Edwards, R.; Azizoddin, D.; Ashcraft, L.; Newhill, C.E.; Hruschak, V. The relationship between emotion regulation and pain catastrophizing in patients with chronic pain. *Pain Med.* **2024**, *25*, 468–477. [CrossRef]
70. Rosenberg, J.C.; Schultz, D.M.; Duarte, L.E.; Rosen, S.M.; Raza, A. Increased pain catastrophizing associated with lower pain relief during spinal cord stimulation: Results from a large post-market study. *Neuromodulation* **2015**, *18*, 277–284, discussion 284. [CrossRef] [PubMed]
71. Pinto, P.R.; McIntyre, T.; Ferrero, R.; Almeida, A.; Araújo-Soares, V. Predictors of acute postsurgical pain and anxiety following primary total hip and knee arthroplasty. *J. Pain* **2013**, *14*, 502–515. [CrossRef] [PubMed]
72. Høvik, L.H.; Winther, S.B.; Foss, O.A.; Gjeilo, K.H. Preoperative pain catastrophizing and postoperative pain after total knee arthroplasty: A prospective cohort study with one year follow-up. *BMC Musculoskelet. Disord.* **2016**, *17*, 214. [CrossRef]
73. Khan, R.S.; Ahmed, K.; Blakeway, E.; Skapinakis, P.; Nihoyannopoulos, L.; Macleod, K.; Sevdalis, N.; Ashrafian, H.; Platt, M.; Darzi, A.; et al. Catastrophizing: A predictive factor for postoperative pain. *Am. J. Surg.* **2011**, *201*, 122–131. [CrossRef]
74. Teunis, T.; Bot, A.G.J.; Thornton, E.R.; Ring, D. Catastrophic Thinking Is Associated with Finger Stiffness after Distal Radius Fracture Surgery. *J. Orthop. Trauma* **2015**, *29*, e414–e420. [CrossRef] [PubMed]
75. Gibson, E.; Sabo, M.T. Can pain catastrophizing be changed in surgical patients? A scoping review. *Can. J. Surg.* **2018**, *61*, 311–318. [CrossRef]
76. Chimenti, R.L.; Pacha, M.S.; Glass, N.A.; Frazier, M.; Bowles, A.O.; Valantine, A.D.; Archer, K.R.; Wilken, J.M. Elevated Kinesiophobia Is Associated with Reduced Recovery from Lower Extremity Musculoskeletal Injuries in Military and Civilian Cohorts. *Phys. Ther.* **2021**, *102*, pzab262. [CrossRef]
77. Örücü Atar, M.; Demir, Y.; Tekin, E.; Kılınç Kamacı, G.; Korkmaz, N.; Aydemir, K. Kinesiophobia and associated factors in patients with traumatic lower extremity amputation. *Turk. J. Phys. Med. Rehabil.* **2022**, *68*, 493–500. [CrossRef]

78. Roelofs, J.; Goubert, L.; Peters, M.; Vlaeyen, J.; Crombez, G. The Tampa Scale for Kinesiophobia: Further examination of psychometric properties in patients with chronic low back pain and fibromyalgia. *Eur. J. Pain* **2004**, *8*, 495–502. [CrossRef]
79. Varallo, G.; Scarpina, F.; Giusti, E.M.; Cattivelli, R.; Guerrini Usubini, A.; Capodaglio, P.; Castelnuovo, G. Does Kinesiophobia Mediate the Relationship between Pain Intensity and Disability in Individuals with Chronic Low-Back Pain and Obesity? *Brain Sci.* **2021**, *11*, 684. [CrossRef]
80. Van Bogaert, W.; Coppieters, I.; Kregel, J.; Nijs, J.; De Pauw, R.; Meeus, M.; Cagnie, B.; Danneels, L.; Malfliet, A. Influence of Baseline Kinesiophobia Levels on Treatment Outcome in People with Chronic Spinal Pain. *Phys. Ther.* **2021**, *101*, pzab076. [CrossRef] [PubMed]
81. Saracoglu, I.; Arik, M.I.; Afsar, E.; Gokpinar, H.H. The effectiveness of pain neuroscience education combined with manual therapy and home exercise for chronic low back pain: A single-blind randomized controlled trial. *Physiother. Theory Pract.* **2022**, *38*, 868–878. [CrossRef] [PubMed]
82. Malfliet, A.; Kregel, J.; Meeus, M.; Roussel, N.; Danneels, L.; Cagnie, B.; Dolphens, M.; Nijs, J. Blended-Learning Pain Neuroscience Education for People with Chronic Spinal Pain: Randomized Controlled Multicenter Trial. *Phys. Ther.* **2018**, *98*, 357–368. [CrossRef]
83. Bodes Pardo, G.; Lluch Girbés, E.; Roussel, N.A.; Gallego Izquierdo, T.; Jiménez Penick, V.; Pecos Martín, D. Pain Neurophysiology Education and Therapeutic Exercise for Patients with Chronic Low Back Pain: A Single-Blind Randomized Controlled Trial. *Arch. Phys. Med. Rehabil.* **2018**, *99*, 338–347. [CrossRef]
84. Kim, H.; Lee, S. Effects of pain neuroscience education on kinesiophobia in patients with chronic pain: A systematic review and meta-analysis. *Phys. Ther. Rehabil. Sci.* **2020**, *9*, 309–317. [CrossRef]
85. Andias, R.; Neto, M.; Silva, A.G. The effects of pain neuroscience education and exercise on pain, muscle endurance, catastrophizing and anxiety in adolescents with chronic idiopathic neck pain: A school-based pilot, randomized and controlled study. *Physiother. Theory Pract.* **2018**, *34*, 682–691. [CrossRef]
86. Lin, L.-H.; Lin, T.-Y.; Chang, K.-V.; Wu, W.-T.; Özçakar, L. Pain neuroscience education for reducing pain and kinesiophobia in patients with chronic neck pain: A systematic review and meta-analysis of randomized controlled trials. *Eur. J. Pain* **2024**, *28*, 231–243. [CrossRef]
87. Wood, L.; Bejarano, G.; Csiernik, B.; Miyamoto, G.C.; Mansell, G.; Hayden, J.A.; Lewis, M.; Cashin, A.G. Pain catastrophising and kinesiophobia mediate pain and physical function improvements with Pilates exercise in chronic low back pain: A mediation analysis of a randomised controlled trial. *J. Physiother.* **2023**, *69*, 168–174. [CrossRef] [PubMed]
88. Savych, B.; Neumark, D.; Lea, R. Do Opioids Help Injured Workers Recover and Get Back to Work? The Impact of Opioid Prescriptions on Duration of Temporary Disability. *Ind. Relat. J. Econ. Soc.* **2019**, *58*, 549–590. [CrossRef]
89. Grattan, A.; Sullivan, M.D.; Saunders, K.W.; Campbell, C.I.; Von Korff, M.R. Depression and Prescription Opioid Misuse among Chronic Opioid Therapy Recipients with No History of Substance Abuse. *Ann. Fam. Med.* **2012**, *10*, 304–311. [CrossRef]
90. Scherrer, J.F.; Ahmedani, B.; Autio, K.; Debar, L.; Lustman, P.J.; Miller-Matero, L.R.; Salas, J.; Secrest, S.; Sullivan, M.D.; Wilson, L.; et al. The Prescription Opioids and Depression Pathways Cohort Study. *J. Psychiatr. Brain Sci.* **2020**, *5*, 9. [CrossRef]
91. Scherrer, J.F.; Salas, J.; Schneider, F.D.; Bucholz, K.K.; Sullivan, M.D.; Copeland, L.A.; Ahmedani, B.K.; Burroughs, T.; Lustman, P.J. Characteristics of new depression diagnoses in patients with and without prior chronic opioid use. *J. Affect. Disord.* **2017**, *210*, 125–129. [CrossRef] [PubMed]
92. Vlaeyen, J.W.S.; Crombez, G.; Linton, S.J. The fear-avoidance model of pain. *Pain* **2016**, *157*, 1588. [CrossRef]
93. Vogel, J.A.; Rising, K.L.; Jones, J.; Bowden, M.L.; Ginde, A.A.; Havranek, E.P. Reasons Patients Choose the Emergency Department over Primary Care: A Qualitative Metasynthesis. *J. Gen. Intern. Med.* **2019**, *34*, 2610–2619. [CrossRef]
94. Rogers, A.H.; Farris, S.G. A meta-analysis of the associations of elements of the fear-avoidance model of chronic pain with negative affect, depression, anxiety, pain-related disability and pain intensity. *Eur. J. Pain* **2022**, *26*, 1611–1635. [CrossRef] [PubMed]
95. Zale, E.L.; Ditre, J.W. Pain-Related Fear, Disability, and the Fear-Avoidance Model of Chronic Pain. *Curr. Opin. Psychol.* **2015**, *5*, 24–30. [CrossRef]
96. Felitti, V.J.; Anda, R.F.; Nordenberg, D.; Williamson, D.F.; Spitz, A.M.; Edwards, V.; Koss, M.P.; Marks, J.S. Relationship of childhood abuse and household dysfunction to many of the leading causes of death in adults. The Adverse Childhood Experiences (ACE) Study. *Am. J. Prev. Med.* **1998**, *14*, 245–258. [CrossRef]
97. Tidmarsh, L.V.; Harrison, R.; Ravindran, D.; Matthews, S.L.; Finlay, K.A. The Influence of Adverse Childhood Experiences in Pain Management: Mechanisms, Processes, and Trauma-Informed Care. *Front Pain Res* **2022**, *3*, 923866. [CrossRef]
98. Fordyce, W.E.; Shelton, J.L.; Dundore, D.E. The modification of avoidance learning pain behaviors. *J. Behav. Med.* **1982**, *5*, 405–414. [CrossRef]
99. Schmidt, A.J. Cognitive factors in the performance level of chronic low back pain patients. *J. Psychosom. Res.* **1985**, *29*, 183–189. [CrossRef]
100. Rachman, S.; Lopatka, C. Accurate and inaccurate predictions of pain. *Behav. Res. Ther.* **1988**, *26*, 291–296. [CrossRef] [PubMed]
101. Rubak, S.; Sandbæk, A.; Lauritzen, T.; Christensen, B. Motivational interviewing: A systematic review and meta-analysis. *Br. J. Gen. Pract.* **2005**, *55*, 305–312.
102. Webster, F.; Connoy, L.; Longo, R.; Ahuja, D.; Amtmann, D.; Anderson, A.; Ashton-James, C.E.; Boyd, H.; Chambers, C.T.; Cook, K.F.; et al. Patient Responses to the Term Pain Catastrophizing: Thematic Analysis of Cross-sectional International Data. *J. Pain* **2023**, *24*, 356–367. [CrossRef]

103. U.P. Foundation. 'Catastrophizing': A Form of Pain Shaming. Available online: https://uspainfoundation.org/blog/catastrophizing-a-form-of-pain-shaming/ (accessed on 24 July 2024).
104. Atkins, N.; Mukhida, K. The relationship between patients' income and education and their access to pharmacological chronic pain management: A scoping review. *Can. J. Pain* **2022**, *6*, 142–170. [CrossRef]
105. Maharaj, A.S.; Bhatt, N.V.; Gentile, J.P. Bringing It in the Room: Addressing the Impact of Racism on the Therapeutic Alliance. *Innov. Clin. Neurosci.* **2021**, *18*, 39–43.
106. Strand, N.H.; Mariano, E.R.; Goree, J.H.; Narouze, S.; Doshi, T.L.; Freeman, J.A.; Pearson, A.C.S. Racism in Pain Medicine: We Can and Should Do More. *Mayo Clin. Proc.* **2021**, *96*, 1394–1400. [CrossRef] [PubMed]
107. Amtmann, D.; Bamer, A.M.; Liljenquist, K.S.; Cowan, P.; Salem, R.; Turk, D.C.; Jensen, M.P. The Concerns About Pain (CAP) Scale: A Patient-Reported Outcome Measure of Pain Catastrophizing. *J. Pain* **2020**, *21*, 1198–1211. [CrossRef] [PubMed]
108. Sullivan, M.J.L.; Tripp, D.A. Pain Catastrophizing: Controversies, Misconceptions and Future Directions. *J. Pain* **2024**, *25*, 575–587. [CrossRef]
109. Raja, S.N.; Carr, D.B.; Cohen, M.; Finnerup, N.B.; Flor, H.; Gibson, S.; Keefe, F.; Mogil, J.S.; Ringkamp, M.; Sluka, K.A.; et al. The Revised IASP definition of pain: Concepts, challenges, and compromises. *Pain* **2020**, *161*, 1976–1982. [CrossRef]
110. U.S. Department of Health and Human Services. Pain Management Best Practices Inter-Agency Task Force Report: Updates, Gaps, Inconsistencies, and Recommendations. Retrieved from U.S. Department of Health and Human Services Website. May 2019. Available online: https://www.hhs.gov/sites/default/files/pain-mgmt-best-practices-draft-final-report-05062019.pdf (accessed on 4 June 2024).
111. Bean, D.J.; Dryland, A.; Rashid, U.; Tuck, N.L. The Determinants and Effects of Chronic Pain Stigma: A Mixed Methods Study and the Development of a Model. *J. Pain* **2022**, *23*, 1749–1764. [CrossRef]
112. Koesling, D.; Bozzaro, C. Chronic pain patients' need for recognition and their current struggle. *Med. Health Care Philos.* **2021**, *24*, 563–572. [CrossRef] [PubMed]
113. Licciardone, J.C.; Tran, Y.; Ngo, K.; Toledo, D.; Peddireddy, N.; Aryal, S. Physician Empathy and Chronic Pain Outcomes. *JAMA Netw. Open* **2024**, *7*, e246026. [CrossRef]
114. Zaman, T.; Striebel, J. *Opioid Refugees: A Diverse Population Continues to Emerge*; California Society of Addiction Medicine: San Francisco, CA, USA, 2015; p. 16.
115. The Georgia Straight. Opioid Refugees: How the Fentanyl Crisis Led to a Backlash against Doctors That's Leaving People in Pain. Available online: https://www.straight.com/news/1043911/opioid-refugees-how-fentanyl-crisis-led-backlash-against-doctors-thats-leaving-people (accessed on 6 May 2020).
116. [Report] | The Pain Refugees, by Brian Goldstone. Available online: https://harpers.org/archive/2018/04/the-pain-refugees/ (accessed on 6 May 2020).
117. Burke, S.E.; Dovidio, J.F.; Przedworski, J.M.; Hardeman, R.R.; Perry, S.P.; Phelan, S.M.; Nelson, D.B.; Burgess, D.J.; Yeazel, M.W.; van Ryn, M. Do Contact and Empathy Mitigate Bias against Gay and Lesbian People among Heterosexual Medical Students? A Report from Medical Student CHANGES. *Acad. Med.* **2015**, *90*, 645–651. [CrossRef]
118. Abd-Elsayed, A.; Heyer, A.M.; Schatman, M.E. Disparities in the Treatment of the LGBTQ Population in Chronic Pain Management. *J. Pain Res.* **2021**, *14*, 3623–3625. [CrossRef]
119. Bailey, Z.D.; Krieger, N.; Agénor, M.; Graves, J.; Linos, N.; Bassett, M.T. Structural racism and health inequities in the USA: Evidence and interventions. *Lancet* **2017**, *389*, 1453–1463. [CrossRef] [PubMed]
120. Hall, W.J.; Chapman, M.V.; Lee, K.M.; Merino, Y.M.; Thomas, T.W.; Payne, B.K.; Eng, E.; Day, S.H.; Coyne-Beasley, T. Implicit Racial/Ethnic Bias among Health Care Professionals and Its Influence on Health Care Outcomes: A Systematic Review. *Am. J. Public. Health* **2015**, *105*, e60–e76. [CrossRef] [PubMed]
121. Atkins, R. Instruments Measuring Perceived Racism/Racial Discrimination: Review and Critique of Factor Analytic Techniques. *Int. J. Health Serv. Plan Adm. Eval.* **2014**, *44*, 711. [CrossRef]
122. Wang, M.L.; Jacobs, O. From Awareness to Action: Pathways to Equity in Pain Management. *Health Equity* **2023**, *7*, 416–418. [CrossRef]
123. Edgoose, J.; Quiogue, M.; Sidhar, K. How to Identify, Understand, and Unlearn Implicit Bias in Patient Care. *FPM* **2019**, *26*, 29–33.
124. Perugino, F.; De Angelis, V.; Pompili, M.; Martelletti, P. Stigma and Chronic Pain. *Pain Ther.* **2022**, *11*, 1085–1094. [CrossRef]
125. Linton, S.J.; Boersma, K.; Vangronsveld, K.; Fruzzetti, A. Painfully reassuring? The effects of validation on emotions and adherence in a pain test. *Eur. J. Pain* **2012**, *16*, 592–599. [CrossRef] [PubMed]
126. Hanssen, M.M.; Peters, M.L.; Vlaeyen, J.W.S.; Meevissen, Y.M.C.; Vancleef, L.M.G. Optimism lowers pain: Evidence of the causal status and underlying mechanisms. *Pain* **2013**, *154*, 53–58. [CrossRef] [PubMed]
127. P. Forum. COVID-19 Pandemic Impact on Patients, Families & Individuals in Recovery from a SUD. Available online: https://www.addictionpolicy.org/post/covid-19-pandemic-impact-on-patients-families-individuals-in-recovery-fromsubstance-use-disorder (accessed on 15 June 2021).
128. Goubert, L.; Crombez, G.; Van Damme, S. The role of neuroticism, pain catastrophizing and pain-related fear in vigilance to pain: A structural equations approach. *Pain* **2004**, *107*, 234. [CrossRef]
129. Levy, B.R.; Slade, M.D.; Kunkel, S.R.; Kasl, S.V. Longevity increased by positive self-perceptions of aging. *J. Pers. Soc. Psychol.* **2002**, *83*, 261–270. [CrossRef] [PubMed]

130. Yamin, J.B.; Meints, S.M.; Edwards, R.R. Beyond pain catastrophizing: Rationale and recommendations for targeting trauma in the assessment and treatment of chronic pain. *Expert. Rev. Neurother.* **2024**, *24*, 231–234. [CrossRef] [PubMed]
131. Maly, A.; Vallerand, A.H. Neighborhood, Socioeconomic, and Racial Influence on Chronic Pain. *Pain. Manag. Nurs.* **2018**, *19*, 14–22. [CrossRef]
132. Cognitive Restructuring: Steps, Technique, and Examples. Available online: https://www.medicalnewstoday.com/articles/cognitive-restructuring (accessed on 19 March 2024).
133. Newman, M.G.; Erickson, T.; Przeworski, A.; Dzus, E. Self-help and minimal-contact therapies for anxiety disorders: Is human contact necessary for therapeutic efficacy? *J. Clin. Psychol.* **2003**, *59*, 251–274. [CrossRef]
134. Mayo-Wilson, E.; Montgomery, P. Media-delivered cognitive behavioural therapy and behavioural therapy (self-help) for anxiety disorders in adults. *Cochrane Database Syst. Rev.* **2013**, *9*, CD005330. [CrossRef]
135. Somatoform Disorders | AAFP. Available online: https://www.aafp.org/pubs/afp/issues/2007/1101/p1333.html (accessed on 7 August 2024).
136. Catastrophizing Misinterpretations Predict Somatoform-Related Symptoms and New Onsets of Somatoform Disorders—ScienceDirect. Available online: https://www.sciencedirect.com/science/article/abs/pii/S0022399915300271 (accessed on 7 August 2024).
137. Seto, H.; Nakao, M. Relationships between catastrophic thought, bodily sensations and physical symptoms. *Biopsychosoc. Med.* **2017**, *11*, 28. [CrossRef]
138. Cate Polacek, M.; Christopher, R.; Michelle Mann, B.S.; Margarita Udall, M.P.H.; Terri Craig, P.; Michael Deminski, M.S.; Nila, A.; Sathe, M.A. Healthcare Professionals' Perceptions of Challenges to Chronic Pain Management. *Am. J. Manag. Care* **2020**, *26*, e135–e139. Available online: https://www.ajmc.com/view/healthcare-professionals-perceptions-of-challenges-to-chronic-pain-management (accessed on 5 August 2024).
139. Woolford, S.J.; Resnicow, K.; Davis, M.M.; Nichols, L.P.; Wasserman, R.C.; Harris, D.; Gebremariam, A.; Shone, L.; Fiks, A.G.; Chang, T. Cost-effectiveness of a motivational interviewing obesity intervention versus usual care in pediatric primary care offices. *Obesity* **2022**, *30*, 2265–2274. [CrossRef] [PubMed]
140. Olmstead, T.A.; Yonkers, K.A.; Forray, A.; Zimbrean, P.; Gilstad-Hayden, K.; Martino, S. Cost and cost-effectiveness of three strategies for implementing motivational interviewing for substance misuse on medical inpatient units. *Drug Alcohol. Depend.* **2020**, *214*, 108156. [CrossRef] [PubMed]
141. Schütze, R.; Rees, C.; Smith, A.; Slater, H.; Campbell, J.M.; O'Sullivan, P. How Can We Best Reduce Pain Catastrophizing in Adults with Chronic Noncancer Pain? A Systematic Review and Meta-Analysis. *J. Pain* **2018**, *19*, 233–256. [CrossRef]
142. Darnall, B.D. Psychological Treatment for Chronic Pain: Improving Access and Integration. *Psychol. Sci. Public. Interest.* **2021**, *22*, 45–51. [CrossRef]
143. Bizzo, B.C.; Almeida, R.R.; Michalski, M.H.; Alkasab, T.K. Artificial Intelligence and Clinical Decision Support for Radiologists and Referring Providers. *J. Am. Coll. Radiol.* **2019**, *16*, 1351–1356. [CrossRef] [PubMed]
144. Hershberger, P.J.; Pei, Y.; Bricker, D.A.; Crawford, T.N.; Shivakumar, A.; Vasoya, M.; Medaramitta, R.; Rechtin, M.; Bositty, A.; Wilson, J.F. Advancing Motivational Interviewing Training with Artificial Intelligence: ReadMI. *Adv. Med. Educ. Pract.* **2021**, *12*, 613–618. [CrossRef]
145. Nurmi, J.; Knittle, K.; Ginchev, T.; Khattak, F.; Helf, C.; Zwickl, P.; Castellano-Tejedor, C.; Lusilla-Palacios, P.; Costa-Requena, J.; Ravaja, N.; et al. Engaging Users in the Behavior Change Process with Digitalized Motivational Interviewing and Gamification: Development and Feasibility Testing of the Precious App. *JMIR Mhealth Uhealth* **2020**, *8*, e12884. [CrossRef]
146. Saiyed, A.; Layton, J.; Borsari, B.; Cheng, J.; Kanzaveli, T.; Tsvetovat, M.; Satterfield, J. Technology-Assisted Motivational Interviewing: Developing a Scalable Framework for Promoting Engagement with Tobacco Cessation Using NLP and Machine Learning. *Procedia Comput. Sci.* **2022**, *206*, 121–131. [CrossRef]
147. Sawyer, C.; McKeon, G.; Hassan, L.; Onyweaka, H.; Martinez Agulleiro, L.; Guinart, D.; Torous, J.; Firth, J. Digital health behaviour change interventions in severe mental illness: A systematic review. *Psychol. Med.* **2023**, *53*, 6965–7005. [CrossRef]

Disclaimer/Publisher's Note: The statements, opinions and data contained in all publications are solely those of the individual author(s) and contributor(s) and not of MDPI and/or the editor(s). MDPI and/or the editor(s) disclaim responsibility for any injury to people or property resulting from any ideas, methods, instructions or products referred to in the content.

MDPI AG
Grosspeteranlage 5
4052 Basel
Switzerland
Tel.: +41 61 683 77 34
www.mdpi.com

Journal of Clinical Medicine Editorial Office
E-mail: jcm@mdpi.com
www.mdpi.com/journal/jcm

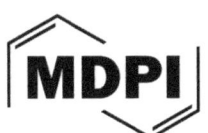

Disclaimer/Publisher's Note: The statements, opinions and data contained in all publications are solely those of the individual author(s) and contributor(s) and not of MDPI and/or the editor(s). MDPI and/or the editor(s) disclaim responsibility for any injury to people or property resulting from any ideas, methods, instructions or products referred to in the content.

www.ingramcontent.com/pod-product-compliance
Lightning Source LLC
LaVergne TN
LVHW072359090526
838202LV00019B/2585